Spinal Tumor Associated Deformity

Daniel M. Sciubba
Editor

Spinal Tumor Associated Deformity

A Guide to Management

Springer

Editor
Daniel M. Sciubba
Neurosurgery
Northwell Health
Great Neck, NY, USA

ISBN 978-3-031-87938-8 ISBN 978-3-031-87939-5 (eBook)
https://doi.org/10.1007/978-3-031-87939-5

This Springer imprint is published by the registered company Springer Nature Switzerland AG
The registered company address is: Gewerbestrasse 11, 6330 Cham, Switzerland

Foreword

The treatment of spinal malignancies—intradural and extradural—often involves extensive soft tissue dissection and resection of bony elements. Disruption of these elements can result in postoperative deformity; tumors of the bony elements can additionally result in spinal deformity, often due to compromise of the load-bearing capacity of the anterior column.

Historically, little attention has been paid to overall alignment in the cancer population, as prognoses are often poor, and emphasis has been placed on maximizing survival and treating preoperative neurological deficits. However, work from the spinal deformity literature has shown the degree to which poor alignment can result in long-term disability. In light of the evolving literature, emphasis on improving quality of life, and improvements in survival outcomes for patients with primary and metastatic spine tumors, increased attention to spinal alignment is warranted.

This book is unique in comparison to prior texts describing the management of spinal malignancies in that it focuses its discussion on the deformity that can occur in the context of spinal malignancy. Topics discussed include coronal plane deformities that can occur in the setting of neurofibromatosis or posterior column primary osseous neoplasms (i.e., osteoid osteoma/osteoblastoma), sagittal plane deformities secondary to intramedullary tumor resection or epidural disease debulking, focal kyphosis from anterior column collapse, and global malalignment in the setting of osseous malignancies of the cervical spine and lumbosacral junction. The text describes fundamental spinal alignment principles and contextualizes them in the setting of spinal tumor management paradigms, illustrating deformity management using specific real-world examples. For relevant pathologies it also discusses nonoperative management, which is often preferable in the spinal oncology population with more pronounced frailty.

No text can describe the management of all potential scenarios; however, the cases described in the present volume represent pathologies likely to be seen by the spinal oncologist. And the fundamentals conveyed here will be invaluable to the practicing spinal oncologist, as it is inevitable that the discussion of spinal alignment within the oncology patient population will only continue to grow.

Durham, NC, USA C. Rory Goodwin

Preface

Conventionally spinal oncology and spinal deformity have been well segregated with regard to the patient whom they treat. With the exception of primary spinal malignancies, for which surgery along oncologic principles can lead to long-term survival, patients with spinal tumors have been defined held to have poor expected survival and thereby distinct from patients with adult spinal deformity, who are offered surgery with the expectation that they will survive years to reap the benefits of surgical correction. However, over the past two decades there have been significant improvements in survival across oncology and many patients seeking care for spinal metastases can now have an expected survival of years. With this blurring of expected survival, it is now possible to see the similarities between the oncologic and adult spinal deformity populations. Both pathologies are most commonly seen in patients in their sixth decade of life and beyond. And patients commonly have multiple medical comorbidities.

In the present text we seek to discuss the management of deformity in the context of spinal oncology. Spinal deformity in this domain can largely be binned into three main domains: (1) deformity caused by the tumor, (2) deformity caused by failure to obey deformity principles during surgical treatment of the tumor, and (3) deformity that results from treatment of the tumor. The first realm is the most obvious and for most practitioners will be the one most frequently encountered. As the tumor develops within the vertebral body, it causes destruction of the normal trabecular bone with a resultant worsening of the load bearing capacity of the vertebra. With continued destruction, patients can present with mechanical pain from the impending instability, and eventually once the destruction reaches a critical threshold, the tumor-invaded vertebra fractures. The resultant fracture can then cause kyphosis, or if the vertebral body collapse is coronal asymmetric, it can cause scoliosis. In these early stages of destruction, cement-augmentation can prevent the development of deformity (assuming the pathology is primary). However, with progression to pathologic fracture, surgery is generally required for stabilization and correction of the focal deformity.

In treating the tumor, however, it is necessary to obey the principles of spinal deformity, focusing on achieving both sagittal and coronal balance. In spinal tumor operations, it is essential that the surgeon not worsen existing deformity or create new deformity. Corpectomy for metastases and en bloc spondylectomy for primary tumors actually provide two of the biggest opportunities for sagittal plane realignment, as an entire segment of the anterior and middle columns is being removed. However, the bone of adjacent levels may be of poor-quality owing to prior radiotherapy or, in the case of metastatic disease, multilevel tumor involvement. Cement augmentation may be helpful in such cases.

Last, deformity may occur following treatment for spinal tumors even where the index operation refrains for placing a construct that creates new deformity. Specifically, most tumors are addressed via a posterior only approach, either to remove an intradural pathology, as is common in the pediatric population, or to debulk epidural disease. In doing so, the posterior tension band is disrupted, and a fraction of patients will experience progressive deformity due to the incompetence of this musculoligamentous complex. Similarly, adjuvant radiotherapy, which has become a staple of treatment for many pathologies, can cause fibrosis and atrophy of the paraspinal musculature. The associated weakening can again lead the posterior tension band to be structurally incompetent with resultant progressive deformity.

Without question the field investigating the intersection of spinal oncology and spinal deformity will continue to progress, but it is our hope that the present text will serve as an effective primer for those treating both intradural and extradural spinal tumors in hopes of maintaining and improving spinal alignment.

Great Neck, NY, USA — Daniel M. Sciubba
Rochester, MN USA — Zach Pennington

Contents

Contributors

Mohamed Abdulkadir Medical Sciences Division, University of Oxford, Oxford, UK

Jetan Badhiwala Cleveland Clinic Center for Spine Health, Cleveland, OH, USA

Ki-Eun Chang Department of Neurosurgery, Brown University, Warren Alpert Medical School/Rhode Island Hospital, Lifespan Health, Providence, RI, USA

Benjamin D. Elder Department of Neurologic Surgery, Mayo Clinic, Rochester, MN, USA

Aladine A. Elsamadicy Department of Neurosurgery, Yale University School of Medicine, New Haven, CT, USA

Ziya L. Gokaslan Department of Neurosurgery, Brown University, Warren Alpert Medical School/Rhode Island Hospital, Lifespan Health, Providence, RI, USA

Danielle Golub Department of Neurosurgery, Northwell Health, Great Neck, NY, USA

Matthew L. Goodwin Department of Orthopedic Surgery, Washington University School of Medicine, St Louis, MO, USA

Jacob Greenberg Cleveland Clinic Center for Spine Health, Cleveland, OH, USA

Mari L. Groves Department of Neurosurgery, Johns Hopkins University School of Medicine, Baltimore, MD, USA

Amit Jain Department of Orthopaedic Surgery, Johns Hopkins University School of Medicine, Baltimore, MD, USA

George I. Jallo Institute for Brain Protection Sciences, Johns Hopkins All Children's Hospital, St Petersburg, FL, USA

Luis Kolb Department of Neurosurgery, Barrow Neurological Institute, Phoenix, AZ, USA

Igor Latich Department of Radiology and Biomedical Imaging, Yale University School of Medicine, New Haven, CT, USA

Darryl Lau Department of Neurosurgery, New York University, New York, NY, USA

Maxwell Laurans Department of Neurosurgery, Yale University School of Medicine, New Haven, CT, USA

Taryn E. LeRoy Department of Orthopedic Surgery, New England Baptist Hospital, Boston, MA, USA

Sheng-Fu Larry Lo Department of Neurosurgery, Donald and Barbara Zucker School of Medicine at Hofstra/Northwell, Great Neck, NY, USA

Department of Neurosurgery, Northwell Health, Great Neck, NY, USA

Daniel G. Lynch Department of Neurosurgery, Northwell Health, Great Neck, NY, USA

Elie Massaad Department of Neurosurgery, Massachusetts General Hospital, Harvard Medical School, Boston, MA, USA

Ehud Mendel Department of Neurosurgery, Yale University School of Medicine, New Haven, CT, USA

Camilo A. Molina Department of Neurosurgery, Washington University School of Medicine, St Louis, MO, USA

Margot Martinez Moreno Department of Neurosurgery, Brown University, Warren Alpert Medical School/Rhode Island Hospital, Lifespan Health, Providence, RI, USA

Tianyi Niu Department of Neurosurgery, Brown University, Warren Alpert Medical School/Rhode Island Hospital, Lifespan Health, Providence, RI, USA

Zach Pennington Department of Neurologic Surgery, Mayo Clinic, Rochester, MN, USA

Thomas A. Pieters Department of Neurosurgery, University of Massachusetts, Worcester, MA, USA

Department of Neurological Surgery, UMass Memorial Health, Worcester, MA, USA

Benjamin C. Reeves Department of Neurosurgery, Barrow Neurological Institute, Phoenix, AZ, USA

Stephanie M. Robert Department of Neurosurgery, Yale University School of Medicine, New Haven, CT, USA

Gabrielle Santangelo Department of Neurosurgery, University of Rochester, Rochester, NY, USA

Jason W. Savage Cleveland Clinic Center for Spine Health, Cleveland, OH, USA

Daniel Schneider Department of Neurosurgery, Northwell Health, Great Neck, NY, USA

Christian Schroeder Department of Neurosurgery, Brown University, Warren Alpert Medical School/Rhode Island Hospital, Lifespan Health, Providence, RI, USA

Joseph H. Schwab Department of Orthopaedic Surgery, Cedars Sinai Medical Center, Los Angeles, CA, USA

Daniel M. Sciubba Department of Neurosurgery, Donald and Barbara Zucker School of Medicine at Hofstra/Northwell Health, Great Neck, NY, USA

Department of Neurosurgery, Zucker School of Medicine at Hofstra, Long Island Jewish Medical Center and North Shore University Hospital, Northwell Health, Great Neck, NY, USA

Department of Neurosurgery, Northwell Health, Great Neck, NY, USA

Nir Shimony Department of Surgery, St Jude's Children's Research Hospital, Le Bonheur Neuroscience Institute, Memphis, TN, USA

John H. Shin Department of Neurosurgery, University of Pennsylvania/Penn Spine Center, Philadelphia, PA, USA

Michael Shost Cleveland Clinic Center for Spine Health, Cleveland, OH, USA

Hesham Soliman Department of Neurosurgery, Donald and Barbara Zucker School of Medicine at Hofstra/Northwell Health, Great Neck, NY, USA

Paul D. Sponseller Department of Orthopaedic Surgery, Johns Hopkins University School of Medicine, Baltimore, MD, USA

Patricia Sullivan Department of Neurosurgery, Brown University, Warren Alpert Medical School/Rhode Island Hospital, Lifespan Health, Providence, RI, USA

Zachary Wilt Cleveland Clinic Center for Spine Health, Cleveland, OH, USA

Grace X. Xiong Department of Orthopaedic Surgery, Stanford University, Redwood City, CA, USA

Amy L. Xu Department of Orthopaedic Surgery, Hospital for Special Surgery, New York, NY, USA

Salim Yakdan Department of Neurosurgery, Washington University, St. Louis, MO, USA

Chapter 1
Management of Deformity Following Intramedullary Tumors

Mohamed Abdulkadir, Mari L. Groves, George I. Jallo, and Nir Shimony

Introduction

Spinal tumors comprise approximately 3–6% all primary central nervous system (CNS) tumors [1]. Tumors can be characterized by histology and location, but are broadly categorized by their anatomical relation to the spinal cord as intradural intramedullary, intradural extramedullary, and extradural. Many tumors invade multiple compartments, though, which can complicate classification. Based on the Central Brain Tumor Registry of the United States (CBTRUS) data, extramedullary lesions are the most common intradural pathology with an incidence of approximately 0.58 per 100,000 persons [2] as compared to 0.37 per 100,000 persons for intramedullary lesions. Overall, ependymomas are the most common primary pathology in adults (20+) [3]; however, astrocytomas are the most common pathology within children (19.7% vs. 19.6% for ependymoma) [3]. Gangliogliomas are also relatively common within children [4].

M. Abdulkadir
Medical Sciences Division, University of Oxford, Oxford, UK
e-mail: abdulkadir.mohamed@st-hughs.ox.ac.uk

M. L. Groves
Department of Neurosurgery, Johns Hopkins University School of Medicine, Baltimore, MD, USA
e-mail: mgroves2@jhmi.edu

G. I. Jallo (✉)
Institute for Brain Protection Sciences, Johns Hopkins All Children's Hospital, St Petersburg, FL, USA
e-mail: gjallo1@jhmi.edu

N. Shimony
Department of Surgery, St Jude's Children's Research Hospital, Le Bonheur Neuroscience Institute, Memphis, TN, USA
e-mail: nshimony@semmes-murphey.com

D. M. Sciubba (ed.), *Spinal Tumor Associated Deformity*,
https://doi.org/10.1007/978-3-031-87939-5_1

The incidence of primary spinal cord tumors is greater in adults than in children, where incidence is between 0.23 and 0.30 per 100,000 persons, as compared to adults, where incidence increases with age to a peak of 2.53 per 100,000 in those aged 70–79 years [2]. However, as a share of all CNS neoplasms, spinal cord tumors comprise a greater proportion of the disease burden as compared to adults (35% compared to 20% in adults) [5]. Despite their lower prevalence within the pediatric population, spinal cord tumors pose additional concerns in the pediatric population. Specifically, surgical intervention within this population necessitates injury to the developing spinal column, which can result in significant deformities and subsequent neurological deficits superimposed on those created by tumor resection and adjuvant oncological treatment. Post-resection spinal deformity is at least twice as common in children as compared to adults, [6] with rates of post-resection scoliosis ranging from 8% to 88% [7] and post-resection deformity ranging from 24% to 100% [8] as compared to 10% in adults [9]. Said deformities can produce significant pain, pose neurological compromise, and ultimately require surgical correction. The increased prevalence of post-resection deformity seen in the pediatric population likely stems from the dynamic nature of the musculoskeletal system in this age group. This can have cosmetic, psychological, and functional consequences, with studies linking deformity to declines in quality-of-life measures and functional scores [10, 11].

Deformity following resection of a spinal cord tumor was first describes in the 1930s by Eiselsberg [12] after resection of a thoracic spinal tumor resulted in the development of kyphoscoliosis, pain, and myelomalacia. Since then, the literature has grown and it is now known that deformities come in many forms, including scoliosis, kyphosis, lordosis, swan neck deformities, and even complex three-dimensional kyphoscoliotic deformities (Fig. 1.1). Not all patients develop such deformities and up-front instrumentation is not preferred given the growing nature of the pediatric spine. Nevertheless, its frequent occurrence merits close follow-up, which must extend through skeletal maturity given the fact that childhood spinal tumor survivors present later and with more severe deformities compared to their counterparts with deformities of other etiologies [13]. Here, we focus on the pathophysiology, diagnosis, and management of post-resection spinal deformity.

Possible Pathological Mechanism

The mechanism of spinal deformity following intradural tumor resection is likely multifactorial and occurs in around a third of patients [14]. Deformity can be caused by direct mechanical injury to the posterior elements or indirectly through anterior horn involvement, [15] with resultant denervation of the paraspinal extensor musculature [16]. These muscles, which include the multifidus, spinalis, longissimus, and iliocostalis, along with the splenius and semispinalis in the cervical spine, are responsible for maintaining normal alignment through extensor forces. This indirect mechanism may partly explain why deformities are more common after resection of

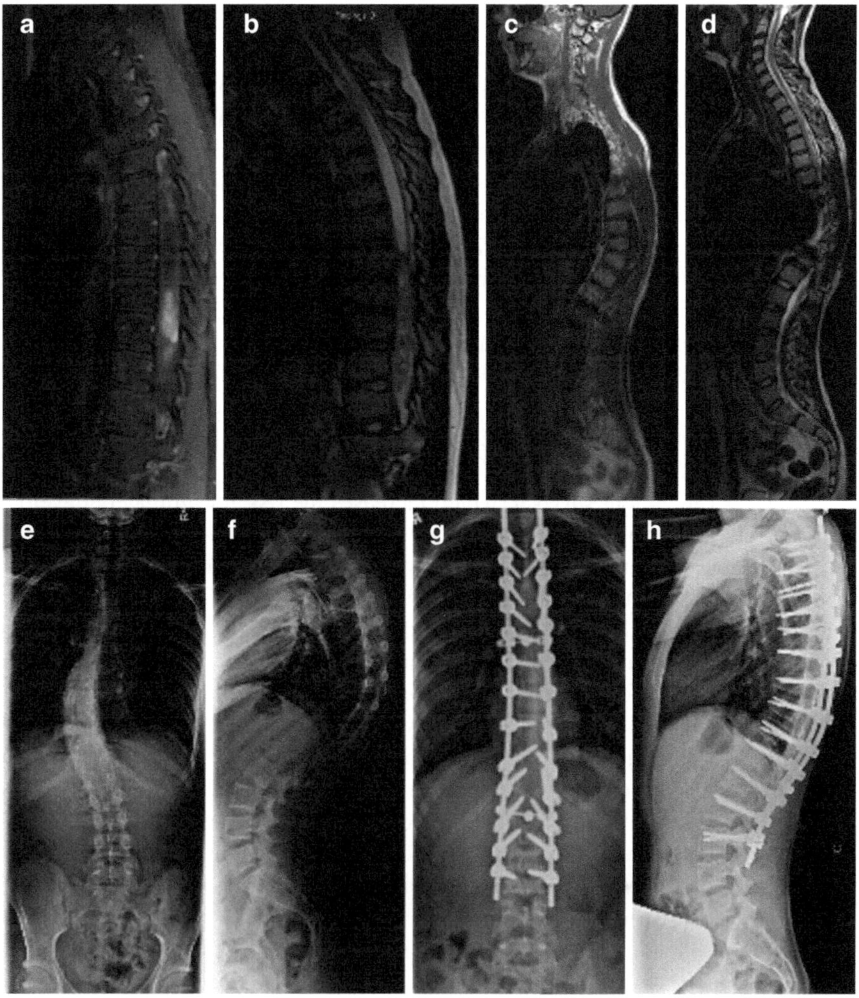

Fig. 1.1 Twelve-year-old male who presented with newly diagnosed and progressive spinal deformity was found to have significant cervicothoracic kyphoscoliosis, and on MRI (**a**—T1 weighted with gadolinium; **b**—T2 weighted), he was seen to have an enhanced intramedullary tumor with associated syringohydromyelia. He went through T8-T10 laminoplasty with gross total resection of pilocytic astrocytoma. Twenty-four months after surgery on routine follow-up, a progressive spinal deformity was diagnosed (**c**—T1 weighted MRI; **d**—T2 weighted MRI; AP and lateral X-rays shown in e and f, respectively), and he was started on conservative treatment without significant improvement. Since the deformity progressed 28 months after his initial surgery, he underwent posterior osteotomies and deformity correction, including instrumentation (g—post-op AP X-ray; h—lateral post-op X-ray). He is 5 years after his initial surgery without any recurrence, associated pain, or progressive deformity

intramedullary spinal cord tumors versus other pathologies, e.g., stenosis [17]. To this end, the denervation mechanism is thought to be particularly important in scoliotic deformities, which commonly occur below the area of decompression and resection and therefore could not be explained by direct mechanical injury. [18]

Direct mechanical injury following surgery for intramedullary lesions stems from the relatively hard-to-access location of these tumors. Biopsy and subsequent radical or subtotal resection (depending on tumor grade) involve dissection and removal of the posterior elements [7, 9]. Subsequently patients may receive adjuvant chemoradiotherapies, which can further contribute to spinal column instability by way of secondary osteoporosis, [19, 20] asymmetrical growth plate cartilage damage with subsequent fibrosis in the pediatric population, [7, 21] and soft tissue and extensor musculature damage [22]. Radiation appears to have a particularly strong association with deformity, with post-radiotherapy deformity risk being reported at 60% in an animal study [23]. These radiotherapies have become increasingly available over the past 30 years. Additionally, patients are experiencing improved post-treatment survival, which increases the risk for ultimately developing deformity requiring intervention.

Mechanistically, laminectomy, which is required to gain access into the spinal cord, involves the removal of posterior bone and soft tissue elements, which leads to a shift in the weight-bearing axis anteriorly along with a greater degree of sagittal plane motion [24]. This is particularly problematic in the cervical spine and at the cervicothoracic junction, which account for 50% of intramedullary tumors [7, 25, 26]. Posterior element resection at these levels leads to a lordotic to kyphotic shift, [27] with a resultant anterior shift in the upper body center of mass, which further alters the force axis and leads to progressive kyphosis. [24] Such progressive kyphosis can lead to “bowstringing” of the cord over the posterior aspect of the cervical vertebrae, causing myelopathy characterized by worsening motor and sensory function [28]. Resection of the facet joints, which is often done for resection of nerve sheath tumors, is particularly impactful, as resection of >50% of the facet has been shown in biomechanical studies to produce instability [29, 30]. Bony element resection is noticeably devastating in the pediatric population since the posterior ligaments are laxer/more cartilaginous and the facet joints have a more horizontal orientation, [17] which makes it easier for the cephalad level to translate anteriorly over the caudad level. This risk appears to increase with the aggressiveness of the posterior element resection [31]. Pediatric patients also have weaker paraspinal muscles and a greater head-to-body mass ratio relative to adults, [32] which further favors progressive kyphosis (Table 1.1). Therefore, if possible, normal anatomy must be preserved to a greater extent within the pediatric population. Beyond age of 23 years—the completion of spine ossification [33]—the relative risk of deformity following facet resection is decreased, though deformity risk can still be in part mitigated by meticulous preservation of the facet capsule to the greatest extent possible.

Minimally invasive (MIS) techniques—those that seek to minimize soft tissue removal—can help reduce the risk of deformity. One such strategy is by employing unilateral hemi-laminectomies versus full laminectomies, thereby preserving the

Table 1.1 Summary of factors that make post-spinal tumor resection spinal deformities more common in the pediatric population compared to adults

Risk factors pertinent to pediatric patients	Evidence and a brief explanation
Lax posterior ligaments	Posterior ligaments are vital for spinal support. Lax ligaments afford less support and a greater chance of deformity [17].
The horizontal orientation of facet joints	The horizontal orientation of facet joints affects the biomechanics and distribution of forces across the spinal column leading to abnormal loading patterns on the spine post-resection and a greater chance of deformity development [17].
Weaker paraspinal musculature	Similar to posterior ligaments, paraspinal musculature supports and stabilizes the spine and allows for movement. Weak muscles afford lesser support [50]. Rehabilitation of paraspinal musculature is something that could offset this problem postoperatively in this demographic [77].
Head-to-body ratio	In children, the head is more extensive and heavier than the rest of the body, placing greater loads on the spinal column [78].
Growing spine	As the spine grows, it is more susceptible to imbalances in muscle tone, position, and mechanical stress in general. Also, the presence of growth plates affords a greater chance of deformity since it is weaker than adjacent bone, and so is increased risk of fracture [17].

posterior tension band contralateral to the resection window. This may not always be possible but may be reasonable for patients with small lesions showing eccentric localization or at non-cord levels, where the roots can be retracted out of the way to visualize the tumor.

Increasing awareness about the impact of posterior element resection on post-resection deformity may help to explain the decreasing rate of postoperative spinal fusion in recent literature [34]. Unfortunately, the literature is still scarce on this topic. Two studies that have suggested a decreased rate of deformity following soft tissue preservice resections are those of Okem et al., Tredway et al., and Oktem et al., [35] described 20 adult patients undergoing 1- to 5-level open unilateral hemi-laminectomy and found no instances of spinal instability up to two years postoperatively; no patients needed spinal instrumentation. Tredway et al. endorsed similarly positive results in their series of six patients with extramedullary tumors treated through a tubular paramedian approach [36]. However, such MIS techniques are useless in tumors spanning >2 spinal vertebral levels [37, 38].

Lastly, the growth rate of the spinal column compounded with surgical adhesions can precipitate tethered cord syndrome with resultant muscular denervation. Hence, there is likely an interplay between the direct and indirect mechanisms of post-resection spinal deformity in pediatric patients [39]. Meticulous surgical technique and close follow-up looking for new-onset deformity are crucial to avoiding its possible ramifications.

Risk Factors for Post-tumor Resection Development of Spinal Deformity

Through years of experience in this known complication for spinal tumor management, an array of risk factors has been noted in the literature. This is useful since, in some, a much closer follow-up is needed with serial imaging given the presence of multiple known risk factors, some more important than others, and are described in further detail below.

The Most Frequently Quoted Risk Factors

1. **Pediatric age** is the most significant risk factor for post-resection deformity [40]—age less than 13 years was the cut-off for increased risk of progressive spinal deformity following intramedullary tumor resection in Yao et al.'s series of 161 pediatric patients [28]. McGirt et al. reported similarl findings, noting age < 13 was associated with a 3.9-fold higher odds of deformity following resection of cervical intramedullary tumors [41]. For comparison, the historical study of Bishara found that adults treated with laminectomy for degenerative pathology rarely experience kyphotic deformity [42].
2. **The number of laminectomies** to be performed is another significant risk factor. Katsumi et al. were one of the earlier groups to describe this, noting ≥4-level laminectomy to be associated with a four-fold higher odds of deformity compared to <4 level laminectomy. [40] However, some debate the association of the extent of decompression with deformity risk [8]. This is the minority opinion though and the current debate is regarding the minimum number of laminectomy levels above which deformity risk is appreciably increased. Papagelopoulos et al. describe increased incidence with >2 level laminectomy [9] and Anakwenze et al. suggest that the threshold is at 3 laminae [43]. Sciubba et al. suggested a geometric relationship between decompression extent and deformity risk with a 3.1-fold increase in the likelihood of instability for every additional lamina removed [44].
3. **The location of laminectomy** is equally as important as the number. The craniocervical, cervicothoracic, and thoracolumbar junctions appear at the highest postresection deformity in pediatric and young adolescent populations [45–47]. Unsurprisingly these are the spinal level subjected to the greatest stresses, especially with motion. Another location described as high risk in a meta-analysis focusing on the cervical spine was C2 laminectomy, [6] which unsurprisingly is linked to an increased incidence of swan neck deformity through kyphotic deformity above C2 and compensatory lordosis below C2 [48]. C2 laminectomy may have this associated risk, as it is a vital attachment point for the suboccipital muscular (rectus capitii, obliquus capitis inferior) that maintains craniocervical extension [40].

4. **Pre-operative deformity,** though not as significant when presenting mildly, is important at a population level. In Yao et al.'s study, 33% of patients presented with deformity prior to resection [28]. Pre-existing deformity conferred a more than two-fold higher risk in a study by Kaptain et al. [49] and even as high as a 27-fold increase in risk as reported by Wang et al. [39] Ahmed and colleagues found that 64% of patients with deformity at the time of presentation ultimately required spinal fusion. [50].

Less Frequently Quoted Risk Factors

1. The need for **facetectomy** for foraminal and extraforaminal tumors. As demonstrated in the biomechanical work of Panjabi et al., [51] injury to the facet joints is associated with a change in motion, which increases risk. However, as reported by Asazuma et al., single-level unilateral facetectomy does not appear to confer a clinically increased risk of deformity [52].
2. Adjuvant or neoadjuvant **radiotherapy** is toxic to bone and related soft tissue and can result in vertebral body growth inhibition, mild tissue fibrosis, and bone necrosis. Paulino [53] looking at pediatric sarcoma radiotherapy, reported that >50% of patients undergoing external beam radiotherapy required surgical procedures for bone deformity (including spinal bone deformity) within 20 years [54]. Advances in radiotherapy, specifically the increased availability of charged particle and focused photon modalities, have lessened this concern by minimizing off-target doses [20]. Nevertheless, the risk remains present.
3. **Method of decompression** also appears to predict risk, with multiple groups reporting laminectomy to have increased risk of deformity relative to osteoplastic laminotomy/laminoplasty. Laminectomy has been reported to confer an approximately seven fold increased risk of postoperative deformity [55] and has also been associated with increased postoperative musculoskeletal pain, [56] longer acute hospitalizations, greater intraoperative risks of CSF leaks [28, 57–59] and greater postoperative risks in revision surgery [60]. However, such findings have not been wholly uniform, with McGirt et al. [58] finding no difference in risk of postoperative deformity between laminoplasty and laminectomy, echoing earlier findings in a meta-analysis by Ratliff and Cooper [61] looking at laminectomy versus laminoplasty in the degenerative population. These studies suggest that the muscle dissection require for laminectomy and laminoplasty is equivalent, and it is the soft tissue atrophy that confers the risk of post-resection of deformity. The etiology of these heterogeneous findings is not entirely clear but may be accounted for by differences in follow-up between studies. Regardless, given the lack of a clearly superior technique, the method of resection should be considered on a case-by-case basis.
4. **Tumor-associated factors** have also been suggested to contribute to deformity. Cited factors include tumor grading, delay in resection, [28] risk of tumor relapse, [57] and the occurrence of asymmetrical paraspinal muscular denerva-

tion secondary to a tumor-associated syrinx [62]. In fact, spinal tumor-associated syrinx is generally underappreciated as a significant risk factor, though the study of Yao et al. [28] noted it to be the second most important risk factor after age, conferring a 3.4-fold higher odds of deformity.

As is clearly evident, there are a multitude of risk factors, with patients differing in the number and types of risk factors they possess. To this end, the study of Katsumi et al. [40] suggested a single risk factor is likely insufficient to precipitate post-resection deformity. They noted that patients in whom deformity did not develop had an average of 1.2 risk factors compared to 2.5 for those who developed deformity and 3 for those developing a deformity severe enough to require surgical stabilization.

The potential for post-resection deformity and the need for intervention should be discussed with the family at the time of counseling about the need for surgical intervention for the tumor. Additionally, follow-up should be tailored to the patient's estimated preoperative risk of subsequent deformity, with those having more risk factors (e.g., preexisting deformity, larger tumors, and tumors with associated syrinxes) requiring more frequent follow-up. Consideration should also be made to obtaining upright scoliosis radiographs at the time of original consultation to be used as baseline references during postoperative surveillance.

Surgical Versus Nonsurgical Bracing Treatment

Bracing

Depending upon patient preference and the severity of the deformity, both operative and nonoperative treatments may be reasonable. External bracing is a form of nonsurgical conservative management that can aid deformity flexibility and muscle adaptation. However, there are few patients that can be reasonably treated with bracing, and bracing is not an operation for cases of severe deformity. Bracing may negatively affect lower limb motor function in neurologically impaired patients, and it is generally accepted that bracing is merely a means of delaying definitive management, and it is incapable of correcting extant deformity [63]. For example, Ahmed et al. noted bracing was effective in only 40% of the 20 patients with deformity; 11 ultimately required surgical intervention (the deformity resolved in the remaining patient) [50]. It is recommended that spinal fusion be considered 1 year post-surgery without adequate efficacy from conservative management [34].

The primary benefit of bracing in patients with post-resection deformity appears to be its ability to delay the need for fusion so as to allow for maximal spinal and pulmonary growth in pediatric patients before fusion [50]. For those being treated with bracing, it has been recommended that brace fitting occur as early as the first postoperative day, [7] as some reports have noted the onset of post-resection deformity to occur within a week post-surgery [7]. Hence, in high-risk patients where the surgeon chose to avoid immediate instrumentation, bracing should be considered. Some advocate for bracing even in the case of performing laminoplasty, as it has been noted that deformity may occur even amongst laminoplasty patients who did not receive postoperative immobilization [7]. There exists not a consensus regarding the duration of bracing that must be pursued; however, one report advocated for 4–6 months of brace immobilization following laminoplasty. [64]

Further, in some patients, the trajectory of the oncological problem is unknown, and in cases of barely ambulatory patients who have a high probability of neurological compromise with spinal fusion, external bracing is something that should be heavily considered, [13] and even if spinal fusion occurs, bracing may be useful to promote bone fusion [7]. Such post-fusion external immobilization has been recommended for 4 months with deformities of the cervical spine and for 6 months with the thoracic [7].

Surgical Management

Surgical management is indicated where there is severe and/or progressive deformity or deformity with associated pain and/or neurological symptoms. Multilevel instability is not directly correlated to the severity of the deformity; hence, the decision should be directed by the Cobb angle and rigidity of the deformity rather than by the length of the deformity [7]. The timing for intervention is sometimes a complex decision, as in many cases, the pediatric patient will still be in a phase where spinal fusion may perturb growth, leading to the loss of growth potential. Additional young patients may have bony anatomy too small to accommodate conventional implants. Another topic that makes the timing for intervention problematic is the oncological phase of the patient. In cases where there is no overt instability and further treatment is needed, which would need to be delayed for surgical intervention (i.e., chemotherapy treatments), the surgeon might decide to let the patient finish the treatment while closely following the deformity.

VEPTR Devices

In recent years, there has been the development of growth-friendly spinal implants (Vertical Expandable Prosthetic Titanium Rib (VEPTR) devices), which allow rib-to-pelvis fixation of the spine, and the length of the implant can be adjusted to afford continued spinal column growth. Additionally, as this device is placed farther from the spinal canal, it affords better surveillance and allows for easier re-accessing of the spinal canal in cases of recurrence (seen in 30% of cases), [65] as compared to conventional instrumented fusion, [66, 67] though the difference is less pronounced for modern titanium instrumentation [68]. The number of adjusting procedures varies by case, with Hell et al. reporting an average of nine lengthening procedures performed biannually in their study focusing on children <10 years [13]. These authors noted significant improvement in scoliosis and kyphosis without a resultant loss of lordosis or increased risk of neurological compromise [13]. Importantly, the use of VEPTR as an initial treatment modality was found to have no deleterious effect on fusion outcomes following definitive management [13]. However, to highlight this point, VEPTR is only meant as a temporizing solution, [28] and fusion is ultimately required for definitive management of the deformity following puberty onset (defined by Risser sign is >2) [69]. In those with overt instability and significant concern for progression, fusion may be required earlier, though it is recommended this be done no earlier than age 10 unless the patient is symptomatic [13].

Despite the potential advantages of VEPTR devices, they have not gained uniform acceptance, which may stem from concerns about the reported high rates of complications. In one series, 49% of cases had complications, including infection, implant rejection, respiratory issues, and spinal cord injury [70]. The relative novelty of VEPTR devices may also dissuade surgeons from using them, as there is limited evidence to support their long term effectiveness, in comparison to spinal fusion, which has been used for many years and is so better understood.

Spinal Fusion

Instrumented fusion is considered definitive management for spinal deformity; it can address underlying instability, correct underlying deformity, and decrease the likelihood of progressive debilitating deformity. As deformity following intradural spine tumor resection is largely thought to result from failure of the posterior tension band, the deformity is often flexible. For this reason, some surgeons employ halo distraction preoperatively to try and reduce the deformity and so lessen the aggressiveness of the correction required intraoperatively, as aggressive correction can be associated with intraoperative neurological injury. However, halo traction is likely to be minimally effective in cases of rigid or severe deformity [13].

Factors favoring prophylactic spinal fusion post-resection of intradural tumors include pre-operative bone erosion, bone resection spanning >2 vertebral segments, utilization of a transpedicular or costovertebral approach, performance of a total fasciectomy, and resection of a high cervical tumor (C1-C3) [71]. The same systematic review noted that a single risk factor is likely an insufficient cause to warrant spinal fusion. As fusion results in loss of spinal motion segments, increases operative time and costs, and increases surgical risks, concurrent fusion is probably best relegated to patients who present with high-risk deformity at the time of tumor resection [43]. For these patients though, concurrent fusion decreases postoperative deformity risk, with one study noting moderate to severe deformity in only 27% of patients treated with concurrent fusion compared with 57% of patients who underwent laminectomy/laminoplasty alone [43]. In another study by Simon and colleagues, 9 of 16 patients who underwent resection alone developed deformity compared to only 1 of 10 treated with concurrent fusion [72]. The protective effect of fusion may be even more significant in skeletally mature children with Anakwenze and colleagues noting postoperative deformity in only 22% of those treated with concomitant fusion compared to 64% who underwent resection alone [43]. However, the protective effects of laminoplasty and fusion are not additive, [72] nor should fusion be seen as a replacement for laminoplasty, as it necessitates the loss of motion segments. Our general approach, based upon clinical experience, is to employ laminoplasty in those without deformity at presentation, taking care to preserve ligamentous structures, joint capsules, and facets during the laminectomy. We reserved concurrent fusion only for those who present with high-risk severe deformity or already proven instability.

Fusion Technique

Anterior, posterior, and combined approaches have all been described. One drawback of posterior instrumentation is that it places metallic hardware immediately adjacent to the spinal cord, with a resultant radiographic artifact that complicates effective radiographic surveillance and radiotherapy treatment planning [73]. Because of this, patients who undergo instrumentation may experience underdosing of the residual tumor and have delayed diagnosis of recurrence. New implant technologies, specifically carbon fiber-reinforced-polyetheretherketone (CFR-PEEK), may help to reduce these effects given their radiolucent nature, [74] though their use in pediatric patients is not thoroughly detailed.

Patients who undergo concurrent fusion still merit radiographic surveillance for subsequent deformity as there are reports of spinal deformity occurring after fusion. This may be secondary to adjacent segment disease, as is thoroughly documented in the adult deformity literature, or may manifest due to tumor progression causing paraspinal denervation and subsequent deformity; this may occur away from the site of initial deformity [72].

Summary of Suggested Paradigm—Flow Chart

To conclude, we advise a generic management plan along the lines of that suggested by Fassett et al., [17] for which a summary is offered below (Fig. 1.2). This includes the need for plain AP and lateral spine radiograph preoperatively, which serve as a baseline alignment film and help to identify preexisting deformity. This latter point allows for risk stratification and identification of patients who may require concurrent fusion at the time of tumor resection. A spinal deformity prediction tool posited by Knafo et al., [75] can be useful to risk stratify further according to other significant risk factors described in this chapter. Dynamic imaging of the spine in flexion and extension can also be useful to assess the mobility of the deformity, and highly mobile deformities can benefit from traction to enable reduction.

For patients with already significant extant kyphosis at the time of initial evaluation, we recommend concurrent stabilization at the time of initial laminectomy to both address the underlying deformity and prevent further deformity. Regular

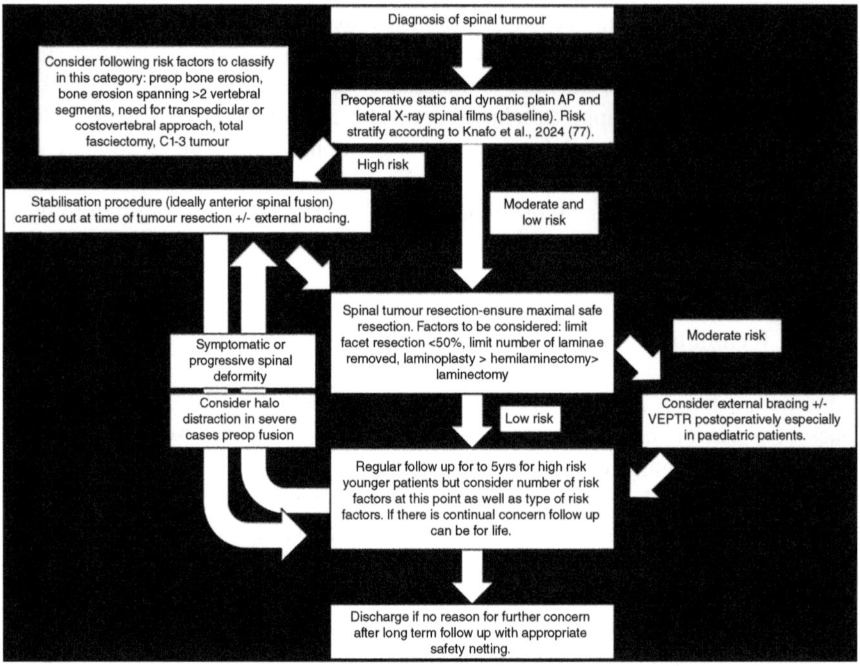

Fig. 1.2 A diagrammatic flow chart summary of our suggested paradigm for the management of spinal tumors that will be managed surgically

radiographic follow-up is warranted for both those who undergo concurrent fusion and those treated with resection alone; the latter may require more frequent surveillance if they undergo resection of a particularly large lesion or one that localizes to a high-risk region, like the cervicothoracic junction.

Intraoperatively, care must be taken to limit facet resection to <50% and avoid injury to the facet capsule [15]. Effort should also be made to limit the number of laminae removed and using a laminoplasty or osteoplastic laminotomy rather than laminectomy, which can partially restore the posterior tension band [7, 22]. For eccentric tumors, or those at non-cord levels, hemilaminectomy may be reasonably possible, [35] as this allows for preservation of the posterior tension band on one side and so may reduce the risk of subsequent deformity. For the patients that are candidates for resection surgery, maximal safe resection should be advocated. Subtotal resection is commonly associated with an increased risk of recurrence, which merits repeat resection that carries with it an increased odds of deformity [28]. Overall, we recommend a surgical strategy that affords the best conditions for tumor resection while preserving the skeletal architecture.

Postoperatively, we recommend follow-up occur at regular intervals for a minimum of 5 years given that deformities can often occur in a delayed fashion [14]. Patients at higher risk of deformity may require shorter follow-up intervals to catch progressive deformity early [76]. The types of risk factors present also likely influence the duration of follow-up required before the patient can be deemed "out of the woods." For example, radiation therapy leads to deformity on average 77 months later (and is seen evidently during rapid pubertal growth) compared to surgical laminectomy, which generally occurs 5–15 months postoperatively [7]. Deformity onset is also generally more rapid for those undergoing resection of cervical or cervicothoracic lesions (5 months) versus thoracic lesions (15 months). However, given the possibility of tumor recurrence to cause delayed-onset deformity, [72] we generally continue clinical follow-up for as long as there is concern for tumor recurrence in low-risk patients (e.g., those treated with gross total resection of ependymoma) and lifelong follow-up for those at high risk (e.g., high-grade astrocytoma).

References

1. Ostrom QT, Patil N, Cioffi G, Waite K, Kruchko C, Barnholtz-Sloan JS (2020) CBTRUS statistical report: primary brain and other central nervous system tumors diagnosed in the United States in 2013–2017. Neuro-Oncology 22:iv1–iv96
2. Duong LM, McCarthy BJ, McLendon RE, Dolecek TA, Kruchko C, Douglas LL, Ajani UA (2012) Descriptive epidemiology of malignant and nonmalignant primary spinal cord, spinal meninges, and cauda equina tumors, United States, 2004-2007. Cancer 118:4220–4227
3. Ostrom QT, Price M, Neff C, Cioffi G, Waite KA, Kruchko C, Barnholtz-Sloan JS (2022) CBTRUS statistical report: primary brain and other central nervous system tumors diagnosed in the United States in 2015–2019. Neuro-Oncology 24:v1–v95
4. Merola AA, Haher TR, Brkaric M et al (2002) A multicenter study of the outcomes of the surgical treatment of adolescent idiopathic scoliosis using the Scoliosis Research Society (SRS) outcome instrument. Spine (Phila Pa 1976) 27:2046–2051
5. Barker DJ, Weller RO, Garfield JS (1976) Epidemiology of primary tumours of the brain and spinal cord: a regional survey in southern England. J Neurol Neurosurg Psychiatry 39:290–296
6. Noh SH, Takahashi T, Inoue T, Park S-M, Hanakita J, Minami M, Kanematsu R, Shimauchi-Ohtaki H, Ha Y (2022) Postoperative spinal deformity and instability after cervical spinal cord tumor resection in adults: a systematic review and meta-analysis. J Clin Neurosci 100:148–154
7. de Jonge T, Slullitel H, Dubousset J, Miladi L, Wicart P, Illés T (2005) Late-onset spinal deformities in children treated by laminectomy and radiation therapy for malignant tumours. Eur Spine J 14:765–771
8. Bell DF, Walker JL, O'Connor G, Tibshirani R (1994) Spinal deformity after multiple-level cervical laminectomy in children. Spine (Phila Pa 1976) 19:406–411
9. Papagelopoulos PJ, Peterson HA, Ebersold MJ, Emmanuel RP, Choudhury SN, Quast LM (1997) Spinal column deformity and instability after lumbar or thoracolumbar laminectomy for Intraspinal tumors in children and young adults. Spine (Phila Pa 1976) 22:442–451
10. Robinson D, Galasko CSB, Delaney C, Williamson JB, Barrie JL (1995) Scoliosis and lung function in spinal muscular atrophy. Eur Spine J 4:268–273
11. Watanabe K, Hasegawa K, Hirano T, Uchiyama S, Endo N (2007) Evaluation of postoperative residual spinal deformity and patient outcome in idiopathic scoliosis patients in Japan using the Scoliosis Research Society outcomes instrument. Spine (Phila Pa 1976) 32:550–554
12. Eiselsberg A (1930) Über eine bemerkenswerte Gestaltsveränderung der Wirbelsäule nach einer ausgedehnten Laminektomie wegen Rückenmarktumors. Arch Orthop Unfallchir 28:132–138

13. Hell AK, Kühnle I, Lorenz HM, Braunschweig L, Lüders KA, Bock HC, Kramm CM, Ludwig HC, Tsaknakis K (2020) Spinal deformities after childhood tumors. Cancers (Basel) 12:3555
14. Lunardi P, Licastro G, Missori P, Ferrante L, Fortuna A (1993) Management of intramedullary tumours in children. Acta Neurochir 120:59–65
15. Epstein JA (1988) The surgical Management of Cervical Spinal Stenosis, spondylosis, and Myeloradiculopathy by means of the posterior approach. Spine (Phila Pa 1976) 13:864–869
16. Nolan JP, Sherk HH (1988) Biomechanical evaluation of the extensor musculature of the cervical spine. Spine (Phila Pa 1976) 13:9–11
17. Fassett DR, Clark R, Brockmeyer DL, Schmidt MH (2006) Cervical spine deformity associated with resection of spinal cord tumors. Neurosurg Focus 20:E2
18. Lonstein JE (1995) Postlaminectomy spinal deformity. In: Bradford DS, Lonstein JE, Ogilvie JW, Winter RB (eds) Moe's Textb. Scoliosis other spinal deform, 3rd edn. Saunders, pp 506–515
19. Arikoski P, Komulainen J, Riikonen P, Parviainen M, Jurvelin JS, Voutilainen R, Kröger H (1999) Impaired development of bone mineral density during chemotherapy: a prospective analysis of 46 children newly diagnosed with cancer. J Bone Miner Res 14:2002–2009
20. Butler MS, Robertson WW, Rate W, D'Angio GJ, Drummond DS (1990) Skeletal sequelae of radiation therapy for malignant childhood tumors. Clin Orthop Relat Res:235–240
21. Dubousset J (1980) Spine deformities induced by irradiation of Wilm's tumors (author's transl). Rev Chir Orthop Reparatrice Appar Mot 66:441–451
22. Joaquim AF, Riew KD (2015) Management of cervical spine deformity after intradural tumor resection. Neurosurg Focus 39:E13
23. Arkin AM, Simon N (1950) Radiation scoliosis; an experimental study. J Bone Joint Surg Am 32A:396–401
24. Goel VK, Clark CR, Harris KG, Schulte KR (1988) Kinematics of the cervical spine: effects of multiple total laminectomy and facet wiring. J Orthop Res 6:611–619
25. Tachdjian MO, Matson DD (1965) Orthopaedic aspects of Intraspinal tumors in infants and children. J Bone Joint Surg Am 47:223–248
26. Constantini S, Houten J, Miller DC, Freed D, Ozek MM, Rorke LB, Allen JC, Epstein FJ (1996) Intramedullary spinal cord tumors in children under the age of 3 years. J Neurosurg 85:1036–1043
27. Pal GP, Sherk HH (1988) The vertical stability of the cervical spine. Spine (Phila Pa 1976) 13:447–449
28. Yao KC, McGirt MJ, Chaichana KL, Constantini S, Jallo GI (2007) Risk factors for progressive spinal deformity following resection of intramedullary spinal cord tumors in children: an analysis of 161 consecutive cases. J Neurosurg Pediatr 107:463–468
29. Zdeblick TA, Abitbol J-J, Kunz DN, Eng M, McCabe RP, Garfin S (1993) Cervical stability after sequential capsule resection. Spine (Phila Pa 1976) 18:2005–2008
30. Zdeblick TA, Zou D, Warden KE, McCabe R, Kunz D, Vanderby R (1992) Cervical stability after foraminotomy. A biomechanical in vitro analysis. J Bone Joint Surg Am 74:22–27
31. White AH, Wiltse LL (1976) Spondylolisthesis after extensive lumbar laminectomy. J Bone Joint Surg Am 58:727
32. Ahmed R, Traynelis VC, Menezes AH (2008) Fusions at the craniovertebral junction. Childs Nerv Syst 24:1209–1224
33. Arey L (1977) Development of the spine and spinal cord. In: Ruge D, Wiltse LL (eds) Spinal Disord. Diagnosis treat, 1st edn. Lea & Febiger, pp 3–13
34. Avila MJ, Walter CM, Skoch J, Abbasifard S, Patel AS, Sattarov K, Baaj AA (2015) Fusion after intradural spine tumor resection in adults: a review of evidence and practices. Clin Neurol Neurosurg 138:169–173
35. Öktem I, Akdemir H, Kurtsoy A, Koç R, Menkü A, Tucer B (2000) Hemilaminectomy for the removal of the spinal lesions. Spinal Cord 38:92–96

36. Tredway TL, Santiago P, Hrubes MR, Song JK, Christie SD, Fessler RG (2006) Minimally invasive resection of Intradural-extramedullary spinal neoplasms. Oper Neurosurg 58:ONS-52–ONS-58
37. Raygor KP, Than KD, Chou D, Mummaneni PV (2015) Comparison of minimally invasive transspinous and open approaches for thoracolumbar intradural-extramedullary spinal tumors. Neurosurg Focus 39:E12
38. Balasubramanian SC, Nair AR, Saphiya NN, Madan A, Mathews SS (2021) Minimally invasive resection of spinal tumors with tubular retractor: case series, surgical technique, and outcome. World Neurosurg 149:e612–e621
39. Wang P, Ma K, Chen T et al (2020) Risk factor analysis for progressive spinal deformity after resection of intracanal tumors— a retrospective study of 272 cases. BMC Neurol 20:34
40. Katsumi Y, Honma T, Nakamura T (1989) Analysis of cervical instability resulting from laminectomies for removal of spinal cord tumor. Spine (Phila Pa 1976) 14:1171–1176
41. McGirt MJ, Chaichana KL, Attenello F, Witham T, Bydon A, Yao KC, Jallo GI (2008) Spinal deformity after resection of cervical intramedullary spinal cord tumors in children. Childs Nerv Syst 24:735–739
42. Bishara SN (1971) The posterior operation in treatment of cervical spondylosis with myelopathy: a long-term follow-up study. J Neurol Neurosurg Psychiatry 34:393–398
43. Anakwenze OA, Auerbach JD, Buck DW, Garg S, Simon SL, Sutton LN, Sponseller PD, Dormans JP (2011) The role of concurrent fusion to prevent spinal deformity after intramedullary spinal cord tumor excision in children. J Pediatr Orthop 31:475–479
44. Sciubba DM, Chaichana KL, Woodworth GF, McGirt MJ, Gokaslan ZL, Jallo GI (2008) Factors associated with cervical instability requiring fusion after cervical laminectomy for intradural tumor resection. J Neurosurg Spine 8:413–419
45. Aronson DD, Kahn RH, Canady A, Bollinger RO, Towbin R (1991) Instability of the cervical spine after decompression in patients who have Arnold-Chiari malformation. J Bone Joint Surg Am 73:898–906
46. Yeh JS, Sgouros S, Walsh AR, Hockley AD (2001) Spinal sagittal malalignment following surgery for primary intramedullary Tumours in children. Pediatr Neurosurg 35:318–324
47. Price C, Makintubee S, Hemdon W, Istre GR (1994) Epidemiology of traumatic spinal cord injury and acute hospitalization and rehabilitation charges for spinal cord injuries in Oklahoma, 1988–1990. Am J Epidemiol 139:37–47
48. Inoue A, Ikata T, Katoh S (1996) Spinal deformity following surgery for spinal cord tumors and tumorous lesions: analysis based on an assessment of the spinal functional curve. Spinal Cord 34:536–542
49. Kaptain GJ, Simmons NE, Replogle RE, Pobereskin L (2000) Incidence and outcome of kyphotic deformity following laminectomy for cervical spondylotic myelopathy. J Neurosurg 93:199–204
50. Ahmed R, Menezes AH, Awe OO, Mahaney KB, Torner JC, Weinstein SL (2014) Long-term incidence and risk factors for development of spinal deformity following resection of pediatric intramedullary spinal cord tumors. J Neurosurg Pediatr 13:613–621
51. Panjabi MM, White AA, Keller D, Southwick WO, Friedlaender G (1978) Stability of the cervical spine under tension. J Biomech 11:189–197
52. Asazuma T, Nakamura M, Matsumoto M, Chibo K, Toyama Y (2004) Postoperative changes of spinal curvature and range of motion in adult patients with cervical spinal cord tumors. J Spinal Disord Tech 17:178–182
53. Paulino AC (2004) Late effects of radiotherapy for pediatric extremity sarcomas. Int J Radiat Oncol 60:265–274
54. Arkin AM, Pack GT, Ransohoff NS, Simon N (1950) Radiation-induced scoliosis; a case report. J Bone Joint Surg Am 32A:401–404
55. McGirt MJ, Chaichana KL, Atiba A, Bydon A, Witham TF, Yao KC, Jallo GI (2008) Incidence of spinal deformity after resection of intramedullary spinal cord tumors in children who underwent laminectomy compared with laminoplasty. J Neurosurg Pediatr 1:57–62

56. Cobb MA, Boop FA (1994) Replacement Laminoplasty in selective dorsal Rhizotomy: possible protection against the development of musculoskeletal pain. Pediatr Neurosurg 21:237–242
57. McGirt MJ, Constantini S, Jallo GI (2008) Correlation of a preoperative grading scale with progressive spinal deformity following surgery for intramedullary spinal cord tumors in children. J Neurosurg Pediatr 2:277–281
58. McGirt MJ, Garcés-Ambrossi GL, Parker SL, Sciubba DM, Bydon A, Wolinksy J-P, Gokaslan ZL, Jallo G, Witham TF (2010) Short-term progressive spinal deformity following Laminoplasty versus laminectomy for resection of Intradural spinal tumors. Analysis of 238 patients. Neurosurgery 66:1005–1012
59. Montano N, Trevisi G, Cioni B, Lucantoni C, Della Pepa GM, Meglio M, Papacci F (2014) The role of laminoplasty in preventing spinal deformity in adult patients submitted to resection of an intradural spinal tumor. Case series and literature review. Clin Neurol Neurosurg 125:69–74
60. Wang Z-C, Li S-Z, Qu X-F, Yin C-Q, Sun Y-L, Wang Y-L, Wang J, Liu C-J, Cao Z-L, Wang T (2021) Application of open-door laminoplasty with ARCH plate fixation in cervical intraspinal tumors. BMC Surg 21:141
61. Ratliff JK, Cooper PR (2003) Cervical laminoplasty: a critical review. J Neurosurg Spine 98:230–238
62. Huebert HT, MacKinnon WB (1969) Syringomyelia and scoliosis. J Bone Joint Surg Br 51:338–343
63. Cattell HS, Clark GL (1967) Cervical kyphosis and instability following multiple laminectomies in children. J Bone Joint Surg Am 49:713–720
64. Ghanem I, Zeller R, Dubousset J (1996) Extra osseous tumors of the spine in children and adolescents. Spinal complications. Rev Chir Orthop Reparatrice Appar Mot 82:313–320
65. Hersh DS, Iyer RR, Garzon-Muvdi T, Liu A, Jallo GI, Groves ML (2017) Instrumented fusion for spinal deformity after laminectomy or laminoplasty for resection of intramedullary spinal cord tumors in pediatric patients. Neurosurg Focus 43:E12
66. Abol Oyoun N, Stuecker R (2014) Bilateral rib-to-pelvis Eiffel tower VEPTR construct for children with neuromuscular scoliosis: a preliminary report. Spine J 14:1183–1191
67. Lorenz HM, Braunschweig L, Schiele S, Tsaknakis K, Hecker MM, Gantner AS, Hell A-K (2018) Surgical treatment of spinal deformities in young paraplegic children with Intraspinal tumors. Pediatr Neurosurg 53:149–152
68. Torpey BM, Dormans JP, Drummond DS (1995) The use of MRI-compatible titanium segmental spinal instrumentation in pediatric patients with intraspinal tumor. J Spinal Disord 8:76–81
69. Risser JC (2010) The classic: the iliac Apophysis: an invaluable sign in the Management of Scoliosis. Clin Orthop Relat Res 468:646–653
70. El-Hawary R, Kadhim M, Vitale M, Smith J, Samdani A, Flynn JM (2017) VEPTR implantation to treat children with early-onset scoliosis without rib abnormalities: early results from a prospective multicenter study. J Pediatr Orthop 37:e599–e605
71. Quiceno E, Hussein A, Pico A et al (2023) Indications for fusion with Intradural spine tumor resection in adults: a systematic review and meta-analysis. World Neurosurg 176:21–30
72. Simon SL, Auerbach JD, Garg S, Sutton LN, Telfeian AE, Dormans JP (2008) Efficacy of spinal instrumentation and fusion in the prevention of Postlaminectomy spinal deformity in children with intramedullary spinal cord tumors. J Pediatr Orthop 28:244–249
73. Garcés-Ambrossi GL, McGirt MJ, Mehta VA, Sciubba DM, Witham TF, Bydon A, Wolinksy J-P, Jallo GI, Gokaslan ZL (2009) Factors associated with progression-free survival and long-term neurological outcome after resection of intramedullary spinal cord tumors: analysis of 101 consecutive cases. J Neurosurg Spine 11:591–599
74. Krätzig T, Mende KC, Mohme M, Kniep H, Dreimann M, Stangenberg M, Westphal M, Gauer T, Eicker SO (2021) Carbon fiber–reinforced PEEK versus titanium implants: an in vitro comparison of susceptibility artifacts in CT and MR imaging. Neurosurg Rev 44:2163–2170
75. Knafo S, Court C, Parker F (2014) Predicting sagittal deformity after surgery for intramedullary tumors. J Neurosurg Spine 21:342–347

76. Yasuoka S, Peterson HA, MacCarty CS (1982) Incidence of spinal column deformity after multilevel laminectomy in children and adults. J Neurosurg 57:441–445
77. Colado JC, Pablos C, Chulvi-Medrano I, Garcia-Masso X, Flandez J, Behm DG (2011) The progression of Paraspinal muscle recruitment intensity in localized and global strength training exercises is not based on instability alone. Arch Phys Med Rehabil 92:1875–1883
78. Hadley MN, Zabramski JM, Browner CM, Rekate H, Sonntag VKH (1988) Pediatric spinal trauma. Review of 122 cases of spinal cord and vertebral column injuries. J Neurosurg 68:18–24

Chapter 2
Neurofibromatosis-Associated Spinal Deformity

Amy L. Xu, Amit Jain, Mari L. Groves, and Paul D. Sponseller

General

Neurofibromatosis type 1 (NF1) is a neurocutaneous disorder rooted in pathologic neural crest cells that manifests with tumors of the brain, nerves, and spinal cord. It is one of the most common single-gene conditions, with an estimated prevalence of 1 in 3000 births [1, 2]. It results from a loss-of-function mutation of the neurofibromin 1 tumor suppressor gene on chromosome 17q11.2. The encoded neurofibromin protein is expressed in a variety of cells, including neurons, oligodendrocytes, astrocytes, and Schwann cells. It works to inactivate the Ras signaling pathway, thereby playing an essential role in the downregulation of cell growth and proliferation [3, 4]. Although considered an autosomal-dominant disorder, NF1 has highly variable expressivity, and disease progression can be difficult to predict [5]. NF1 is the only type of neurofibromatosis associated with orthopedic complications, with approximately 10–60% of patients developing spinal deformities during their lifetime [6–8]. For patients with NF1, age-related disease progression is a key consideration, thereby emphasizing the value of early detection and treatment [9]. In this chapter,

A. L. Xu
Department of Orthopaedic Surgery, Hospital for Special Surgery, New York, NY, USA
e-mail: amyxu@alumni.stanford.edu

A. Jain · P. D. Sponseller (✉)
Department of Orthopaedic Surgery, Johns Hopkins University School of Medicine, Baltimore, MD, USA
e-mail: ajain24@jhmi.edu; psponse1@jhmi.edu

M. L. Groves
Department of Neurosurgery, Johns Hopkins University School of Medicine, Baltimore, MD, USA
e-mail: mgroves2@jhmi.edu

D. M. Sciubba (ed.), *Spinal Tumor Associated Deformity*, https://doi.org/10.1007/978-3-031-87939-5_2

we will discuss the characteristics of neurofibromatosis-associated spinal deformity and principles to approach its diagnosis, evaluation, and management.

Deformity Types in Neurofibromatosis

Scoliosis

Early-onset scoliosis (EOS, defined as a spinal curvature of >10° in the coronal plane in patients who are <10 years of age) is the most common skeletal manifestation seen in patients with NF1, with 2% of pediatric scoliosis estimated to occur secondary to the diagnosis [10]. NF1-associated EOS can be classified as nondystrophic versus dystrophic. Most children with NF1 who present with scoliosis have the nondystrophic variant, which behaves similar to and requires treatment like that employed for adolescent idiopathic scoliosis (AIS) (Fig. 2.1a). However, nondystrophic vertebrae in NF1 are more likely to have abnormal pedicles, including smaller transverse pedicle widths that lead to increased risk of screw misplacement during correction surgeries [11]. Additionally, close follow-up is necessary given that nondystrophic curves can acquire dystrophic features [12]. This phenomenon, termed "modulation," is unique to NF1 and has been reported to occur in 81% of children who present with scoliosis before age seven and in 25% who develop deformity after age 7 [13]. Compared with AIS, surgical correction of nondystrophic NF1-associated deformity is also associated with higher rates of pseudarthrosis and revision [14].

Dystrophic curves are less common but more likely to progress rapidly than nondystrophic curves. While there are no existing diagnostic criteria for dystrophic scoliosis, the following nine radiographic characteristics have been described: rib penciling, vertebral rotation, vertebral scalloping, vertebral wedging in either the sagittal or coronal plane, spindling of the transverse process, widened interpedicular distance, and enlarged intervertebral foramina [13, 15] (Fig. 2.1b). The most frequently observed pattern involves one thoracic curve across four to six vertebrae with sharp angulation and severe apical rotation in association with the typical bony features noted above. These changes are thought to result from primary bone dysplasia via disordered chondrogenesis and osteogenesis, which manifests in pathologic growth plate properties on the curve concavity. In contrast, the convex side retains adequate proliferation, differentiation, and osteogenesis [16]. This growth pattern—along with continued load on the spine as well as the presence of intraspinal neurofibromas, pseudomeningoceles, and dural ectasia—contributes to growth asymmetry and deformity development [6, 17]. The abnormal tissue can also erode the surrounding bony structures, leading to significant destabilization of the spine, vertebral collapse, and a resultant deterioration of pulmonary and neurologic function [15].

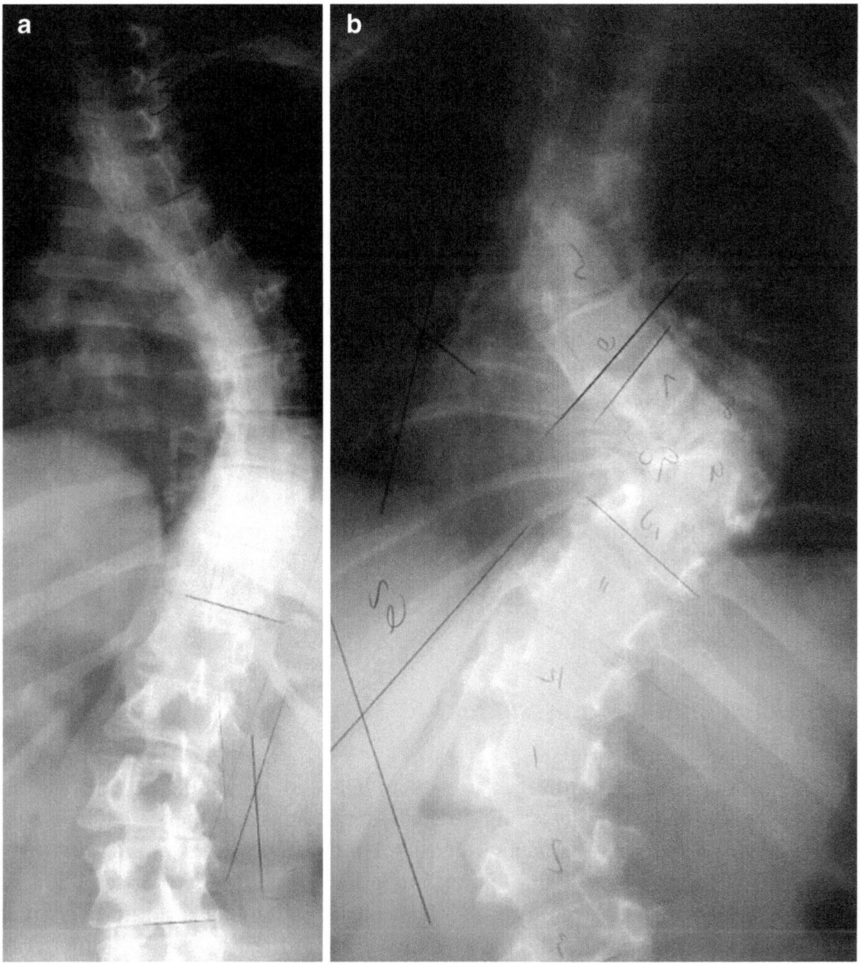

Fig. 2.1 Radiographs of (**a**) nondystrophic deformity, (**b**) dystrophic deformity

Risk factors for the rapid progression of dystrophic curves have been postulated, one of which is the co-occurrence of multiple signs of vertebral dysplasia [18]. These signs, which are concerning for progression, include high Cobb angle, abnormal kyphosis, anterior vertebral scalloping, severe (>11°) apical rotation of the curve, a mid to lower thoracic curve apex, penciling of ≥1 rib bilaterally or on the curve concavity, and penciling of ≥4 ribs [7, 13, 19]. In contrast, curves with lordotic wedging are slower to progress [19]. These is currently no clear consensus on how the number of involved vertebrae impacts curve progression [7, 20].

Regardless of type, NF1-associated EOS most frequently presents in the thoracic region, and the lumbosacral region is uncommonly affected. The deformity often spans multiple spinal regions, but whole spine involvement is rare [21]. Deformity is also not limited to the coronal plane. Apical rigid kyphosis has been reported in up to 50% of patients with scoliosis, and lordoscoliosis is seen in a small subset of patients [7, 22].

Cervical Kyphosis

Cervical deformity is reported in up to 30% of NF1 patients, yet the precise rate of occurrence is not well-defined because most patients are asymptomatic [23]. Patients' higher tolerance for cervical deformity may stem from the larger spinal canal size and an increased ability for adjacent vertebrae to compensate for the deformity, as compared with the thoracolumbar spine [24]. Children with thoracic scoliosis frequently have concurrent subtle dystrophic changes in the cervical spine, and frank cervical deformity is more likely to develop in these patients. The most common presentation is cervical kyphosis, which can progress to instability and atlantoaxial dislocation in severe cases [24–26]. Despite the lower prevalence of symptoms in NF1 cervical deformity, the risk of severe neurologic complications, including paraplegia, is higher than that associated with thoracolumbar deformities [18, 23, 27].

Associated Spinal Manifestations

NF1-associated spinal deformities rarely occur in isolation. Findings often observed in conjunction with the deformity include dural ectasia, Chiari malformation, meningocele, syrinx, and paraspinal and intraspinal tumors. [21] Dural ectasia—expansion of the dural sac—and tumor burden have both been correlated with the development of spinal deformity [28–30]. It has been hypothesized that vertebral bone in NF1 may respond differently to local stimuli, [31] thereby fostering more severe morphological changes. Shah and George [32] described an NF1-specific grading system for dural ectasia that considers the vertebral element involved with modifiers based on the extent of bony destruction: grade 1—vertebral body (1A— $< 1/3$ destruction, 1B— $1/3-2/3$ destruction, 1C— $> 2/3$ destruction), grade 2—pedicle (2A—partial destruction, 2B—complete destruction), and grade 3—posterior elements (3A—partial destruction, 3B—complete destruction). The modifier "0" refers to no destruction at the indicated element. Patients with paraspinal neurofibromas have been shown to have higher degrees of apical vertebral rotation than those without. They are also more likely to have rotatory subluxation, vertebral scalloping, and dysplastic pedicles [33]. Overall, these associated skeletal manifestations are most common in the thoracic region, though spinal tumors more commonly localize to the cervical or lumbar spine in NF1 [21, 34, 35].

Additionally, atraumatic costovertebral joint dislocation can occur in dystrophic cases, resulting in direct cord impression and potential neurological compromise [36, 37]. When it occurs, rib head dislocation localizes to the convexity of the curve's apex, customarily in the mid- to lower ribs. While multiple ribs can be involved, a single rib head dislocation is seen in most cases [37, 38]. Recently, the Haleem–Marks–Botchu classification was created to quantify rib head penetration in neurofibromatosis. The computed tomography (CT)-based system describes four grades: grade 0—normal rib head position, grade 1—subluxed extracanal rib head position, grade 2—rib head at pedicle, and grade 3—intracanal rib head. Grade 3 is further subdivided based on the depth of rib head penetration into the spinal canal: grade 3A—proximal third, grade 3B—middle third, and grade 3C—distal third [39]. Here the third describes the location of the rib head in the axial plane with the ipsilateral foramen defining the proximal end.

Patient Screening and Surveillance

Due to the high risk for spinal deformity and progressive nature of NF1, early detection is essential for maximizing the opportunity for timely intervention and the prevention of complications. Despite recognition of the importance of screening in this population, there are currently no consensus guidelines on this topic. This includes the 2019 American Academy of Pediatrics guidelines for monitoring major manifestations of NF1, which did not address spinal deformity [40].

However, a recent Delphi study utilizing a committee of multidisciplinary NF1 experts, including the authors of the present chapter, provided best practice guidelines on screening and surveillance of spinal deformity [41]. Based on a median of 11 years of independent practice, the group recommended initial screening with physical examination for all patients at the time of diagnosis with NF1. Repeat physical exams were recommended on an annual basis for patients with previously normal exams and 6–12-month intervals for those with abnormal exams. The spine exam should include, but is not limited to, the following: general inspection, paraspinal palpation, Adam's forward bend test, sensory and motor examination, and reflex testing. For patients with clinical concern for spinal deformity, diagnostic imaging should be performed using radiographs. Magnetic resonance imaging (MRI) can also be utilized as appropriate for each case. Once pathology is established, surveillance imaging should be performed every 6–12 months to monitor progression, with shorter interval follow-up for dystrophic cases. Of note, whole body MRI can be a useful tool for neuro-oncologists in the initial screening for tumor burden and gross spinal characteristics. However, detail is restricted due to the large area assessed, thereby limiting adequate surveillance and the proper evaluation of focal intraspinal lesions.

Nonoperative Management

Nonoperative treatment of NF1-associated spinal deformity should only be considered in nondystrophic cases, as dystrophic deformity can rapidly progress and lead to neurologic dysfunction. Nondystrophic curves tend to behave similarly to AIS and have comparable responses to treatment. For nondystrophic or dystrophic deformity magnitude up to 20°, it is reasonable to observe the patient closely at 6-month intervals using physical examination and appropriate imaging [29]. Brace management is recommended for nondystrophic scoliosis or kyphosis measuring between 20° and 40° in children who are skeletally immature [18, 42]. A full-time Rigo Cheneau brace is a good option until the patient reaches skeletal maturity [26]. It must be noted that there is a significantly higher rate of subsequent surgical intervention in patients with NF1-associated nondystrophic deformity (27%) versus AIS (14%) [43, 44]. Three-year outcomes for bracing have shown nondystrophic curve progression of >5° in all patients [45]. This difference in brace effectiveness has been attributed in part to the challenges in compliance for patients with NF1, who are more often compromised by cognitive dysfunction, attention deficit disorders, seizures, and suffer social, emotional, and psychological problems at higher rates than the general population [46, 47]. Bracing is rarely successful for dystrophic cases [15, 18].

Preoperative Evaluation

The NF1 spine is complex; multiplanar thoracolumbar and cervical deformity, occult vertebral dysplasia, and paraspinal and intraspinal tumors frequently co-occur. Given the high likelihood of having comorbid pathologies, a comprehensive preoperative evaluation is essential to guide surgical planning. In addition to preoperative radiographs, preoperative MRI of the spinal region of interest should be obtained, with particular focus on the apex to assess for dural ectasia and the extent of paravertebral tumors [48]. In severely dystrophic cases, preoperative CT is a valuable tool to evaluate vertebral morphology and identify appropriate fixation techniques. CT is also important for diagnosing rib head dislocation in patients with clinical suspicion, as MRI has low specificity for identifying intraspinal penetration of rib heads [26, 49].

Operative Management

Early and aggressive surgical intervention is an essential treatment principle of dystrophic deformity in NF1. Pedicle screw constructs are preferred as they offer the advantages of providing a strong anchor, deformity correction in all three planes, and reduced long-term loss of correction [50, 51]. However, successful surgical fixation can be difficult to achieve in NF1 due to significantly diminished bone mineral density and dysplastic pedicles [52, 53]. Pedicle morphology in NF1 can be classified based on the middle of the narrowest transverse pedicle on CT: type A—a cancellous channel of >4 mm, type B—a cancellous channel of 2–4 mm, type C—a cancellous channel of <2 mm with an entirely cortical channel of ≥2 mm, grade D—a cortical channel of <2 mm, and grade E—pedicle absence. This system relays the ease of pedicle screw insertion; only grade A is considered normal [54]. The prevalence of abnormal pedicles (grades B-E) in NF1 is estimated at 67% and is significantly higher for dystrophic (70%) versus nondystrophic spines (59%). For reference, the prevalence of abnormal pedicles in AIS is only 22% [55].

Vertebral morphology dictates the fixation techniques that can be applied, as severely dysplastic pedicles are not suitable for pedicle screws. The incidence of improper pedicle screw placement is threefold higher for dysplastic versus normal pedicles, with an incidence rate as high as 31% (10% medial breach and 21% lateral breach) with freehand insertion for NF1-associated deformity [11, 55, 56]. Intraoperative navigation holds promise to reduce the misplacement rate, although over 20% of screws are still malpositioned even with image guidance [57]. Misplacement is correlated with pedicle transverse diameter and can cause neurologic injury if breaching occurs, especially in the case of medial breaches. Thus, there is value in obtaining preoperative CTs for surgical planning; pedicle screws should be used with caution for grade C and D pedicles and should be avoided in grade E (i.e., absent) pedicles. Another principle that must be considered is that of implant density. While its benefit is not clear for AIS, higher implant density is associated with greater initial curve correction and less loss of correction for dystrophic deformity [58]. As a result, hybrid constructs that maximize implant density are favored for NF1. This involves the utilization of pedicle screws at all amenable segments and hooks (laminar, pedicle, and transverse process), laminar bands, and wires at levels with severe pedicle dysplasia, regardless of whether definitive spinal fusion or growth-friendly constructs are pursued.

Spinal Fusion

Spinal fusion is the mainstay of surgical management for NF1-associated deformity. Generally, posterior spinal fusion (PSF) is indicated for patients with nondystrophic curves measuring >40° in any plane. In dystrophic cases, PSF is recommended for scoliotic curves measuring between 20° and 40° with less than 50° kyphosis, whereas anteroposterior spinal fusion (APSF) with segmental instrumentation is the preferred approach for curves measuring >40° or with associated kyphosis exceeding 50° [59].

Compared with the early 2000s, there has been a significant rise in the volume of spinal fusions being performed for NF1, with a shift away from APSF and preference toward using PSF alone in recent years (Fig. 2.2) [60]. These trends likely

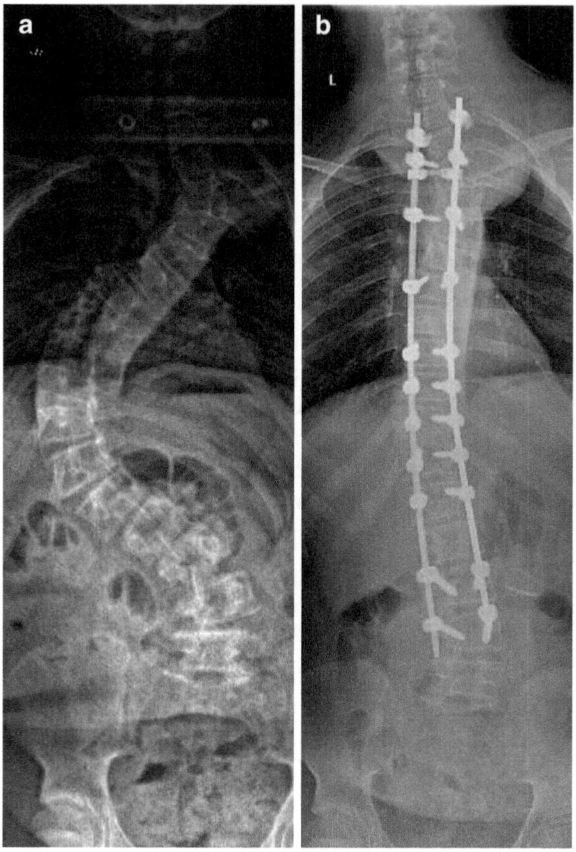

Fig. 2.2 13-year-old male with NF1 presenting with 100-degree main thoracic and 55-degree proximal thoracic curves; (**a**) preoperative radiograph, (**b**) radiograph status post T2-L4 PSF

reflect an increase in surgeons' familiarity with pedicle screw constructs and posterior column osteotomies, which allow for three-column fixation without reliance on anterior approach. There has also been an increase in the availability of intraoperative image guidance, which increases the odds of successful pedicle screw placement [57]. Recent meta-analyses have shown that one-stage PSF using third-generation instrumentation (e.g., hook- or screw-rod systems and hybrid constructs) can stabilize scoliosis as effectively as APSF in patients with NF1 who are older than 10 years old and with curves as high as 90° in magnitude [51, 61]. This can be accomplished with minor loss of deformity correction for up to 15 years post-operatively, although long-term data is sparse [51, 61]. In recent years, posterior-only vertebral column resection (pVCR) at the apical level has been explored as an effective adjunct to PSF for severe, rigid deformities (Fig. 2.3). This technique, along with improved bone grafting and other osteotomy techniques, facilitates solid fusion and better alignment. pVCR can be performed safely in dystrophic NF1 when necessary and is recommended when flexibility is less than 35% or the Cobb angle measures >90° [62]. It should be noted that historical failure rates for PSF were estimated near 50% when used for dystrophic cases [63]. However,

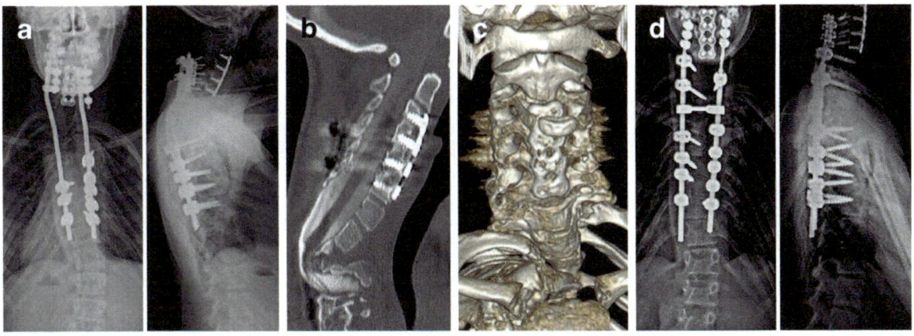

Fig. 2.3 16-year-old male with a history of multiple surgeries for NF1-associated kyphoscoliosis presenting with lower extremity numbness and weakness; (**a**) preoperative radiographs showing sharp kyphotic deformity with apex at T3, T2–3 dislocation, and loss of proximal fixation, (**b**) preoperative CT showing severe cord impingement, (**c**) 3D CT reconstruction showing apical dislocation, (**d**) radiographs status post revision C4-T9 PSF with pVCR at T3

these complications have decreased significantly with the adoption of modern techniques.

APSF has traditionally been favored for NF1-associated deformity due to concern for pseudarthrosis with earlier fixation techniques [64]. Compared with PSF, the combined approach typically requires an extensive procedure with longer lengths of stay and higher costs [60]. It is also associated with a 23% failure rate, which is comparable to or worse than that of modern PSF. [63] Hence, APSF has decreased in popularity. However, it remains the standard for cervical kyphosis (Fig. 2.4) [65]. APSF is also an option for complex thoracolumbar deformities, including dystrophic kyphotic curvatures >50° that tend to respond poorly to posterior instrumentation alone (Fig. 2.5) [15, 18]. Kyphosis creates pathologic spinal cord deformation that is more likely to give rise to neurological symptoms than scoliosis, where canal widening allows greater tolerance of deformity in the coronal plane. This situation requires anterior or posterior decompression via vertebrectomy, as laminectomy is ineffective in relieving the ventral cord compression [66]. Reinforcement using anterior strut grafts, either rib or fibula autograft, as well as posterior augmentation with autologous iliac crest bone, is recommended for sharply angulated kyphosis in NF1 [29]. Additional allograft augmentation may be beneficial in cases with severe anterior and posterior scalloping. Preoperative halo traction may be considered to maximize correction, though it is likely minimally effective for rigid deformities [29, 67]. Postoperative bracing may also be utilized to prevent pseudarthrosis, especially in cases where dysplastic vertebrae are noted to be weak intraoperatively and there is concern for implant dislodgement [10, 68]. Some surgeons have reported success with modern PSF and pVCR in correcting sagittal balance with comparable effectiveness as APSF, although outcomes are extremely heterogeneous.

Regardless of the chosen approach, a key consideration is the selection of fusion levels. Fusion of fewer vertebral segments has the benefits of preserving mobility, avoiding early degeneration, and reducing the incidence of back pain. However, this

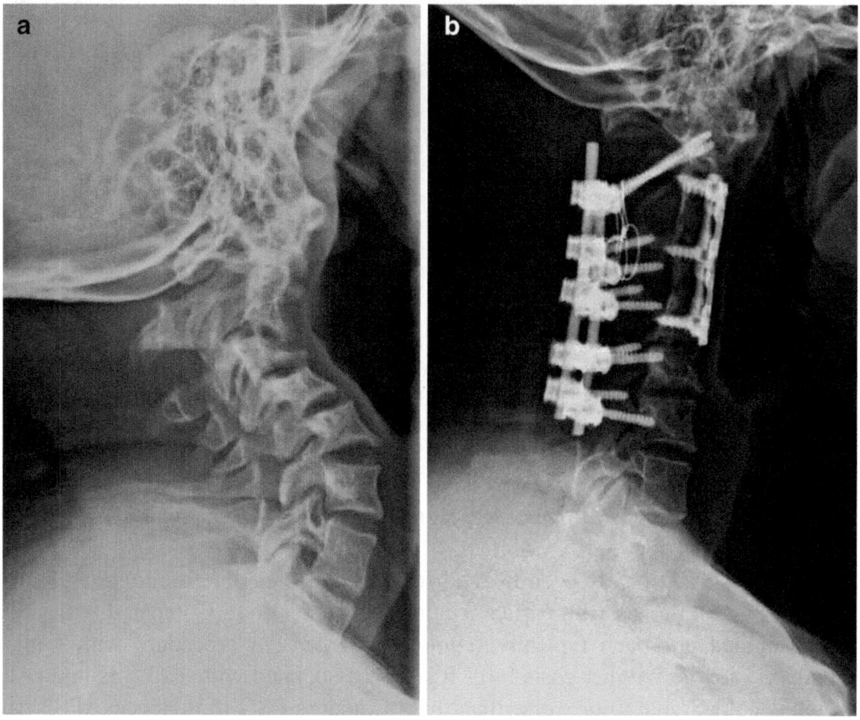

Fig. 2.4 16-year-old male with NF1 presenting with 90-degree cervical kyphosis; (**a**) preoperative radiograph, (**b**) radiograph status post C2–6 APSF with C3 corpectomy, anterior rib strut, and posterior iliac crest autograft

technique is not recommended in patients with NF1, as they are at higher risk of postoperative decompensation and revision procedures for adding-on (progressive increase in the number of vertebrae included in the main curvature) following PSF. [51] Thus, proximal and distal fusion should reach stable vertebrae rather than end vertebrae in dystrophic scoliosis. This principle is essential in both the coronal and sagittal planes. Since dystrophic deformities—especially those with an early age of onset—tend to progress even after achieving solid arthrodesis (Figs. 2.6 and 2.7), [10, 69] some surgeons recommend including any areas of the spine that exhibit dystrophic change within the fusion length, even if these sections are straight at the time of surgery [70].

Growth-Friendly Options

In skeletally immature patients younger than 10 years of age, deformity correction must be balanced with the preservation of growth [71]. Early fusion for NF1-associated EOS carries the risk of thoracic insufficiency syndrome, in which truncal

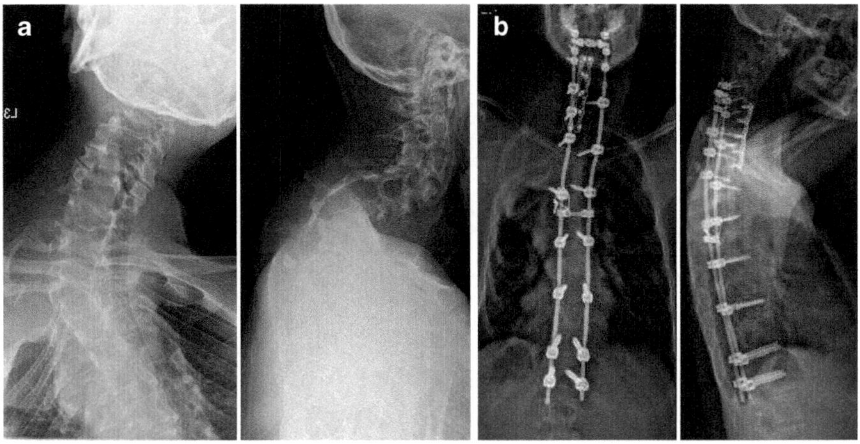

Fig. 2.5 18-year-old male presenting with proximal thoracic NF1-associated kyphoscoliosis (50-degree coronal, 90-degree sagittal deformity); (**a**) preoperative radiographs, (**b**) radiographs status post C4-T12 APSF with iliac crest autograft

height loss can result in poor pulmonary function. To minimize this risk, early fusion should be performed on as few vertebral levels as possible, and reports have demonstrated successful outcomes with fusion up to five levels at a mean 14 years follow-up [70]. Yet, effective correction may require APSF to protect against the crankshaft phenomenon, and the progressive nature of dystrophic deformities frequently necessitates augmentation with bone grafting at regular intervals. With these limitations, growth-friendly options (i.e., growing rods and vertical expandable prosthetic titanium rib [VEPTR]) have been explored for the treatment of NF1-associated EOS.

Early studies have shown that traditional growing rods (TGRs) can achieve coronal correction averaging 31%–53% and yearly T1-S1 height gain measuring 11.2–13.6 mm in patients with NF1 [72–74]. This is similar to the normal spine growth per year for a healthy child. The majority of this growth occurs outside of the thoracic spine, however, suggesting that it may be difficult to achieve an increase in length at T1-T12, where dystrophic changes tend to concentrate [75]. These constructs are associated with a high rate of implant-related complications (IRCs), though, with as many as 65% of patients treated with TGRs experiencing IRCs, predominantly at the proximal end of the construct [72, 75–78]. The most common presentations are proximal hook dislodgment or screw pullout as well as adding-on (Fig. 2.8). Occurrence is reportedly lower for patients who receive combined halo-gravity traction and dual TGR constructs [74]. TGRs have the disadvantage of repeated rod distraction surgeries at 6-month to 1-year intervals, which carry substantial risk for wound infection, general anesthesia complications, and psychosocial problems. Magnetically controlled growing rods (MCGRs) are being increasingly utilized (Fig. 2.9), although studies reporting their outcomes in NF1 are sparse. Available data for MCGRs demonstrate 43% curve correction and

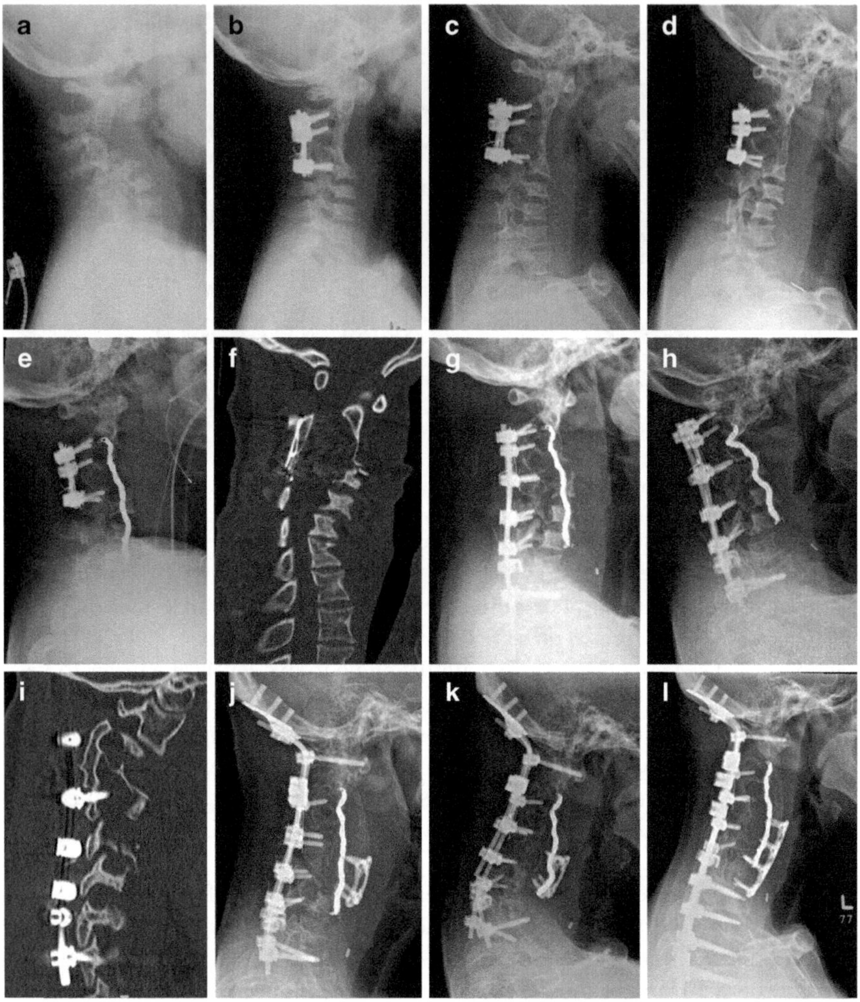

Fig. 2.6 4-year-old female with NF1 presenting with early-onset 70-degree cervical kyphosis; (**a**) preoperative radiograph, (**b**) radiograph 1 year status post C2–5 APSF with C4–5 corpectomies, anterior rib strut, and posterior iliac crest autograft, (**c–d**) radiographs showing progressive lucency of rib strut and C6–7 dystrophic scalloping at 5 and 10 years postoperatively, (**e–f**) radiograph and CT showing anterior fusion fracture and C6 anterolisthesis at 14 years postoperatively, (**g**) radiograph status post revision C2-T2 PSF (revision #1), (**h–i**) radiograph and CT showing loss of C2 alignment and C2 pedicle lysis at 1 week after revision #1, (**j**) radiograph status post revision C2–6 ASF and occiput-C4 PSF (revision #2), (**k**) radiograph showing C6 anterior subluxation and posterior rod fracture at 9 months after revision #2, (**l**) radiograph status post revision C6-T2 ASF and occiput-T5 PSF with iliac crest autograft (revision #3)

approximately 7 mm/year of T1-T12 growth at up to 7 years postoperatively [26, 79]. At least three years of growth-friendly treatment is recommended prior to definitive fusion. Conversion to final fusion should be pursued when patients no

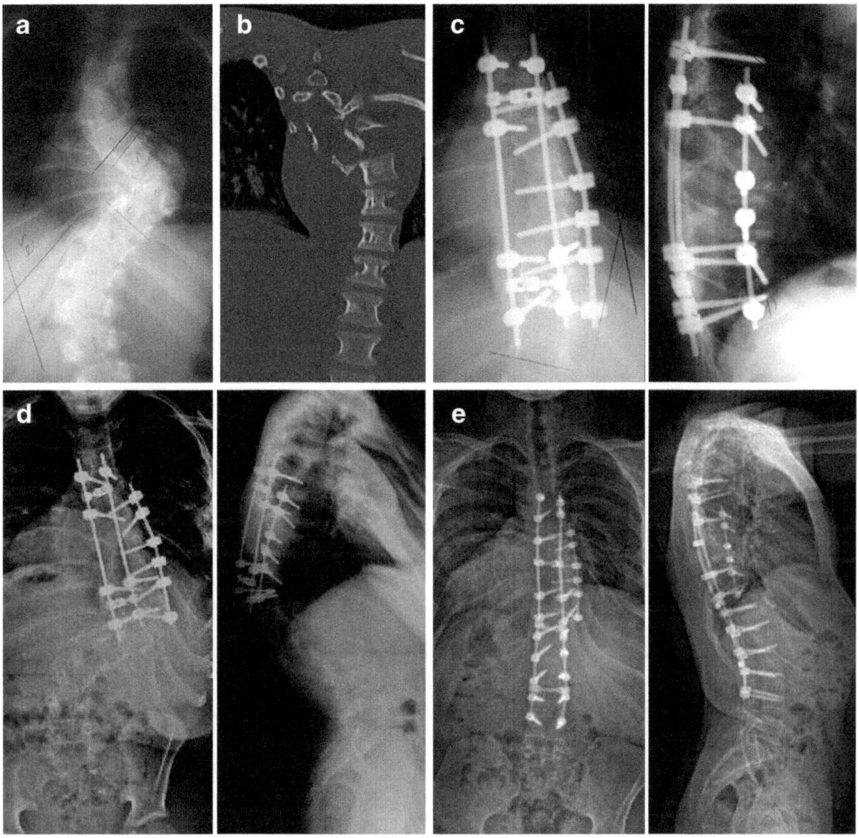

Fig. 2.7 8-year-old male with NF1 presenting with early-onset 45-degree thoracic curve with rotation and T7–8 dislocation; (**a**) preoperative radiograph, (**b**) preoperative CT showing 4.4x7.5x5.6 cm paravertebral tumor spanning apex on concave side, (**c**) radiographs status post T5–11 APSF, (**d**) radiographs showing progressive kyphoscoliosis with distal adding-on at 5 years postoperatively, (**e**) radiographs status post revision T4-L4 PSF with T12 vertebral body excision (revision #1)

longer acquire length with distraction or sustain multiple implant-related complications.

To date, only one study has reported on the use of rib-based distraction (i.e., VEPTR) in patients with NF1-associated EOS. The 12-patient case series concluded that all patients experienced T1-S1 height gain after an average of 5 years of follow-up, and deformity progression can be effectively mediated during the primary growth spurt [80]. In non-NF1 EOS, VEPTR has demonstrated similar coronal correction and spinal growth as TGRs, but it is significantly less effective in controlling thoracic kyphosis [81]. Thus, rib-based systems may not be optimal for patients with severe sagittal plane deformity. Because rib dysplasia is a defining

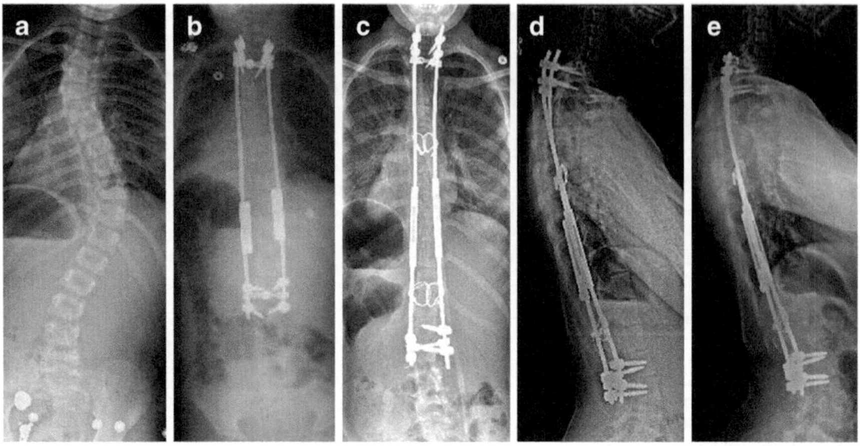

Fig. 2.8 7-year-old female with NF1-associated early-onset scoliosis; (**a**) preoperative radiograph, (**b**) radiograph status post TGR insertion, (**c**) radiograph status post 7 distraction surgeries and conversion to T4-L4 PSF at 7.5 years postoperatively, (**d**) radiograph showing proximal fixation failure with T1–3 pseudarthrosis at 1 year after final fusion, (**e**) radiograph status post proximal construct repair (revision #1)

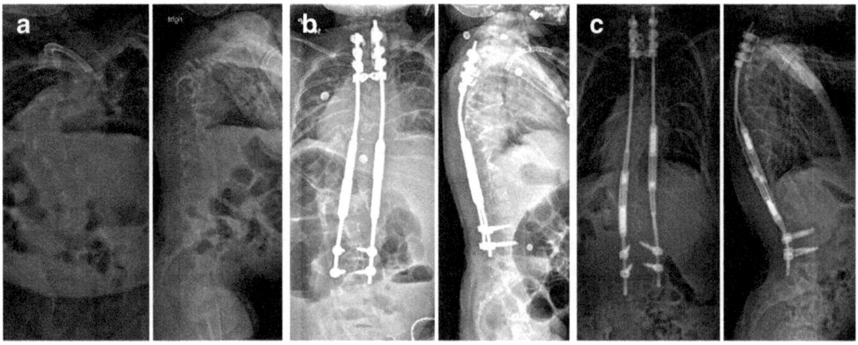

Fig. 2.9 3-year-old female with NF1-associated early-onset kyphoscoliosis; (**a**) preoperative radiographs, (**b**) radiographs status post preoperative halo traction and MCGR insertion, (**c**) radiographs status post 1 MCGR exchange at 4.5 years postoperatively

characteristic of dystrophic NF1, these constructs can be complicated by progression causing rib migration and are rarely used in modern practice.

Overall, there is still controversy regarding whether early definitive fusion or growth-friendly techniques are the superior option for NF1-associated EOS. The decision is patient dependent. Early fusion may be favored for patients with short, sharp curves who are approaching skeletal maturity or who are ≥10 years old with long curves [48]. While the preference for growth-friendly options cites the preservation of thoracic height, surgeons must understand that the dystrophic characteristics of NF1 may prevent appropriate thoracic development. Consequently, patients with NF1 undergoing early fusion and growth-friendly options both have shorter trunk height and lower lung functional vital capacity than the general population. Complication rates are similar; growth-friendly procedures have more implant-related complications, and early fusion has more anterior surgery-related issues. Growth-friendly techniques also achieve less, albeit still substantial, deformity correction. Despite these limitations, they effectively lengthen T1-S1 spinal height and may be preferred in young patients <10 years with extensive deformity.

Spinal Tumor Resection and Other Associated Procedures

As stated earlier in this chapter, NF1-associated spinal deformity rarely occurs in isolation. Preoperative MRI is recommended in all patients to assess for the extent of associated pathologies, including dural ectasia, plexiform neurofibromas, and intraspinal rib head dislocation. These areas are more prone to dystrophic changes and should be taken into consideration when choosing instrumentation levels during surgical planning. If these pathologies are present, surgeons must decide on the value of performing adjunct procedures.

Surgical resection of spinal tumors should be considered when there is suspicion for malignancy, the tumor is causing neural element compression with or without associated symptoms, or where the tumor impairs access to the spine for deformity correction. Even in patients who are asymptomatic, there is substantial benefit to resection of paraspinal and intraspinal tumors to prevent continued pressure erosion of the adjacent vertebral elements. Plexiform neurofibromas are typically located on the concavity of the curve apex, which can lead to vertebral morphological changes and deformity progression [33]. These most frequently develop in the cervical spine, which can preclude gross total resection due to anatomic constraints posed by the vertebral artery and brachial plexus. Since the extent of resection is often limited, recurrence rates are high [82]. Resection can be pursued safely and effectively in the same procedure as deformity correction. Intradural lesions require laminectomy, though hemilaminectomy, where possible, is preferred so as to preserve the posterior elements as grafting surfaces.

There is currently no consensus on the management of intraspinal rib dislocations. It is essential to recognize the presence of rib head protrusion preoperatively, as cord impingement can develop or worsen with manipulation of the spine during deformity correction. In patients with deformity, the cord sits toward the concave side of the curve and away from the convex side where rib heads may translate into the canal. Correction of vertebral rotation and angulation centralizes the cord, thereby increasing the probability of impingement by the protruding rib head [37]. This is more likely to happen with the superior three-dimensional correction employed by modern instrumentation than with earlier systems [83]. For patients with neurological deficits or signs of cord indentation on preoperative imaging, the preferred option is complete or partial rib head resection during deformity correction, which should be performed prior to any surgical manipulation of the spine. In this procedure, a rib segment is resected distal to the tip of the transverse process. The intracanal fragment may be removed or purposely retained if adhesions to the cord are noted intraoperatively. For patients who are neurologically intact, the risk-benefit profile does not favor resection of the intracanal portion of the rib head. The intracanal procedure lengthens operative time and increases surgical complexity. It additionally exposes patients to a higher risk of neurological injury without contributing additional correction of the primary deformity [37]. In these cases, surgeons can safely pursue correction of NF1-associated deformity with intraoperative neurophysiological monitoring.

Perioperative Complications

Common perioperative complications tend to be secondary to the inherent complexity of NF1 and the features that characterize the condition's associated deformity. Of patients with NF1 undergoing surgical correction of dystrophic scoliosis, 14% experienced at least one complication according to a recent systematic review [84]. The most common complications in this population are wound infections (4.2%) and cerebrospinal fluid (CSF) leaks (2.4%). Over 25% of patients with dystrophic scoliosis also have associated dural ectasia, which predisposes these patients to intraoperative CSF leakage [44]. When encountered, tears can be difficult to repair in these patients due to the structural weakness of the dura, leaving the patients at greater risk for postoperative septic and aseptic meningitis [84]. In addition, compared with the general population, patients with NF1 undergoing spinal fusion are at elevated risk of experiencing intraoperative bleeding [85]. Accidental vessel lacerations may be more likely to occur due to the need for high-grade osteotomies to facilitate deformity correction, tumors' close vicinity to spinal vasculature, and intrinsic vessel wall lesions that are characteristic of the condition. The increased vascularity of neurofibromatous tissue can also inhibit visualization, especially for anterior approaches, as well as contribute to a greater risk of postoperative bleeding and hematoma formation. When significant, hematomas can cause cord compression and lead to neurologic deficits. Thoracic cavity tumors, pulmonary arterial hypertension, and lateral thoracic meningoceles also contribute to this risk [86].

More significantly, the rates of immediate postoperative and permanent neurologic deficits are reported at 2.1% and 1.2%, respectively. These rates may be falsely low, as these complications are infrequently reported in the available literature [84]. Such deficits are likely due to the correction of large, rigid deformities that place greater tension on the neural elements. Patients with NF1 also have a higher baseline risk of other central nervous system complications, including hydrocephalus and seizures, which may manifest in the postoperative period. Thus, close postoperative monitoring is critical. Revision surgery is required in approximately 22% of patients, largely due to IRCs [84].

Postoperative Surveillance

Postoperative MRIs are limited by artifact presenting as a halo around metal instrumentation, which makes it difficult to ascertain the accuracy of implant placement and the surrounding structures. Since MRI is the preferred modality for screening and surveillance of spinal tumors, this raises concern for spine visualization and tumor surveillance after instrumentation is placed. Need for routine MRI surveillance is often considered a contraindication to surgical correction of spinal deformity in patients with NF1, as the high risk for malignancy can outweigh other concerns in this population. However, surgical correction should be pursued when indicated, especially in dystrophic cases that can rapidly decompensate. Multidetector CT has been shown to be superior to MRI for evaluation of the postoperative NF1 spine, as there is less interference from metal artifacts and gross changes can be effectively monitored [33, 87]. However, it is not an effective replacement for tumor surveillance.

Conclusion

Neurofibromatosis has a high prevalence of complex three-dimensional deformities throughout the entire spine. Early detection is important, and bracing may have a delaying role. Growth-friendly treatments are beneficial if they become severe early in the first decade. For severe deformities, posterior-based correction is the mainstay of modern treatment, after comprehensive imaging of the neuraxis and surrounding regions. Nevertheless, NF1-associated deformity is rapidly progressive and may continue to evolve after appropriate management.

References

1. Lammert M, Friedman JM, Kluwe L, Mautner VF (2005) Prevalence of Neurofibromatosis 1 in German children at elementary school enrollment. Arch Dermatol 141:71–74
2. Gutmann DH, Ferner RE, Listernick RH, Korf BR, Wolters PL, Johnson KJ (2017) Neurofibromatosis type 1. Nat Rev Dis Prim 3:17004
3. Hirbe AC, Gutmann DH (2014) Neurofibromatosis type 1: a multidisciplinary approach to care. Lancet Neurol 13:834–843
4. Bergoug M, Doudeau M, Godin F, Mosrin C, Vallée B, Bénédetti H (2020) Neurofibromin structure, functions and regulation. Cells 9:2365
5. Viskochil D (2002) Review article : genetics of Neurofibromatosis 1 and the NF1 gene. J Child Neurol 17:562–570
6. Akbarnia BA, Gabriel KR, Beckman E, Chalk D (1992) Prevalence of scoliosis in Neurofibromatosis. Spine (Phila Pa 1976) 17:244–248
7. Funasaki H, Winter RB, Lonstein JB, Denis F (1994) Pathophysiology of spinal deformities in neurofibromatosis. An analysis of seventy-one patients who had curves associated with dystrophic changes. J Bone Jt Surg 76:692–700

8. Rossi SE, Erasmus JJ, McAdams HP, Donnelly LF (1999) Thoracic manifestations of neurofibromatosis-I. Am J Roentgenol 173:1631–1638
9. Pasmant E, Vidaud M, Vidaud D, Wolkenstein P (2012) Neurofibromatosis type 1: from genotype to phenotype. J Med Genet 49:483–489
10. Vitale MG, Guha A, Skaggs DL (2002) Orthopaedic manifestations of Neurofibromatosis in children: an update. Clin Orthop Relat Res 401:107–118
11. Yang N, Luo M, Zhao S, Wang W, Xia L (2020) Morphological differences between the pedicles in nondystrophic scoliosis secondary to Neurofibromatosis type 1 and those in adolescent idiopathic scoliosis. World Neurosurg 144:e9–e14
12. Crawford AH (1978) Neurofibromatosis in the pediatric patient. Orthop Clin North Am 9:11–23
13. Durrani AA, Crawford AH, Chouhdry SN, Saifuddin A, Morley TR (2000) Modulation of spinal deformities in patients with Neurofibromatosis type 1. Spine (Phila pa 1976) 25:69
14. Crawford AH (1989) Pitfalls of spinal deformities associated with neurofibromatosis in children. Clin Orthop Relat res 29–42
15. Crawford AH, Herrera-Soto J (2007) Scoliosis associated with Neurofibromatosis. Orthop Clin North Am 38:553–562
16. Zaidman A, Zaidman M, Mikhailovsky M, Suzdalov V, Zavyalova E, Sadovoy M (2012) Morphology of spinal deformity with Neurofibromatosis - type 1. Orthop Proc 94-B:21–21
17. Crawford AH, Bagamery N (1986) Osseous manifestations of Neurofibromatosis in childhood. J Pediatr Orthop 6:72–88
18. Winter RB, Moe JH, Bradford DS, Lonstein JE, Pedras CV, Weber AH (1979) Spine deformity in neurofibromatosis. A review of one hundred and two patients. J Bone Joint Surg Am 61:677–694
19. Calvert P, Edgar M, Webb P (1989) Scoliosis in neurofibromatosis. The natural history with and without operation. J Bone Joint Surg Br 71-B:246–251
20. Chaglassian JH, Riseborough EJ, Hall JE (1976) Neurofibromatous scoliosis. Natural history and results of treatment in thirty-seven cases. J Bone Joint Surg Am 58:695–702
21. Sial M, George KJ (2023) A review of spinal lesions in Neurofibromatosis type 1 in a large Neurofibromatosis type 1 center. World Neurosurg 169:e157–e163
22. Crawford AH, Schorry EK (1999) Neurofibromatosis in children: the role of the Orthopaedist. J Am Acad Orthop Surg 7:217–230
23. Yong-Hing K, Kalamchi A, MacEwen GD (1979) Cervical spine abnormalities in neurofibromatosis. J Bone Joint Surg Am 61:695–699
24. Crawford AH, Gr HC, Schumaier AP, Mangano FT (2018) Management of Cervical Instability as a complication of Neurofibromatosis type 1 in children: a historical perspective with a 40-year experience. Spine Deform 6:719–729
25. Isu T, Miyasaka K, Abe H, Ito T, Iwasaki Y, Tsuru M, Kitaoka K, Tsunoda M (1983) Atlantoaxial dislocation associated with neurofibromatosis. Report of three cases J Neurosurg 58:451–453
26. Mladenov KV, Spiro AS, Krajewski KL, Stücker R, Kunkel P (2020) Management of spinal deformities and tibial pseudarthrosis in children with neurofibromatosis type 1 (NF-1). Childs Nerv Syst 36:2409–2425
27. Curtis BH, Fisher RL, Butterfield WL, Saunders FP (1969) Neurofibromatosis with paraplegia. Report of eight cases. J Bone Joint Surg Am 51:843–861
28. Khong P-L, Goh WHS, Wong VCN, Fung C-W, Ooi G-C (2003) MR imaging of spinal tumors in children with Neurofibromatosis 1. Am J Roentgenol 180:413–417
29. Tsirikos AI, Saifuddin A, Noordeen MH (2005) Spinal deformity in neurofibromatosis type-1: diagnosis and treatment. Eur Spine J 14:427–439
30. Curtis-Lopez CM, Soh C, Ealing J, Gareth Evans D, Burkitt Wright EMM, Vassallo G, Karabatsou K, Joshi George K (2020) Clinical and neuroradiological characterisation of spinal lesions in adults with Neurofibromatosis type 1. J Clin Neurosci 77:98–105
31. Alwan S, Tredwell S, Friedman J (2005) Is osseous dysplasia a primary feature of neurofibromatosis 1 (NF1)? Clin Genet 67:378–390

32. Shah S, George KJ (2019) The association of spinal deformity with dural ectasia in neurofibromatosis type 1. Br J Neurosurg 33:620–623
33. Hu Z, Liu Z, Qiu Y, Xu L, Yan H, Zhu Z (2016) Morphological differences in the vertebrae of scoliosis secondary to Neurofibromatosis type 1 with and without Paraspinal Neurofibromas. Spine (Phila Pa 1976) 41:598–602
34. Thakkar SD, Feigen U, Mautner V-F (1999) Spinal tumours in neurofibromatosis type 1: an MRI study of frequency, multiplicity and variety. Neuroradiology 41:625–629
35. Well L, Careddu A, Stark M, Farschtschi S, Bannas P, Adam G, Mautner V-F, Salamon J (2021) Phenotyping spinal abnormalities in patients with Neurofibromatosis type 1 using whole-body MRI. Sci Rep 11:16889
36. DeLucia TA, Yohay K, Widmann RF (2011) Orthopaedic aspects of neurofibromatosis: update. Curr Opin Pediatr 23:46–52
37. Gao R, Guo D, Zhang X, Sun B, Yao Z, Cao J, Long CY, Bai Y, Liu H (2022) Surgical treatment of the Intraspinal rib head dislocation in children with dystrophic scoliosis secondary to type 1 Neurofibromatosis. J Pediatr Orthop 42:e242–e249
38. Ton J, Stein-Wexler R, Yen P, Gupta M (2010) Rib head protrusion into the central canal in type 1 neurofibromatosis. Pediatr Radiol 40:1902–1909
39. Haleem S, Malik M, Azzopardi C, Botchu R, Marks DS (2021) The Haleem–Marks–Botchu classification: a novel CT-based classification for intracanal rib head penetration. Spine Deform 9:1651–1657
40. Miller DT, Freedenberg D, Schorry E et al (2019) Health supervision for children with Neurofibromatosis type 1. Pediatrics 143:e20190660
41. Xu AL, Suresh KV, Gomez JA et al (2023) Consensus-based best practice guidelines for the Management of Spinal Deformity and Associated Tumors in pediatric Neurofibromatosis type 1: screening and surveillance, surgical intervention, and medical therapy. J Pediatr Orthop 43:e531–e537
42. Cai S, Tian Y, Qiu G, Zhang J, Shen J, Zhao H, Zhao Y (2020) Neurofibromatosis type <scp>1</scp> with severe dystrophic kyphosis: surgical treatment and prognostic analysis of <scp>27</scp> patients. Orthop Surg 12:1923–1940
43. Rigo M, Reiter C, Weiss H-R (2003) Effect of conservative management on the prevalence of surgery in patients with adolescent idiopathic scoliosis. Pediatr Rehabil 6:209–214
44. Toro G, Santoro C, Ambrosio D et al (2021) Natural history of scoliosis in children with NF1: an observation study. Healthcare 9:881
45. Shi B-L, Li Y, Zhu Z-Z, Mao S-H, Liu Z, Sun X, Qiu Y (2021) Curve evolution during bracing in children with scoliosis secondary to early-onset neurofibromatosis type 1: indicators of rapid curve progression. Chin Med J 134:1983–1987
46. Van Es S, North KN, McHugh K, De Silva M (1996) MRI findings in children with neurofibromatosis type 1: a prospective study. Pediatr Radiol 26:478–487
47. Johnson NS, Saal HM, Lovell AM, Schorry EK (1999) Social and emotional problems in children with neurofibromatosis type 1: evidence and proposed interventions. J Pediatr 134:767–772
48. Yao Z, Guo D, Li H, Bai Y, Sun B, Zhang X, Li C, Qi X (2019) Surgical treatment of dystrophic scoliosis in Neurofibromatosis type 1. Clin Spine Surg A Spine Publ 32:E50–E55
49. Gkiokas A, Hadzimichalis S, Vasiliadis E, Katsalouli M, Kannas G (2006) Painful rib hump: a new clinical sign for detecting intraspinal rib displacement in scoliosis due to neurofibromatosis. Scoliosis 1:10
50. Lee S-M, Suk S-I, Chung E-R (2004) Direct vertebral rotation: a new technique of three-dimensional deformity correction with segmental pedicle screw fixation in adolescent idiopathic scoliosis. Spine (Phila Pa 1976) 29:343–349
51. Wang Z, Fu C, Leng J, Qu Z, Xu F, Liu Y (2015) Treatment of dystrophic scoliosis in neurofibromatosis type 1 with one-stage posterior pedicle screw technique. Spine J 15:587–595
52. Illés T, Halmai V, de Jonge T, Dubousset J (2001) Decreased bone mineral density in Neurofibromatosis-1 patients with spinal deformities. Osteoporos Int 12:823–827

53. Kuorilehto T, Pöyhönen M, Bloigu R, Heikkinen J, Väänänen K, Peltonen J (2005) Decreased bone mineral density and content in neurofibromatosis type 1: lowest local values are located in the load-carrying parts of the body. Osteoporos Int 16:928–936
54. Li Y, Luo M, Wang W, Shen M, Xu G, Gao J, Xia L (2017) A Computed Tomography–Based Comparison of Abnormal Vertebrae Pedicles Between Dystrophic and Nondystrophic Scoliosis in Neurofibromatosis Type 1. World Neurosurg 106:898–904
55. Sarwahi V, Suggs W, Wollowick AL, Kulkarni PM, Lo YT, Amaral TD, Thornhill B (2014) Pedicle screws adjacent to the great vessels or viscera a study of 2132 pedicle screws in pediatric spine deformity. J Spinal Disord Tech 27:64–69
56. Li S, Mao S, Du C, Zhu Z, Shi B, Liu Z, Qiao J, Qiu Y (2021) Assessing the unique characteristics associated with surgical treatment of dystrophic lumbar scoliosis secondary to neurofibromatosis type 1: a single-center experience of more than 10 years. J Neurosurg Spine 34:413–423
57. Jin M, Liu Z, Liu X, Yan H, Han X, Qiu Y, Zhu Z (2016) Does intraoperative navigation improve the accuracy of pedicle screw placement in the apical region of dystrophic scoliosis secondary to neurofibromatosis type I: comparison between O-arm navigation and free-hand technique. Eur Spine J 25:1729–1737
58. Li Y, Yuan X, Sha S, Liu Z, Zhu W, Qiu Y, Wang B, Yu Y, Zhu Z (2017) Effect of higher implant density on curve correction in dystrophic thoracic scoliosis secondary to neurofibromatosis type 1. J Neurosurg Pediatr 20:371–377
59. Crawford AH, Schorry EK (2006) Neurofibromatosis update. J Pediatr Orthop 26:413–423
60. Kurucan E, Bernstein DN, Thirukumaran C, Jain A, Menga EN, Rubery PT, Mesfin A (2018) National Trends in spinal fusion surgery for Neurofibromatosis. Spine Deform 6:712–718
61. Li M, Fang X, Li Y, Ni J, Gu S, Zhu X (2009) Successful use of posterior instrumented spinal fusion alone for scoliosis in 19 patients with neurofibromatosis type-1 followed up for at least 25 months. Arch Orthop Trauma Surg 129:915–921
62. Stoker GE, Lenke LG, Dorward IG (2012) Posterior vertebral column resection for the treatment of dystrophic kyphosis associated with Type-1 Neurofibromatosis. Spine (Phila Pa 1976) 37:E1659–E1664
63. Parisini P, Di Silvestre M, Greggi T, Paderni S, Cervellati S, Savini R (1999) Surgical correction of dystrophic spinal curves in Neurofibromatosis. Spine (Phila pa 1976) 24:2247
64. Halmai V, Domán I, de Jonge T, Illés T (2002) Surgical treatment of spinal deformities associated with neurofibromatosis type 1. J Neurosurg Spine 97:310–316
65. Helenius IJ, Sponseller PD, Mackenzie W et al (2016) Outcomes of spinal fusion for cervical kyphosis in children with Neurofibromatosis. J Bone Jt Surg 98:e95
66. Winter RB, Lonstein JE, Anderson M (1988) Neurofibromatosis hyperkyphosis: a review of 33 patients with kyphosis of 80 degrees or greater. J Spinal Disord 1:39–49
67. Kim HW, Weinstein SL (1997) The Management of Scoliosis in Neurofibromatosis. Spine (Phila Pa 1976) 22:2770–2776
68. Shufflebarger HL (1989) Cotrel-Dubousset instrumentation in neurofibromatosis spinal problems. Clin Orthop Relat Res 245:24–28
69. Wilde PH, Upadhyay SS, Leong JCY (1994) Deterioration of operative correction in dystrophic spinal Neurofibromatosis. Spine (Phila Pa 1976) 19:1264–1270
70. Tauchi R, Kawakami N, Castro MA, Ohara T, Saito T, Morishita K, Yamauchi I (2020) Long-term surgical outcomes after early definitive spinal fusion for early-onset scoliosis with Neurofibromatosis type 1 at mean follow-up of 14 years. J Pediatr Orthop 40:42–47
71. Crawford AH, Parikh S, Schorry EK, Von Stein D (2007) The immature spine in Type-1 Neurofibromatosis. J Bone Jt Surg 89:123–142
72. Jain VV, Berry CA, Crawford AH, Emans JB, Sponseller PD (2017) Growing rods are an effective Fusionless method of controlling early-onset scoliosis associated with Neurofibromatosis type 1 (NF1): a multicenter retrospective case series. J Pediatr Orthop 37:e612–e618
73. Carbone M, Vittoria F, Del Sal A (2019) Treatment of early-onset scoliosis with growing rods in patients with neurofibromatosis-1. J Pediatr Orthop B 28:278–287

74. Xu E, Gao R, Jiang H, Lin T, Shao W, Zhou X (2019) Combined halo gravity traction and dual growing rod technique for the treatment of early onset dystrophic scoliosis in Neurofibromatosis type 1. World Neurosurg 126:e173–e180
75. Tauchi R, Kawakami N, Suzuki T, Uno K, Yamaguchi T, Yanagida H, Yamamoto T, Murakami H, Demura S, Kotani T (2020) Comparison of early definitive fusion and traditional growing rods in early-onset dystrophic scoliosis in Neurofibromatosis type 1: a preliminary report. J Pediatr Orthop 40:569–574
76. Akbarnia BA, Marks DS, Boachie-Adjei O, Thompson AG, Asher MA (2005) Dual growing rod technique for the treatment of progressive early-onset scoliosis: a multicenter study. Spine (Phila pa 1976) 30:S57
77. Yao Z, Li H, Zhang X, Li C, Qi X (2018) Incidence and risk factors for instrumentation-related complications after scoliosis surgery in pediatric patients with NF-1. Spine (Phila Pa 1976) 43:1719–1724
78. Bouthors C, Dukan R, Glorion C, Miladi L (2020) Outcomes of growing rods in a series of early-onset scoliosis patients with neurofibromatosis type 1. J Neurosurg Spine 33:373–380
79. Nnadi C, Thakar C, Wilson-MacDonald J, Milner P, Rao A, Mayers D, Fairbank J, Subramanian T (2018) An NIHR-approved two-year observational study on magnetically controlled growth rods in the treatment of early onset scoliosis. Bone Joint J 100-B:507–515
80. Heflin JA, Cleveland A, Ford SD, Morgan JV, Smith JT (2015) Use of rib-based distraction in the treatment of early-onset scoliosis associated with Neurofibromatosis type 1 in the young child. Spine Deform 3:239–245
81. Chen Z, Li S, Qiu Y, Zhu Z, Chen X, Xu L, Sun X (2017) Evolution of the postoperative sagittal spinal profile in early-onset scoliosis: is there a difference between rib-based and spine-based growth-friendly instrumentation? J Neurosurg Pediatr 20:561–566
82. Safaee M, Parsa AT, Barbaro NM, Chou D, Mummaneni PV, Weinstein PR, Tihan T, Ames CP (2015) Association of tumor location, extent of resection, and neurofibromatosis status with clinical outcomes for 221 spinal nerve sheath tumors. Neurosurg Focus 39:E5
83. Yalcin N, Bar-on E, Yazici M (2008) Impingement of spinal cord by dislocated rib in dystrophic scoliosis secondary to Neurofibromatosis type 1. Spine (Phila Pa 1976) 33:E881–E886
84. Neifert SN, Khan HA, Kurland DB, Kim NC, Yohay K, Segal D, Samdani A, Hwang S, Lau D (2022) Management and surgical outcomes of dystrophic scoliosis in neurofibromatosis type 1: a systematic review. Neurosurg Focus 52:E7
85. Price G, Martini ML, Caridi JM, Lau D, Oermann EK, Neifert SN (2023) A Nationwide study characterizing the risk and outcome profiles of multilevel fusion procedures in neuromuscular scoliosis patients with Neurofibromatosis type 1. World Neurosurg 171:e620–e630
86. Zamora AC, Collard HR, Wolters PJ, Webb WR, King TE (2006) Neurofibromatosis-associated lung disease: a case series and literature review. Eur Respir J 29:210–214
87. Debnam JM, Mahfouz YM, Ketonen L, Slopis JM, McCutcheon IE, Guha-Thakurta N (2014) Multidetector CT with 3-dimensional volume rendering in the evaluation of the spine in patients with Neurofibromatosis type 1: a retrospective review in 73 patients. Scoliosis 9:15

Chapter 3
Management of Deformity in Osteoid Osteoma and Osteoblastoma

Hesham Soliman, Daniel M. Sciubba, and Zach Pennington

Introduction and Epidemiology

Osteoid osteoma (OO) and osteoblastoma are benign primary bone tumors affecting both the appendicular and axial skeleton [1]. First described in 1930 by Bergstrand [2] and later characterized by Jaffe in 1935 [3]. Osteoblastoma, a related lesion, was also subsequently described by Jaffe [4] and Lichtenstein [5] and shared many histological similarities to OO, though OO are four to ten times more common than osteoblastoma [6, 7].

OO is the third most common benign primary neoplasm, [8] comprising approximately 11% of benign tumors and 3% of all primary bone tumors [2]. OOs most commonly localize to the lower extremity long bones, with the femur being the most common location, [3] but in a minority of cases can also arise from the spine. It is estimated that only 20% of OO and 40% of osteoblastoma localize to the spine, [7] and OO is thought to comprise only 10% of primary spine tumors and 1% of all spine neoplasms [9]. Most osteoid osteomas in the spine are located in the posterior elements, with 70–100% involving the neural arch [1, 9]. Isolated vertebral body involvement is described as occurring in only 3% of cases [10].

H. Soliman · D. M. Sciubba (✉)
Department of Neurosurgery, Donald and Barbara Zucker School of Medicine at Hofstra/Northwell Health, Great Neck, NY, USA
e-mail: hsoliman1@northwell.edu; dsciubba1@northwell.edu

Z. Pennington
Department of Neurologic Surgery, Mayo Clinic, Rochester, MN, USA
e-mail: pennington.zachary@mayo.edu

D. M. Sciubba (ed.), *Spinal Tumor Associated Deformity*,
https://doi.org/10.1007/978-3-031-87939-5_3

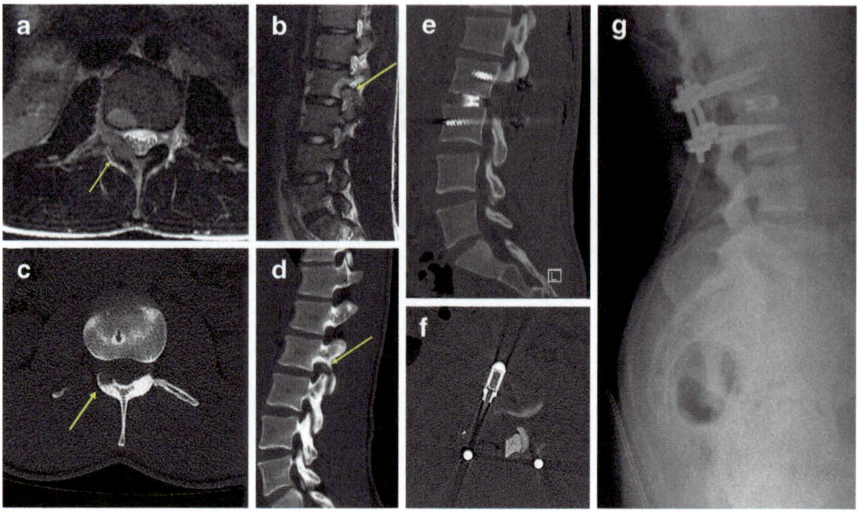

Fig. 3.1 A 21-year-old college athlete presented with severe right sided flank pain of insidious onset. Patient ultimately underwent MR (**a**, **b**) that demonstrated a T2-hyperintense mass of the L2 vertebra involving the posterior body, right pedicle, and lamina. (**c**, **d**) Noncontrast CT demonstrated a lytic lesion involving the right lateral hemilamina. (**e**–**g**) The patient was taken for right-sided hemilaminectomy, facetectomy and excision of the mass. The resultant instability was managed with a L2/3 transforaminal lumbar interbody fusion. The specimen was removed *en bloc*

When they occur in the vertebral body, they appear to show a predilection for the lumbar spine (59%, Fig. 3.1), followed by the thoracic spine (Fig. 3.2). OO of the cervical spine and sacrum are uncommon. However, it has been reported in some series that osteoblastomas of the vertebral body show a predilection for the cervical spine [10, 11].

Both OO and osteoblastoma predominantly affect patients in the first two decades of life, and patients are predominantly male with a reported 2–4:1 male:female preponderance for osteoid osteoma and 1.8–4.5:1 for osteoblastoma [2, 7, 10].

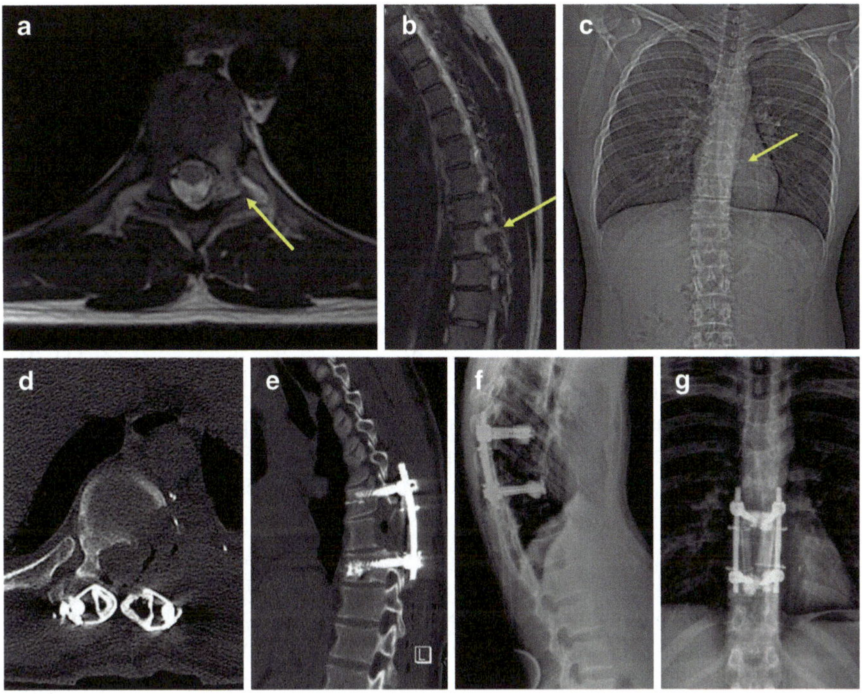

Fig. 3.2 A 26-year-old male presented with persistent mid-back pain progressive over multiple months that had proven refractory to nonoperative interventions. (**a, b**) Patient underwent MR that showed T2-hyperintense mass involving the left T9 pedicle, superior articular process, transverse process, and vertebral body without significant epidural disease. (**c**) Radiographs showed a mild levoscoliosis with its apex near the level of the lesion. Patient was taken for a left T9 hemilaminectomy, pediculectomy and posterolateral partial corpectomy (**d, e**). He underwent reconstruction with a T8–10 instrumented fusion with fenestrated pedicle screws at T8 and T10 that underwent cement augmentation (**f**). The construct was reinforced with fibular strut graft cabled to the rods. (**g**) Postoperative upright radiographs showed restoration of neutral coronal alignment at the treated segment

Clinical Presentation, Radiologic Features, and Histology

Clinical Presentation

Patients with OO and osteoblastoma commonly present with neck or back pain (80–100% of cases) of insidious onset with an average reported prodrome of 15–20 months [6, 7]. Pain is usually focal but may be accompanied by a radicular component [7] where the lesion approximates one of the exiting nerve roots. Pain is commonly reported as being worse at night [1, 2, 7] and infrequently has a mechanical component. Classically, pain in OO is relieved with the administration of aspirin or nonsteroidal anti-inflammatory drugs (NSAIDs), which reduce the production of prostaglandin PGE_2. PGE_2 production is thought to be the primary driver of pain [2] in OO, and histologic staining of nidus osteoblasts shows diffuse positive staining for cyclooxygenase-2 (COX-2) [2]. Prostaglandins are thought to mediate pain through vasodilation and sensitization of unmyelinated nerve fibers adjacent to the lesion. The vasodilation allows for greater vessel permeability and increases in local concentrations of bradykinin and histamine, to which prostaglandins PGE_2 and PGI_2 may also sensitize the unmyelinated afferents. Osteoblastoma appears to have a less robust response to aspirin and NSAIDs as compared to OO, though pain at presentation is also often reported as less severe [10].

The production of prostaglandins is also thought to contribute to scoliosis that can be seen in patients with OO and osteoblastoma [2]. In comparison to adolescent idiopathic scoliosis (AIS), the scoliosis associated with OO and osteoblastoma is painful. The scoliosis localizes with the lesion at the concavity of the curve apex [1]. The mechanism by which the lesion causes scoliosis is thought to be through inflammation of the paraspinal musculature surrounding the lesion. PGE_2 production instigates the inflammation and causes muscle spasm, flexing the spine away from the lesion. Consistent with this, lesions that localize to the spinous process do not appear to cause scoliosis [12, 13]. Similar to the observed association of lesion location and scoliotic curve directionality in thoracic tumors, eccentric cervical lesions can lead children to present with a painful torticollis, where the child's head turns away from the lesion. Overall deformity is more common in osteoblastoma, but scoliosis also appears common in OO [7, 10, 13]. Curves most commonly localize to the thoracic spine, and there is a marked male predominance, with males presenting with scoliosis at a rate nearly five times higher than females [7, 14]. In rare cases, the OO-associated scoliosis has been reported to precede the onset of pain [15–17].

Neurological symptoms can occur in both OO and osteoblastoma, though at a lower rate than axial pain [1, 7]. Neurological symptoms are more common in osteoblastoma (25–70% of cases) given the larger size and occur when there is epidural invasion by the lesion or compression of the nerve root at the level of the foramen. It has been reported that such an invasion may occur in more than 50% of cases [18]. Neurological deficits occur in a fraction of OO cases as well (0–30%) [7]. Myelopathy, which results from epidural invasion by the tumor, is uncommon, and weakness occurs in only one-third of cases [10].

Radiographic Features

On plain radiographs, OO and osteoblastoma appear as round radiolucent lesions with intranidal calcifications and a surrounding reactive sclerosis [1]. Radiographs are relatively insensitive for diagnosis of OO and osteoblastoma, though, and are predominately acquired to assess any concurrent deformity. On MR, osteoid osteomas have low-to-intermediate T1-weighted signal and high T2-weighted signal [1]. They are commonly heterogeneous due to intranidal calcifications, and the surrounding reactive sclerosis is low intensity on T1- and T2-weighted sequences [7]. The vascular nidus may demonstrate avid vascular enhancement. In osteoblastoma, the bony trabeculae can be visualized as irregular, linear signal voids, and the vascular nidus shows high T1-weighted signal. In both lesions, the surrounding edema shows high signal on T2-weighted images [7]. On CT, lesions show a lytic/lucent nidus, often with scattered intranidal calcifications and a sclerotic rim, which corresponds to the surrounding reactive bone [19]. The presence of sclerosis may vary, especially if the nidus is subchondral. Radiographically, the size of the lesion nidus is used to differentiate OO and osteoblastoma; osteoblastoma is defined by a nidus $\geq$2 cm in diameter, whereas OO has a nidus <2 cm [1, 10]. Others have suggested a nidus size cutoff of 1.5 cm though [20].

Technitium-99 m bone scans can be useful for identifying small lesions, as OO and osteoblastoma both show avid radiotracer uptake [2, 7]. It is the most sensitive tool for lesion detection and can be used when other detection modalities have failed to identify the lesion [7, 10]. Classically, spinal OOs demonstrate a "double density" on scintigraphy [2].

Histopathology

Histologically OO and osteoblastoma have similar features. OO has a nidus that is grossly yellow to red in appearance [7]. Within the lesions are osteoblasts, which produce osteoid and woven bone, the latter of which corresponds to the calcifications seen on CT [1, 6, 21]. The lesions are well-circumscribed and osteoblasts stain diffusely for COX-2 [2]. In osteoblastoma, there are also large vascular spaces containing reactive giant cells, which can give a radiological impression similar to aneurysmal bone cysts, especially in the case of aggressive lesions [10]. In 10–15% of cases, histological evaluation may also reveal components of aneurysmal bone cysts [10]. Average nidus size for osteoblastoma is 3–4 cm [10] and the surrounding reactive bone varies in thickness, though it is often thinner than in OO, consistent with the more aggressive nature of these lesions. Histologically, it has been suggested that osteoblastoma can be further differentiated into aggressive and conventional lesions [22]. Aggressive lesions have histopathological grades intermediate to conventional lesions and osteosarcoma. They show invasion of surrounding cortical bone, [23] have larger epithelioid osteoblasts, and show increased alkaline phosphatase synthesis compared to conventional osteoblastomas [22]. The aggressive lesions also show more cellular pleomorphism, larger, more irregular trabeculae, and possess osteoclast-like cells [10].

Evaluation

Evaluation of patients with OO and osteoblastoma should begin with thorough radiographic characterization. This includes contrast-enhanced MR to define lesion morphology and potential invasion of the epidural space. Computed tomography should also generally be obtained to analyze the extent of surrounding osteolysis and because MR features can often be misleading due to inflammatory changes in the surrounding tissues [24, 25]. Patients should also undergo upright posterior-anterior and lateral scoliosis radiographs to assess spinal alignment. Though not all patients present with scoliosis, baseline alignment should be appreciated for follow-up and in the case of surgical intervention. For those presenting with scoliosis, we generally obtain lateral bending films as well to demonstrate the flexibility of the curve. A definitive diagnosis is made through fine needle aspiration or CT-guide biopsy.

Tumor Management

OO shows the potential for spontaneous regression, [1, 2] and consequently, initial management is nonoperative in neurologically intact patients. Pain relief is chiefly through the administration of aspirin or NSAIDs, to which both lesions classically show good response [6]. In these patients, care must be taken to assess baseline deformity, which, while generally nonstructural, can become structural with delayed treatment [10].

Operative Management

Most patients with OO and patients with osteoblastoma ultimately proceed to surgical resection [2]. Indications for resection include pain refractory to medical management, tumor growth, deformity progression, and the onset of neurological symptoms; patient preference for oncologic cure is also an indication for resection [7]. As OO and osteoblastoma are both benign lesions, *en bloc* resection is not required, and surgical resection of the nidus is curative [7, 26]. Some groups recommend gross total resection for osteoblastoma, describing superior long-term local control as compared to subtotal resection with adjuvant radiotherapy [10].

Preoperative planning should include upright scoliosis films to assess baseline alignment and advanced imaging—CT and MR—to morphologically define the lesion and the position of the tumor nidus. CT is also useful for evaluating the extent of bony erosion; significant erosion of the facet joints or pars interarticularis is indicative of likely underlying instability and the need for concurrent fusion [10]. For patients with scoliosis on upright radiographs, we generally recommend lateral bending films to assess whether the lesion is structural or not.

As tumors generally arise from the posterior elements, a posterior approach is advantageous for most tumors. Given the vascular nature of osteoblastomas, some authors have described the use of preoperative embolization to reduce intraoperative blood loss [27–30]. If this is pursued, care must be taken during angiography to look for shared feeders with the spinal cord, which is a contraindication to embolization. Meticulous extracapsular dissection is important to help reduce intraoperative bleeding in the case of osteoblastoma. For osteoid osteoma, intralesional curettage of the nidus may be sufficient, though some authors also recommend excision of the surrounding sclerotic bone [7]. More than 90% of patients endorse pain relief with excision of the lesion, and pain relief may occur as rapidly as hours after the surgical resection [7].

Various ablative options are available for OO, including radiofrequency ablation (RFA), cryoablation, laser, microwave, and ultrasound-mediated MRI-guided ablations [31]. However, due to the limitations posed by spine lesions, CT-guided RFA is generally the more commonly used option in these cases. However, when the lesion is located in the posterior elements of the spine, close to the nerve roots, the application of ablative options can be challenging [31, 32]. For patients who have subtotal resection of their osteoblastoma (e.g., due to technical difficulty), adjuvant radiotherapy has been recommended by some groups, with Yin et al. [22] reporting a regimen of 30–50 Gy delivered over 20 fractions. However, there is the concern for malignant/sarcomatous transformation of the lesion, [10] which must be weighed against the potential complications associated with repeat resection.

Management of the Curve

Given the young age of most patients undergoing surgery for osteoid osteoma and osteoblastoma, surgeons must consider the potential impact of fusion on the growing spine. With historical instrumentation systems, specifically hook constructs, selective posterior fusion could result in a crankshaft phenomenon as the anterior column continues to elongate while the posterior column is fixed at the fused level. However, the incidence appears to have decreased with modern instrumentation systems, even in skeletally immature patients [33].

As mentioned previously, the scoliotic curve is nonstructural in most cases of OO and osteoblastoma. Rather, the painful scoliotic deformity results from long-standing inflammation (myositis) due to prostaglandin production by the lesion nidus. This inflammation can instigate muscle spasm and, in rare cases, even myolysis of the erector spinae muscle [34]. Resection of the lesion is associated with improvement of the scoliosis in 70–90% of cases, [7, 15, 35–38] and instrumentation planning consequently need not consider correction of the curve. For example, in the series of 22 patients described by Ozaki et al., [18] 17 presented with deformity, and in 16 of these patients (94%), it resolved with resection of the lesion alone. In most cases (50–80%), it has been reported that concurrent fusion is not even required. Our general preference is to avoid fusion in patients who are skeletally immature. If there is evidence of instability (e.g., osteolysis of the pars leaving <5 mm or complete facet joint destruction), [25] we prefer to minimize the number of segments included in the construct and feel that single-level fusion may be reasonable for lesions of the thoracic spine with preserved pedicles above and below the level of the lesion. There are at present no descriptions of growth-sparing technologies (e.g., vertical expandable prosthetic titanium rib/VEPTR and growing rods) being used in this clinical population.

The response of the scoliotic curve to resection alone appears to be proportional to the duration it has been present. In one series by Pettine and Klassen [39] reported outcomes for 42 patients treated for osteoid osteoma or osteoblastoma of the spine, in whom 26 presented with scoliosis. Of these patients, 11 of the 12 patients who had symptoms for less than 15 months at the time of clinical presentation experienced improvement or resolution of the scoliotic deformity as compared to only 1 of the 11 patients with symptoms present for more than 15 months at the time of diagnosis. It is posited that the chronic inflammation associated with long-standing lesions may be associated with injury to the growth plate on the curve concavity; there may also be degeneration and fibrosis of the paraspinal musculature [7, 13]. In this case, the curve may be structural and so require operative intervention [40].

For patients presenting with scoliotic curves, our initial approach is to examine the degree to which the curve is rigid on preoperative scoliosis films. If these films demonstrate a rigid curve and the patient is skeletally mature, our preference is to correct the curve at the time of lesion resection. To minimize the motion segments fused, we generally select the end vertebra as the upper and lower instrumented vertebrae. In skeletally immature patients and those with flexible curves, we opt initially for conservative management with bracing. This strategy has been successfully used by others [18, 25, 40] and is reasonable given the mild curvature reported in most cases—mean 19.1° for thoracic lesions and 18.6° for lumbar lesions in the review of Saifuddin et al. [13] It has been reported that deformity correction with conservative management typically occurs within the first 6 months of lesion excision [41].

The timing of when the functional deformity transitions into a fixed structural deformity is subject to debate. This transition is thought to be driven by vertebral rotation and inhibited end plate growth on the concave side, ultimately requiring more extensive corrective surgery. Historically, Ransford et al. [42] proposed 15 months of symptoms as the cut-off for improvement, but there have been case reports of deformity improvement even after years of pain and scoliosis following OO resection [43].

There have been reports of OO-associated scoliosis preceding the onset of pain [15–17]. In such cases, it is important to differentiate OO from other causes of painless deformity in adolescence, particularly idiopathic adolescent scoliosis. The latter may exhibit features such as hemivertebra, butterfly vertebra, or a rotational element in the vertebral bodies. A failed attempt at bracing may prompt further investigation, leading to the correct diagnosis. Other causes of painless scoliosis in adolescents include Chiari malformation (early-onset, long C-curve), neurofibromatosis I (NF-1) (short, sharp angular curve), and Marfan's syndrome (associated with increased kyphosis across the thoracic/lumbar junction) [16].

Conclusions

Osteoid osteoma and osteoblastoma are benign primary bone lesions that can cause painful scoliosis due to inflammation of the adjacent paraspinal tissue. Failure to address the lesion early can potentially lead to endplate cartilage injury, bony erosion, and fibrosis of the paraspinal musculature, converting a functional deformity into a structural deformity that requires surgical correction. In the majority of cases, surgical excision of the lesion is sufficient to allow for correction of the underlying deformity. Given the young age of most patients and the mild nature of the curve, surgical excision followed by trials on nonoperative therapy is reasonable. Failure of the curve to correct with these interventions may suggest a curve that has progressed to become structural or an alternative cause of the scoliosis that merits further investigation.

References

1. Pennington Z, Goodwin CR, Ahmed AK, Sciubba DM (2019) Primary Tumors of the thoracic spinal column. In: Baaj AA, Kakarla UK, Kim HJ (eds) Surgery of the thoracic spine, 1st edn. Georg Thieme, Stuttgart, pp 154–173
2. Lee EH, Shafi M, Hui JHP (2006) Osteoid osteoma. A current review. J Pediatr Orthop 26:695–700
3. Jaffe HL (1935) "Osteoid-Osteoma." a benign osteoblastic tumor composed of osteoid and atypical bone. Arch Surg 31:709–728
4. Jaffe HL (1956) Benign osteoblastoma. Bull Hosp Joint Dis 17:141–151
5. Lichtenstein L (1956) Benign osteoblastoma. A category of osteoid- and bone-forming tumors other than classical osteoid osteoma, which may be mistaken for giant-cell tumor or osteogenic sarcoma. Cancer 9:1044–1052
6. Ropper AE, Cahill KS, Hanna JW, McCarthy EF, Gokaslan ZL, Chi JH (2011) Primary vertebral tumors: a review of epidemiologic, histological, and imaging findings, part I: benign tumors. Neurosurgery 69:1171–1180
7. Kan P, Schmidt MH (2008) Osteoid osteoma and osteoblastoma of the spine. Neurosurg Clin N Am 19:65–70
8. Frassica FJ, Waltrip RL, Sponseller PD, Ma LD, McCarthy EF (1996) Clinicopathologic features and treatment of osteoid osteoma and osteoblastoma in children and adolescents. Orthop Clin North Am 27:559–574
9. Mallepally AR, Mahajan R, Pacha S, Rustagi T, Marathe N, Chhabra HS (2020) Spinal osteoid osteoma: surgical resection and review of literature. Surg Neurol Int 11:308
10. Galgano MA, Goulart CR, Iwenofu H, Chin LS, Lavelle W, Mendel E (2016) Osteoblastomas of the spine: a comprehensive review. Neurosurg Focus 41:E4
11. Schwartz HS, Pinto M (1990) Osteoblastomas of the cervical spine. J Spinal Disord 3:179–182
12. Azouz EM, Kozlowski K, Marton D, Sprague P, Zerhouni A, Asselah F (1986) Osteoid osteoma and osteoblastoma of the spine in children. Pediatr Radiol 16:25–31
13. Saifuddin A, White J, Sherazi Z, Shaikh MI, Natali C, Ransford AO (1998) Osteoid osteoma and osteoblastoma of the spine. Factors associated with the presence of scoliosis. Spine (Phila Pa 1976) 23:47–53
14. Nemoto O, Moser RP, Van Dam BE, Aoki J, Gilkey FW (1990) Osteoblastoma of the spine. A review of 75 cases. Spine (Phila Pa 1976) 15:1272–1280
15. Pourfeizi HH, Tabrizi A, Bazavar M, Sales JG (2014) Clinical findings and results of surgical resection of thoracolumbar osteoid osteoma. Asian Spine J 8:150–155
16. Uehara M, Takahashi J, Kuraishi S, Shimizu M, Ikegami S, Futatsugi T, Kato H (2015) Osteoid osteoma presenting as thoracic scoliosis. Spine J 15:e77–e81
17. Zhang H, Niu X, Wang B, He S, Hao D (2016) Scoliosis secondary to lumbar osteoid osteoma. Medicine (Baltimore) 95:e5362
18. Ozaki T, Liljenqvist U, Hillmann A, Halm H, Lindner N, Gosheger G, Winkelmann W (2002) Osteoid osteoma and osteoblastoma of the spine: experiences with 22 patients. Clin Orthop Relat Res 397:394–402
19. Chai JW, Hong SH, Choi J-Y, Koh YH, Lee JW, Choi J-A, Kang HS (2010) Radiologic diagnosis of osteoid osteoma: from simple to challenging findings. Radiographics 30:737–749

20. McLeod R, Dahlin D, Beabout J (1976) The spectrum of osteoblastoma. Am J Roentgenol 126:321–325
21. Zileli M, Çagli S, Basdemir G, Ersahin Y (2003) Osteoid osteomas and osteoblastomas of the spine. Neurosurg Focus 15:1–7
22. Yin H, Zhou W, Yu H, Li B, Zhang D, Wu Z, Liu T, Xiao J (2014) Clinical characteristics and treatment options for two types of osteoblastoma in the mobile spine: a retrospective study of 32 cases and outcomes. Eur Spine J 23:411–416
23. Lucas DR, Krishnan Unni K, McLeod RA, O'Connor MI, Sim FH (1994) Osteoblastoma: clinicopathologic study of 306 cases. Hum Pathol 25:117–134
24. Shaikh MI, Saifuddin A, Pringle J, Natali C, Sherazi Z (1999) Spinal osteoblastoma: CT and MR imaging with pathological correlation. Skeletal Radiol 28:33–40
25. Burn SC, Ansorge O, Zeller R, Drake JM (2009) Management of osteoblastoma and osteoid osteoma of the spine in childhood. J Neurosurg Pediatr 4:434–438
26. Quraishi NA, Boriani S, Sabou S et al (2017) A multicenter cohort study of spinal osteoid osteomas: results of surgical treatment and analysis of local recurrence. Spine J 17:401–408
27. Wang J, Du Z, Yang R, Tang X, Yan T, Guo W (2021) Surgical strategy of pediatric benign sacral tumors. J Pediatr Orthop 41:227–235
28. Schur S, Camlioglu E, Jung S, Powell T, Gutman G, Golan J (2017) Preoperative embolization and complete tumoral resection of a cervical aggressive epithelioid osteoblastoma. World Neurosurg 106:1051.e1–1051.e4
29. Jiang L, Liu X, Wang C, Yang S, Liu C, Wei F, Wu F, Zhou H, Dang L, Liu Z (2015) Surgical treatment options for aggressive osteoblastoma in the mobile spine. Eur Spine J 24:1778–1785
30. Ruggieri P, Huch K, Mavrogenis AF, Merlino B, Angelini A (2014) Osteoblastoma of the sacrum: report of 18 cases and analysis of the literature. Spine (Phila Pa 1976) 39:E97–E103
31. Parmeggiani A, Martella C, Ceccarelli L, Miceli M, Spinnato P, Facchini G (2021) Osteoid osteoma: which is the best mininvasive treatment option? Eur J Orthop Surg Traumatol 31:1611–1624
32. Sagoo NS, Haider AS, Chen AL et al (2022) Radiofrequency ablation for spinal osteoid osteoma: a systematic review of safety and treatment outcomes. Surg Oncol 41:101747
33. Murphy RF, Mooney JF (2017) The crankshaft phenomenon. J Am Acad Orthop Surg 25:e185–e193
34. Kawahara C, Tanaka Y, Kato H, Watanabe S, Kokubun S (2002) Myolysis of the erector spinae muscles as the cause of scoliosis in osteoid osteoma of the spine. Spine (Phila Pa 1976) 27:E313–E315
35. Raskas DS, Graziano GP, Herzenberg JE, Heidelberger KP, Hensinger RN (1992) Osteoid osteoma and osteoblastoma of the spine. J Spinal Disord 5:204–211
36. Gasbarrini A, Cappuccio M, Bandiera S, Amendola L, van Urk P, Boriani S (2011) Osteoid osteoma of the mobile spine: surgical outcomes in 81 patients. Spine (Phila Pa 1976) 36:2089–2093
37. Pan X, Qiao J, Liu Z, Sun X, Zhu Z (2022) Spontaneous correction of scoliosis after curettage of spinal osteoid osteoma: how and when? J Orthop Surg Res 17:534
38. Etemadifar MR, Hadi A (2015) Clinical findings and results of surgical resection in 19 cases of spinal osteoid osteoma. Asian Spine J 9:386
39. Pettine KA, Klassen RA (1986) Osteoid-osteoma and osteoblastoma of the spine. J Bone Joint Surg Am 68:354–361
40. Zairi M, Nessib MN (2023) Structural scoliosis secondary to thoracic osteoid osteoma: a case report of delayed diagnosis. Spine Deform 11:247–251
41. Gaike C, Lalwani K, Panat M (2022) Osteoid osteoma of lumbar vertebra presenting as low back ache and scoliosis in a young child – a case report. J Orthop Case Rep 12:95–97
42. Ransford A, Pozo J, Hutton P, Kirwan E (1984) The behaviour pattern of the scoliosis associated with osteoid osteoma or osteoblastoma of the spine. J Bone Joint Surg Br 66-B:16–20
43. Sapkas G, Efstathopoulos NE, Papadakis M (2009) Undiagnosed osteoid osteoma of the spine presenting as painful scoliosis from adolescence to adulthood: a case report. Scoliosis 4:9

Chapter 4
De novo Kyphosis from Pathological Compression Fractures

Taryn E. LeRoy, Camilo A. Molina, and Matthew L. Goodwin

Introduction

Vertebral compression fractures can result from a combination of osteoporosis, primary and metastatic spine tumors, trauma, and infection, including osteomyelitis, discitis, and Pott's disease. Although all compression fractures have some underlying pathology, pathologic vertebral compression fractures are traditionally thought to be fractures that result from primary or metastatic spine tumors. Most neoplastic pathologic fractures are secondary to metastatic disease rather than primary bone tumors, which are overall uncommon. The incidence of metastatic pathologic compression fractures continues to rise due to improvements in the diagnosis and treatment of metastatic disease and resultant longer patient survivals.

T. E. LeRoy
Department of Orthopedic Surgery, New England Baptist Hospital, Boston, MA, USA
e-mail: tleroy@nebh.org

C. A. Molina (✉)
Department of Neurosurgery, Washington University School of Medicine, St Louis, MO, USA
e-mail: cmolina@wustl.edu

M. L. Goodwin
Department of Orthopedic Surgery, Washington University School of Medicine, St Louis, MO, USA
e-mail: matthewlgoodwin@wustl.edu

D. M. Sciubba (ed.), *Spinal Tumor Associated Deformity*,
https://doi.org/10.1007/978-3-031-87939-5_4

Anatomy and Biomechanics

The spine is the most common site of skeletal metastases. Erosion of healthy bone by the pathologic lesion alters the skeletal biomechanics by reducing the load-bearing capacity of the vertebra and rendering it susceptible to fracture, even under normal physiologic stress. The risk of fracture is related to the extent of bony destruction, lesion location, and inherent bone quality [1]. The structure of the spine and regional variations in spinal anatomy expose the upper cervical, subaxial cervical, thoracic, and lumbar regions to different mechanical forces, resulting in a variety of fracture types. The thoracic spine is the most common region involved in spinal metastases, with the cervical and lumbar regions being less commonly affected.

The vertebral body is the most common site for metastatic lesions within the spine, with the dorsal elements rarely affected. Bony destruction of the vertebral body by tumor can decrease the load-bearing capacity of the vertebral body and when a critical point is reached, the vertebral body becomes prone to fracture under normal physiologic load resulting in a pathologic fracture [2]. In cadaveric models, both Dimar et al. [3] and Windhagen et al. [4] showed that the threshold for pathologic fractures can be predicted by measuring the remaining intact vertebral body cross-sectional area and the bone mineral density. The critical threshold of tumor involvement beyond which patients are at risk of pathologic fracture has been reported to be between 51% and 96% of the cross-sectional area; less tumor involvement is necessary for patients with poor underlying bone mineral density. Once the critical threshold is reached, the vertebral body is prone to pathologic fracture.

The two major fracture patterns are wedge/compression fractures, characterized by anterior column failure, and burst fractures, which are characterized by concurrent anterior and middle column failure. Compromise of the middle column in burst fractures can be associated with bony retropulsion and resultant spinal canal compromise with compression of the neural elements that requires surgical decompression. Compression versus burst fracture morphology is the result of the force generated in relation to the instantaneous axis of rotation (IAR) of the spinal segment. In a compression fracture, the force is placed ventral to the IAR, whereas in a burst fracture, the force is in line with the IAR [5]. Compression fractures are more common in the thoracic spine due to the inherent kyphosis, whereas burst morphology appears more common in the cervical and lumbar spine due to the baseline lordotic alignment. If there is concurrent posterior column involvement, pathologic dislocation or translation can occur.

Clinical Evaluation

A thorough history and physical are essential when evaluating patients with pathologic compression fractures. It is important to differentiate pathologic fractures from osteoporotic/fragility fractures, as the subsequent diagnostic workup and therapeutic plan will differ substantially. Furthermore, if suspicious for pathologic vertebral compression fractures, workup also varies based on the patient's oncologic history; patients without known oncologic disease required more extensive workup given the possibility the fracture may represent a primary bone tumor.

Most pathologic fractures are secondary to metastatic disease, with the five most common primary pathologies being breast, lung, thyroid, renal, and prostate. If the patient has no known history of malignancy, the history should include questions about prodromal pain, "B" symptoms (e.g., fevers, night sweats, and unintentional weight loss), as well as questions specific to primary carcinomas (e.g., hematochezia and melena in patients with concern for colorectal cancer and hemoptysis, chest pain, dyspnea, and cough in patients with concern for lung cancer) [6, 7]. Patients may also have signs or symptoms of hypercalcemia of malignancy, including fatigue, altered mental status, gastrointestinal abnormalities, cardiac arrhythmia, and/or renal failure.

In the setting of kyphotic deformity secondary to pathologic fracture, proper characterization of the pain and associated neurological symptoms (e.g., weakness and sensory changes) is important, as are details regarding progression of the deformity. Characterization of the patient's neurological deficits should include questions about fine motor tasks, gait instability, imbalance, and difficulties with bowel or bladder incontinence. Neurological symptoms can occur secondary to concurrent epidural disease, which requires decompression, or due to draping of the spinal cord over the kyphotic segment. Symptom severity and the timing of symptom onset are both important and help to determine the urgency of surgical intervention.

On physical examination, it is important to evaluate the patient's global coronal and sagittal balance, palpate over painful areas, and complete a thorough neurologic examination. The neurologic examination should include a full assessment of strength, sensation, reflexes, ± rectal examination. In cervicothoracic lesions, examination may also include assessment for signs and symptoms of myelopathy, including spasticity, hyperreflexia, and abnormal reflexes, including Babinski, clonus, inverted radial reflex, and/or Hoffman's sign. However, it must be noted that these may be absent in the case of acute compression.

Radiographic Evaluation

Conventional Radiographs

Radiographic evaluation of de novo kyphosis from pathologic compression fractures is made using long-cassette 36-inch posteroanterior (PA) and lateral standing radiographs. Patients should stand with the elbows flexed approximately 45°, the fingers positioned along the clavicles, with the head facing forward. This position captures the degree of deformity (sagittal and coronal) and recruitment of compensatory mechanisms without the influence from supports. In some patients this may not be possible, e.g., in the case of baseline immobility or severe mechanical pain. Patients precluded from undergoing standing radiographs due to mechanical pain likely have underlying instability.

PA radiographs are used to assess coronal alignment and lateral radiographs demonstrate sagittal alignment. Coronal alignment is quantified using the coronal vertical axis—the horizontal distance between plumb lines drawn caudally from the center of the C7-plumb line (C7PL) and cranially from the center of the sacrum (CSVL). A C7PL that falls to the left or right of the CSVL is designated with negative or positive values, respectively, and coronal malalignment is commonly defined by a C7PL more than 3 cm displaced from the CSVL [8]. In the sagittal plane, the sagittal vertical axis (SVA) is measured as the distance between the C7PL and the posterosuperior corner of S1; an SVA greater than 5 cm is generally used as the threshold for sagittal imbalance.

Areas of kyphosis, lordosis, and scoliosis are measured utilizing the Cobb method [9]. For coronal curves, the angulation is defined by parallel lines drawn at the superior endplate of the most tilted vertebra above the apex of the curve and the inferior endplate of the most tilted vertebra below the apex of the curve. Cobb angles are also used to describe angulation in the sagittal plane with kyphosis being designated by positive values and lordosis by negative values. Typical angles measured are the T4–12 kyphosis, L1-S1 lordosis, and L4-S1 lordosis. In the context of compression fractures, the focal kyphotic angle can also be measured, which is the angle defined by lines drawn parallel to the superior endplate of one vertebra above the fracture and the inferior endplate of the vertebra one level below the fracture (Fig. 4.1).

Other radiographic measurements that may be utilized include the vertebral body translation percentage, to express traumatic anterolisthesis and the anterior vertebral body compression percentage, to assess vertebral body compression. Parameters used to assess the degree of concurrent compression include the sagittal-to-transverse canal diameter ratio, the canal total cross-sectional area, and the percent canal occlusion, to assess canal dimensions [10].

The vertebral body translation percentage is determined by drawing lines along the posterior borders of the superior and inferior vertebral bodies and dividing this distance by the sagittal diameter of the cranial/slipped vertebra [10]. The anterior vertebral body compression percentage is defined using the anterior vertebral body heights of the injured level (V_2) and two adjacent levels (V_1, V_3), where compression percentage = $[(V_1 + V_3)/2 - V_2]/(V_1 + V_3)/2$. For the spinal canal dimensions, the trans-axial CT is used to measure the sagittal and transverse canal diameters. These measurements provide the sagittal-to-transverse canal diameter ratio. Utilizing the sagittal canal diameter and comparing the injured level to an uninjured level can provide the percent canal occlusion.

To assess the rigidity of the kyphotic deformity, a comparison should be made between the degree of deformity on weight-bearing (standing) and non-weight-bearing (supine) radiographs, utilizing Cobb angles. Rigid deformities will show minimal changes in the focal kyphotic angle between standing and supine radiographs, which likely indicate the need for more extensive osteotomy work intraoperatively. Additional radiographs over a bolster may help to further assess the stiffness of the deformity.

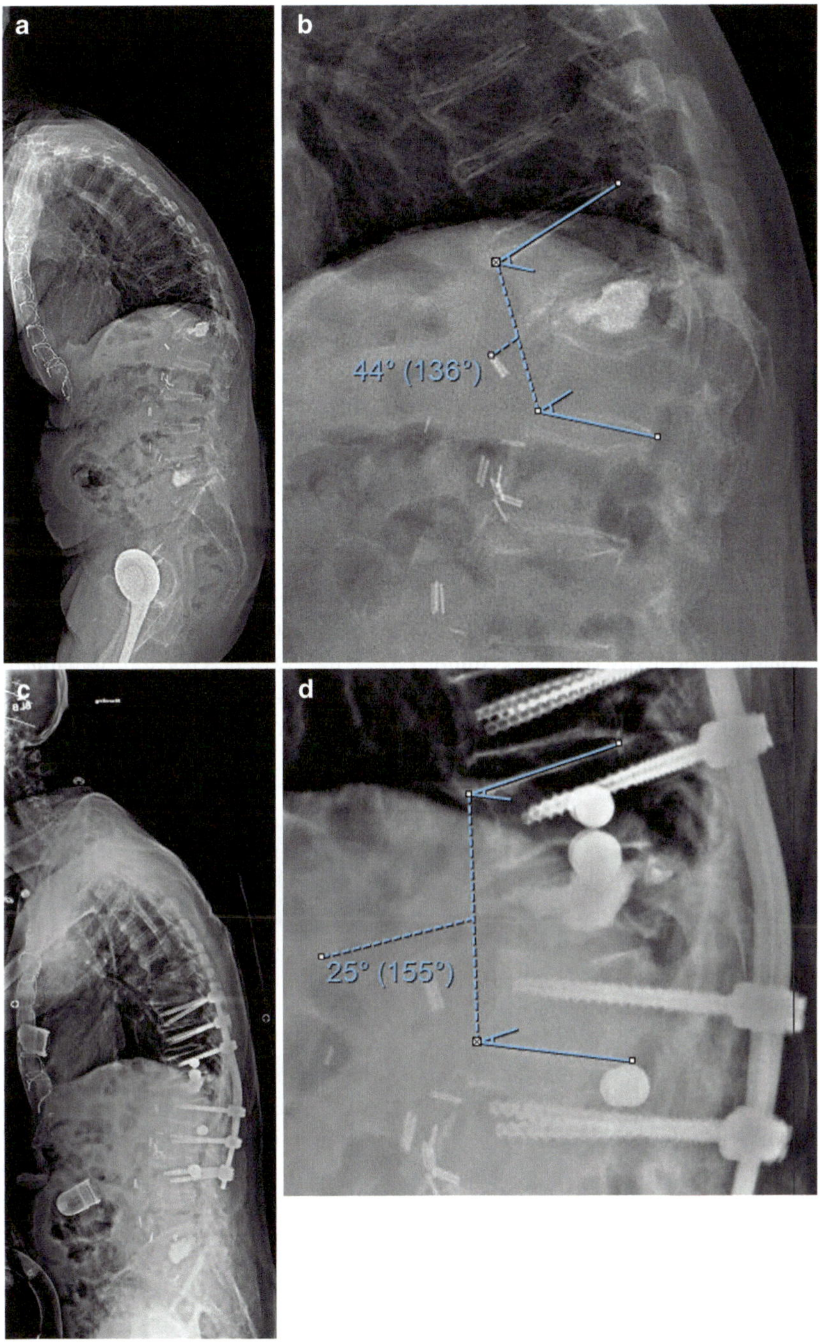

Fig. 4.1 (**a**). Standing scoliosis lateral radiograph demonstrating marked positive sagittal balance, T12 pathologic compression fracture status post vertebroplasty in the setting of renal cell carcinoma with collapse and focal kyphosis resulting in spinal cord compression. (**b**). Focal kyphotic angle. (**c**). Postoperative scoliosis radiographs. (**d**). Focal kyphotic angle revealing improvement in kyphosis by 19°

Advanced Imaging

Advanced imaging has become standard of care in the evaluation of patients with spinal deformity and is routinely obtained in patients with concern for neoplastic disease. MR and CT are the most common advanced modalities seen in the clinical setting, though CT myelogram, CT angiography (CTA), and MR angiography (MRA) may also be available depending upon the patient's clinical history. CT is the modality of choice for defining bony anatomy; it can be used to assess degree of vertebral body collapse and estimate the quality of the bone. It is also useful for preoperative planning when instrumented fusion is being considered. MRI should be obtained in all cases with concern for neurologic compromise, unless contraindicated, in which case CT myelogram should be obtained (Fig. 4.2). CTA and MRA are useful in the evaluation of vascular anatomy and may be utilized for surgical planning and approach considerations.

Spinal Instability Neoplastic Score

In 2010, the Spinal Oncology Study Group developed the Spinal Instability Neoplastic Score (SINS) to assess tumor-related intervertebral instability (Table 4.1) [11]. This classification system defines lesions as stable, potentially unstable, or unstable, and has been previously validated and found to have excellent inter- and intra-observer reliability [12, 13]. Tumor-related instability is assessed by assigning

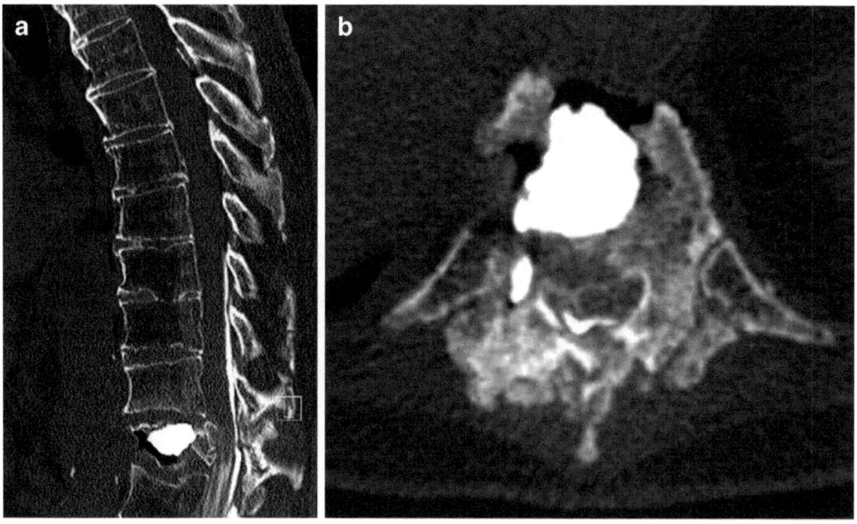

Fig. 4.2 (**a**). Sagittal CT myelogram demonstrating pathologic T12 compression fracture status post vertebroplasty with bony retropulsion. (**b**). Axial view of CT myelogram demonstrating severe stenosis at T12

Table 4.1 The spinal instability neoplastic score

Component	Score
Location	
Junctional (O-C2; C7-T2; T11-L1; L5-S1)	3
Mobile spine (C3–6; L2–4)	2
Semi-rigid (T3–10)	1
Rigid (S2-S5)	0
Mechanical pain	
Yes	3
No	2
Pain-free lesion	1
Bone lesion	
Lytic	2
Mixed (lytic/blastic)	1
Blastic	0
Radiographic spinal alignment	
Subluxation/translation present	4
Deformity (kyphosis/scoliosis)	2
Normal	0
Vertebral body collapse	
> 50% collapse	3
< 50% collapse	2
No collapse with >50% body involved	1
None of the above	0
Posterolateral involvement	
Bilateral	3
Unilateral	1
None of the above	0

points based on five imaging and one clinical component: lesion location, the presence and type of pain, bone lesion quality, spinal alignment, the extent of vertebral body collapse, and posterolateral involvement. The maximum number of points is 18, where a score of 0–6 denotes stability, 7–12 denotes a lesion of "indeterminate" stability, and 13–18 indicates instability. Surgical consultation is recommended for any patient with a score greater than or equal to 7 and prior work has suggested surgery to be beneficial for lesions with an SINS ≥10 [14, 15].

Treatment

Treatment Options

Both nonoperative and surgical interventions can be considered for compression fractures resulting in kyphotic deformity. These interventions include medical management/analgesics for pain, bracing, radiation therapy, vertebroplasty/kyphoplasty, and surgical management. Patients generally benefit from having their care guided by a multidisciplinary team including their primary oncologist, along with a radiation oncologist, spine surgeon, diagnostic and interventional radiologist, and/or pain specialist.

Nonoperative Treatment

Nonoperative management is a reasonable first choice for patients with minimal pain and those without any neurologic compromise. The traditional first-line treatment includes oral medications and bracing. Medications follow the World Health Organization analgesic ladder, beginning with nonsteroidal anti-inflammatory medications and escalating to muscle relaxants, and/or opioids. Bisphosphonates may also be utilized in pathologic compression fractures with severe, worsening pain. By inhibiting osteoclasts, they can help with pain palliation and decrease the risk of future fractures [16, 17]. Mild-to-moderate compression fractures may initially be treated with bracing for 6–12 weeks, undergoing regular radiographic follow-up. As the patient's pain subsides the brace may be discontinued; pain progression or radiographic progression of the deformity should be considered grounds for escalation to cementoplasty or surgical stabilization.

Radiation therapy is a common treatment for lesions with oncologic [vs mechanical] pain and is a preferred option in the absence of instability or concurrent neurologic deficits. Advantages include its noninvasive nature, ability to provide local tumor control, and significant pain relief. It cannot provide stabilization though and should not be considered as a replacement for surgery in unstable lesions. Furthermore, radiation itself can be considered an independent risk factor for vertebral compression fractures, with reported rates ranging from 5% to 39% depending on the modality employed [18, 19]. Focused modalities, such as stereotactic body radiotherapy (SBRT), are preferred due to the lower rate of off-target toxicities relative to conventional therapy. The American Society of Therapeutic Radiation Oncology developed guidelines for SBRT in 2011 and patients with mechanical instability are not considered candidates for SBRT [20]. Therefore, radiation therapy should be used with caution in patients with pathologic compression fractures and may need to be delayed in patients with kyphotic deformity until after surgical stabilization has been performed.

Cement augmentation procedures, including vertebroplasty and kyphoplasty, are increasingly recognized as safe and effective methods for pain control and preventing disability in carefully selected patients [21]. Vertebroplasty (VP) with polymethylmethacrylate (PMMA) was first introduced as a technique for treatment of vertebral hemangiomas in 1984 [22]. It is performed by obtaining transpedicular access to the vertebral body and injecting PMMA into the collapsed vertebral body under continuous fluoroscopic visualization. Kyphoplasty differs in that an inflatable balloon catheter is first inserted within the vertebral body and expanded, with the goal being to restore vertebral body height, correct any underlying kyphotic deformity, and create a receiving area for the cement. Indications for vertebroplasty and kyphoplasty are similar and include painful pathologic fractures and tumor-invaded vertebrae at risk of collapse [23]. Cement augmentation procedures can also be considered for patients with spinal instability who are not deemed surgical candidates. The goal of these procedures is pain palliation, and the cement augmentation may offer a low level of instability; it is not a replacement for surgical stabilization in unstable segments though. Contraindications to cementoplasty include sepsis, osteomyelitis of the target vertebra, and uncorrectable coagulopathy [23]. Relative contraindications include radiculopathy, retropulsion of a fracture fragment with signs or symptoms of neurologic compromise, epidural tumor extension leading to significant encroachment of the spinal canal, ongoing systemic infection, pain improvement at the time of evaluation, and pregnancy [23].

Operative Treatment

For patients with progressive neurologic deficit, spinal instability, progressive deformity, or symptoms refractory to conservative treatment, surgical intervention is indicated. Prior to surgical intervention, it is necessary to diagnose the etiology of the pathologic fracture. Additionally, a patient's ability to tolerate and have a successful outcome from surgery should be assayed, taking stock of the patient's age, medical comorbidities, bone quality, primary cancer type, preoperative ambulatory status, and baseline functionality.

The primary goals of surgery are to treat the offending pathology, decompress the neural elements, stabilize the spine, and correct deformity. Correcting deformity can prevent future failure and decrease patient disability caused by sagittal imbalance; however, one must also balance this with the patient's age, bone quality, medical comorbidities, and ultimate ability to tolerate deformity correction.

Effective surgical planning necessitates thorough understanding of the deformity, including assessment of the curve magnitude, characterization of the length and flexibility of the kyphotic segment, and evaluation of the patient's overall coronal and sagittal balance. Both clinical and radiographic assessment of the patient's balance and alignment are crucial in surgical planning. To assess curve flexibility, upright and supine films should be obtained; supine radiographs obtained over a bolster can also be considered, though this is uncommon in the oncology population. Deformities that appear flexible on preoperative imaging may require minimal osteotomy work, whereas rigid deformities may require multilevel osteotomies or more aggressive osteotomies, including vertebral column resection. While developing the surgical plan, it is also necessary to identify regions of neural element compression, as this should be addressed prior to correction of the deformity.

Depending upon the spinal level involved, surgery can employ an anterior-only, posterior-only, or combined approach. Factors influencing the selection of an anterior versus posterior approach include the level being treated, severity of the focal deformity, extent of ventral cord compression, and the patient's ability to tolerate surgery. The anterior approach in the thoracic and lumbar spine is considered to provide the best visualization of the ventral spinal cord, can provide a more direct and complete decompression of the canal in the case of vertebral tumor, and allows the surgeon to restore the load-bearing anterior column. However, anterior approaches to the thoracolumbar spine can be morbid and may be contraindicated in the case of patients with prior abdominal surgeries. Furthermore, for thoracic lesions—the region most common affected by pathologic fracture—pulmonary complications are common, and it is therefore important to assess preoperative lung function, especially in patients with a history of smoking or chronic lung disease.

Anterior approaches for the thoracic spine can be divided into two techniques: transthoracic and transdiaphragmatic. The transthoracic approach provides exposure from T2 to T12; however, exposure in the upper thoracic spine, T3-T5, may require a transsternal approach [24], performed in conjunction with a thoracic surgeon. The transdiaphragmatic approach provides access to the upper lumbar spine and thoracolumbar junction; it can theoretically be used to access lesions as cephalad as T6. To gain adequate exposure with this technique, one requires dissection of the psoas and diaphragmatic crus in the lumbar spine, incision of the diaphragm at the thoracolumbar junction, and reflection of the parietal pleura in the thoracic spine. As with anterior approaches to the upper thoracic spine, transdiaphragmatic approaches are relatively morbid and carry a nontrivial risk of respiratory complications (atelectasis, pneumonia, pneumothorax). Other complications include deep infection (including empyema), thoracic duct injury, injury to the great vessels, ventral durotomy, and spinal cord ischemia secondary to injury of the radicular artery giving rise to the artery of Adamkiewicz. Additional risks with the transdiaphragmatic approach include abdominal and diaphragmatic hernias. Anterior approaches to the thoracic spine are on the whole relatively morbid and almost never indicated in the case of metastatic lesions.

Anterior approaches for the lumbar spine can be performed via a paramedian retroperitoneal approach or using an oblique trajectory. The paramedian approach is better for lower lumbar vertebra and the chief advantage of this approach is direct access to the vertebral column for anterior column reconstruction. Sagittal correction using interbody fusion via an anterior approach is also associated with reduced blood loss relative to an all-posterior approach but necessitates a complimentary posterior approach. Such circumferential fusion may be too great a physical insult for frail patients with metastatic disease. Downsides of the anterior approach include the need for a vascular access surgeon and the risks of vascular injury, retrograde ejaculation, ileus, peritoneal injury, ureteral injury, retroperitoneal hematoma, arterial thrombosis, DVT, rectus muscle paresis, and hernia.

The posterior approach is historically more familiar to surgeons. This approach allows direct posterior decompression and instrumentation. Ventral decompression and anterior column reconstruction can be achieved via a posterior-only technique though it may require a more aggressive approach, such as a transpedicular approach, costotransversectomy (CTE), or lateral extracavitary approach (LECA). The transpedicular approach, if performed bilaterally, can be used to perform a vertebrectomy and minimally invasive versions of this technique have been described for metastases by Chou and others [25]. CTE and LECA provide more extensive access to the ventral spine, with LECA affording the ability to achieve decompression of midline ventral lesions. However, the soft tissue dissection required by the costotransversectomy and LECA is far more extensive than the midline and transpedicular approaches and again may be too aggressive for patients with metastatic disease. In general, most patients are adequately treated with a conventional midline approach that exposes laterally to the transverse processes. A chief advantage of the posterior-only approach is the ability to treat all pathology through a single stage. It also removes the risk posed to the thoracic and abdominal viscera and offers the ability to perform osteotomy work for the correction of rigid deformity. Anterior stages generally require a complementary posterior stage to support the anterior construct. However, for cervical and high thoracic lesions, anterior column reconstruction requires an anterior stage due to the risk posed to the spinal cord and nerve roots by attempting vertebral column resection from a posterior approach. Posterior-only procedures are also challenged by the large cantilever stresses placed on the spinal instrumentation during deformity correction; this may lead to hardware failure in patients with weak bone, such as those with prior radiation, osteoporosis, or multilevel metastatic disease.

Osteotomies

Osteotomies are required to correct rigid deformity, though the aggressiveness of the osteotomy performed depends on the focality and severity of the deformity. The most common osteotomy techniques described in the literature for deformity correction are posterior column osteotomies, including Smith-Petersen osteotomy (SPO) and Ponte osteotomy. Pedicle subtraction osteotomy and vertebral column resections are also described in the deformity literature, though their use in patients with metastatic disease is less common given concern regarding the ability of patients with metastatic disease to tolerate the associated morbidity.

When evaluating the osteotomy required, the patient's spine will fall into one of the three categories: totally flexible, partially correctable, and totally inflexible, with no correction on supine imaging. Bridwell as well as Dorward and Lenke proposed algorithms to aid in decision making between posterior column osteotomies and three-column osteotomies [26, 27]. These algorithms consider the angularity, flexibility, and location of the deformity, as well as surgeon and patient characteristics.

A posterior column osteotomy includes removal of the facet joints, the lamina, and the posterior ligamentous structures. A posterior column osteotomy corrects the deformity by shortening the posterior column; concomitant anterior column lengthening can also be achieved with concurrent placement of an interbody in the corresponding disc space. Although PCOs are commonly employed, there is much confusion surrounding the nomenclature and technique for Smith-Petersen and Ponte osteotomies. Smith-Petersen osteotomy was first described for patients with rheumatologic conditions and ankylosing spondylitis; however, this method involved violation of the anterior longitudinal ligament and posed significant risk to the anterior vascular structures [28]. The Ponte osteotomy was later described for kyphotic deformity in patients with Scheuermann's disease and involved posterior compression along unfused spinal segments [29]. The amount of kyphotic correction obtained in these osteotomies has been reported to range from 9.3 to 10.7° per level [30, 31].

For patients with rigid, focal deformities, pedicle subtraction osteotomy (PSO) allows for aggressive sagittal place correction. The PSO is a three-column osteotomy that removes the pedicles and a wedge-shaped portion of the vertebral body. An extended-PSO extends the wedge-shaped cut into the cranial disc space and includes exenteration of this adjoining disc space. Kyphosis is corrected by compressing across the PSO, which results in shortening of the posterior column. If performed asymmetrically, one can not only acquire sagittal deformity correction, but also gain coronal correction. The extended PSO can include placement of a Harms cage or interbody in the exenterated disc space. This serves as a fulcrum and can allow for some anterior column lengthening as compression is being performed across the screws. Clinical studies have shown relative uniformity in the degree of kyphosis correction ranging from 26.2 to 40.1°, averaging 32° across multiple studies [32–44]. It must be noted that in order for the PSO to be successful, the patient's bone must be strong enough to tolerate the compression maneuver without dislodgement of the pedicle screws.

Vertebral column resection is the most aggressive and powerful method for focal deformity correction and involves resection of all posterior elements, the facet joints at the levels above and below, the entire vertebral body, and the supra-adjacent and subjacent discs. A cage or bone strut graft is placed in the defect and the height selected for the graft determines the degree of anterior lengthening achieved. The use of narrow footprint cages increases the risk of implant subsidence and postoperative kyphotic deformity [45], and the height of the anterior column graft should not exceed the height of the adjacent normal vertebrae.

Due to the variable use of osteotomy terminology, the SRS-Schwab classification system was devised and provides consistent descriptions of the above osteotomies [46]. Six grades are outlined based on the extent of bone and disc resection. Grade 1 osteotomies involve resection of the inferior facets. Grade 2 osteotomies include resection of both the superior and inferior facets and other posterior ligamentous and osseous structures. Grade 3 osteotomies involve removal of posterior elements, the pedicles, and part of the vertebral body. Grade 4 osteotomies involve wider resections, including at least a portion of the adjacent disc. Grade 5 osteotomies involve the complete removal of one vertebra and adjacent discs. Grade 6 osteotomies involve any resection that exceeds a Grade 5. It should be noted that frail cancer patients may be unable to tolerate the morbidity associated with higher-grade osteotomies (grades 3–6), which can significantly prolong operative times and result in notable increases in intraoperative blood loss [47]. Such three-column osteotomies must be judicially employed in the oncology population and are likely best reserved for the following patient populations: (1) patients with primary tumors who are already undergoing significant bony resection as part of the attempt at oncologic cure, (2) patients with benign lesions (e.g., hemangioma) in whom treatment of the underlying deformity is a chief goal of surgery, and (3) metastatic lesions in patients with good overall health (minimal frailty) and good life expectancy (likely ≥1 year given the time required to heal a three-column osteotomy).

Conclusion

In summary, kyphotic deformity resulting from pathologic compression fractures requires a multidisciplinary approach to management. The primary indications for surgical intervention include progressive neurologic deficit, spinal instability, progressive deformity, and symptoms refractory to conservative treatment. However, the benefits of surgical correction must be weighed against the risks of surgical intervention, which can be particularly morbid in the frail metastatic tumor population. If one is to proceed with surgical intervention, it is imperative to understand the patient's global alignment as well as understand the nature of the kyphotic deformity, including curve magnitude, curve flexibility, and the length of the kyphotic segment. Both anterior and posterior procedures can be utilized. Posterior-only approaches are more popular and are reasonable for thoracolumbar lesions with flexible or mild multilevel deformities. Cervical, upper thoracic, and lumbar lesions with fixed, rigid deformities may require an anterior approach for corpectomy so as to allow for anterior column reconstruction and correction of the deformity.

References

1. Pennington Z, Ahmed AK, Sciubba DM (2020) Deformity secondary to vertebral body metastases. In: Ramakrishna R, Magge RS, Baaj AA, Knisely JPS (eds) Central nervous system metastasis, 1st edn. Springer International Publishing, Cham, pp 583–601
2. Krishnaney AA, Steinmetz MP, Benzel EC (2004) Biomechanics of metastatic spine cancer. Neurosurg Clin N Am 15:375–380
3. Dimar JR, Voor MJ, Zhang YM, Glassman SD (1998) A human cadaver model for determination of pathologic fracture threshold resulting from tumorous destruction of the vertebral body. Spine 23:1209–1214
4. Windhagen HJ, Hipp JA, Silva MJ, Lipson SJ, Hayes WC (1997) Predicting failure of thoracic vertebrae with simulated and actual metastatic defects. Clin Orthop Relat Res 344:313–319
5. Benzel EC, Kayanja M, Fleischman A, Roy S (2006) Spine biomechanics: fundamentals and future. Clin Neurosurg 53:98–105
6. Gridelli C, Rossi A, Carbone DP, Guarize J, Karachaliou N, Mok T, Petrella F, Spaggiari L, Rosell R (2015) Non-small-cell lung cancer. Nat Rev Dis Prim 1:15009
7. Kuipers EJ, Grady WM, Lieberman D, Seufferlein T, Sung JJ, Boelens PG, van de Velde CJH, Watanabe T (2015) Colorectal cancer. Nat Rev Dis Prim 1:15065
8. Zuckerman SL, Chanbour H, Hassan FM et al (2022) Evaluation of coronal alignment from the skull using the novel orbital–coronal vertical axis line. J Neurosurg Spine 37:410–419
9. De Smet AA (1985) Radiographic evaluation. In: De Smet AA (ed) Radiology spinal curvature, 1st edn. Mosby, p 23

10. Keynan O, Fisher CG, Vaccaro A et al (2006) Radiographic measurement parameters in thoracolumbar fractures: a systematic review and consensus statement of the spine trauma study group. Spine 31:E156–E165
11. Fisher CG, DiPaola CP, Ryken TC et al (2010) A novel classification system for spinal instability in neoplastic disease: an evidence-based approach and expert consensus from the spine oncology study group. Spine 35:E1221–E1229
12. Fourney DR, Frangou EM, Ryken TC et al (2011) Spinal instability neoplastic score: an analysis of reliability and validity from the spine oncology study group. J Clin Oncol 29:3072–3077
13. Pennington Z, Ahmed AK, Cottrill E, Westbroek EM, Goodwin ML, Sciubba DM (2019) Intra- and interobserver reliability of the spinal instability neoplastic score system for instability in spine metastases: a systematic review and meta-analysis. Ann Transl Med 7:218
14. Pennington Z, Ahmed AK, Westbroek EM, Cottrill E, Lubelski D, Goodwin ML, Sciubba DM (2019) SINS score and stability: evaluating the need for stabilization within the uncertain category. World Neurosurg 128:e1034–e1047
15. Hussain I, Barzilai O, Reiner AS, DiStefano N, McLaughlin L, Ogilvie S, Bilsky M, Laufer I (2018) Patient-reported outcomes after surgical stabilization of spinal tumors: symptom-based validation of the spinal instability neoplastic score (SINS) and surgery. Spine J 18:261–267
16. Lopez-Olivo MA, Shah NA, Pratt G, Risser JM, Symanski E, Suarez-Almazor ME (2012) Bisphosphonates in the treatment of patients with lung cancer and metastatic bone disease: a systematic review and meta-analysis. Support Care Cancer 20:2985–2998
17. Body J-J, Diel IJ, Lichinitser MR, Kreuser ED, Dornoff W, Gorbunova VA, Budde M, Bergström B (2003) Intravenous ibandronate reduces the incidence of skeletal complications in patients with breast cancer and bone metastases. Ann Oncol 14:1399–1405
18. Leone A, Cianfoni A, Zecchi V, Cortese MC, Rumi N, Colosimo C (2019) Instability and impending instability in patients with vertebral metastatic disease. Skeletal Radiol 48:195–207
19. Pennington Z, Mikula AL, Lakomkin N et al (2023) Comparison of Hounsfield units and vertebral bone quality score for the prediction of time to pathologic fracture in mobile spine metastases treated with radiotherapy. J Neurosurg Spine 40:19–27
20. Lutz S, Berk L, Chang E et al (2011) Palliative radiotherapy for bone metastases: an ASTRO evidence-based guideline. Int J Radiat Oncol 79:965–976
21. Barr JD, Jensen ME, Hirsch JA et al (2014) Position statement on percutaneous vertebral augmentation: a consensus statement developed by the Society of Interventional Radiology (SIR), American Association of Neurological Surgeons (AANS) and the Congress of Neurological Surgeons (CNS), American college of radiology (ACR), American society of neuroradiology (ASNR), American society of spine radiology (ASSR), Canadian interventional radiology association (CIRA), and the society of NeuroInterventional surgery (SNIS). J Vasc Interv Radiol 25:171–181
22. Deramond H, Depriester C, Toussaint P, Galibert P (1997) Percutaneous vertebroplasty. Semin Musculoskelet Radiol 1:285–295
23. Baerlocher MO, Saad WE, Dariushnia S, Barr JD, McGraw JK, Nikolic B (2014) Quality improvement guidelines for percutaneous Vertebroplasty. J Vasc Interv Radiol 25:165–170
24. Pennington Z, Westbroek EM, Lo S-FL, Sciubba DM (2021) Surgical approaches to tumors of the Occipito-cervical, subaxial cervical, and Cervicothoracic spine: an algorithm for standard versus extended anterior cervical access. World Neurosurg 156:e41–e56
25. Chou D, Lu DC (2011) Mini-open transpedicular corpectomies with expandable cage reconstruction. J Neurosurg Spine 14:71–77
26. Bridwell KH (2006) Decision making regarding Smith-Petersen vs. pedicle subtraction osteotomy vs. vertebral column resection for spinal deformity. Spine 31:S171–S178
27. Dorward IG, Lenke LG (2010) Osteotomies in the posterior-only treatment of complex adult spinal deformity: a comparative review. Neurosurg Focus 28:E4
28. Smith-Petersen MN, Larson CB, Aufranc OE (1969) Osteotomy of the spine for correction of flexion deformity in rheumatoid arthritis. Clin Orthop Relat Res 66:6–9
29. Ponte A (1985) Surgical treatment of Scheuermann's hyperkyphosis. Orthop Trans 9:127

30. Cho K-J, Bridwell KH, Lenke LG, Berra A, Baldus C (2005) Comparison of Smith-Petersen versus pedicle subtraction osteotomy for the correction of fixed sagittal imbalance. Spine 30:2037
31. Geck MJ, Macagno A, Ponte A, Shufflebarger HL (2007) The Ponte procedure: posterior only treatment of Scheuermann's kyphosis using segmental posterior shortening and pedicle screw instrumentation. J Spinal Disord Tech 20:586–593
32. Berven SH, Deviren V, Smith JA, Emami A, Hu SS, Bradford DS (2001) Management of fixed sagittal plane deformity: results of the transpedicular wedge resection osteotomy. Spine 26:2036–2043
33. Bridwell KH, Lewis SJ, Lenke LG, Baldus C, Blanke KM (2003) Pedicle subtraction osteotomy for the treatment of fixed sagittal imbalance. J Bone Joint Surg Am 85:454–463
34. Murrey DB, Brigham CD, Kiebzak GM, Finger F, Chewning SJ (2002) Transpedicular decompression and pedicle subtraction osteotomy (eggshell procedure). Spine 27:2338–2345
35. Thomasen E (1985) Vertebral osteotomy for correction of kyphosis in ankylosing spondylitis. Clin Orthop Relat Res:142–152
36. Yang BP, Ondra SL, Chen LA, Jung HS, Koski TR, Salehi SA (2006) Clinical and radiographic outcomes of thoracic and lumbar pedicle subtraction osteotomy for fixed sagittal imbalance. J Neurosurg Spine 5:9–17
37. Chen I-H, Chien J-T, Yu T-C (2001) Transpedicular wedge osteotomy for correction of thoracolumbar kyphosis in ankylosing spondylitis. Spine 26:E354–E360
38. Danisa OA, Turner D, Richardson WJ (2000) Surgical correction of lumbar kyphotic deformity: posterior reduction "eggshell" osteotomy. J Neurosurg Spine 92:50–56
39. Ikenaga M, Shikata JJ, Takemoto M, Tanaka C (2007) Clinical outcomes and complications after pedicle subtraction osteotomy for correction of thoracolumbar kyphosis. J Neurosurg Spine 6:330–336
40. Kim K-T, Suk K-S, Cho Y-J, Hong G-P, Park B-J (2002) Clinical outcome results of pedicle subtraction osteotomy in ankylosing spondylitis with kyphotic deformity. Spine 27:612–618
41. Kim YJ, Bridwell KH, Lenke LG, Cheh G, Baldus C (2007) Results of lumbar pedicle subtraction osteotomies for fixed sagittal imbalance. Spine 32:2189–2197
42. Lazennec J-Y, Neves N, Rousseau M-A, Boyer P, Pascal-Mousselard H, Saillant G (2006) Wedge osteotomy for treating post-traumatic kyphosis at thoracolumbar and lumbar levels. J Spinal Disord Tech 19:487–494
43. Lehmer SM, Keppler L, Biscup RS, Enker P, Miller SD, Steffee AD (1994) Posterior transvertebral osteotomy for adult thoracolumbar kyphosis. Spine 19:2060–2066
44. Mummaneni PV, Dhall SS, Ondra SL, Mummaneni VP, Berven S (2008) Pedicle substraction osteotomy. Neurosurgery 63:A171–A176
45. Stinchfield T, Vadapalli S, Pennington Z, Sivagnanam R, Prevost J, Schroeder G, Sciubba DM (2019) Improvement in vertebral endplate engagement following anterior column reconstruction using a novel expandable cage with self-adjusting, multiaxial end cap. J Clin Neurosci 67:249–254
46. Schwab F, Blondel B, Chay E et al (2014) The comprehensive anatomical spinal osteotomy classification. Neurosurgery 74:112–120
47. Pennington Z, Ehresman J, Feghali J, Schilling A, Hersh A, Hung B, Lubelski D, Sciubba DM (2021) A clinical calculator for predicting intraoperative blood loss and transfusion risk in spine tumor patients. Spine J 21:302–311

Chapter 5
Pathologic Burst Fracture and De Novo Scoliosis from Pathological Burst Fractures

Zach Pennington, Elie Massaad, and John H. Shin

Introduction

The bony spine is a common site of metastatic spread in patients with solid tumors, with a reported prevalence of 40–70% of patients in older cadaveric series [1, 2] and 16% of patients in newer cohort studies [3]. While most patients are asymptomatic, patient can become symptomatic from progressive tumor involvement leading to: (1) epidural disease compression of the neural elements, (2) distortion of the periosteum and alterations in the microenvironment around sensory neurons innervating the periosteum, and (3) mechanical destabilization of the tumor-infiltrated element. For those with progressive symptoms, there are potentially multiple options depending upon the nature of the patient's clinical complaints. For those with persistent, oncologic-type pain, radiotherapy can be an effective option [2, 4–6]. However, with increased tumor involvement of the vertebral body, there is often mechanical axial pain—pain that worsens when the spinal column is subjected to loading. These patients may benefit from undergoing a stabilization procedure, which may be a percutaneous cement augmentation in the case of mild instability, or an instrumented fusion in the case of gross instability [2, 7].

Z. Pennington (✉)
Department of Neurologic Surgery, Mayo Clinic, Rochester, MN, USA
e-mail: pennington.zachary@mayo.edu

E. Massaad
Department of Neurosurgery, Massachusetts General Hospital, Harvard Medical School, Boston, MA, USA

J. H. Shin
Department of Neurosurgery, University of Pennsylvania/Penn Spine Center, Philadelphia, PA, USA
e-mail: shin.john@mgh.harvard.edu

D. M. Sciubba (ed.), *Spinal Tumor Associated Deformity*,
https://doi.org/10.1007/978-3-031-87939-5_5

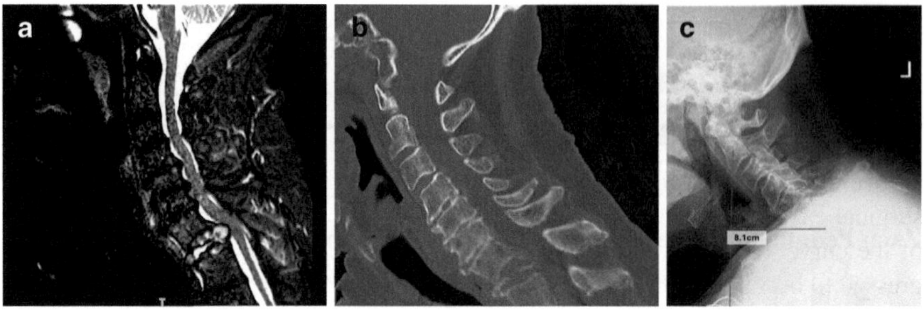

Fig. 5.1 Illustration of deformity following pathologic fracture. Patient with a known history of metastatic cancer and complaints of mechanical neck pain worsened with upright posture. (**a**) MR demonstrated a pathologic T1 burst fracture with significant retropulsion causing cord compression. (**b**) CT demonstrated near-complete collapse of the anterior and middle columns and (**c**) upright radiographs showed

With continued progression of the tumor-involved vertebral body, there can be vertebral body fracture with resultant height loss. Most common are anterior column structural failures, resulting in a compression fracture with vertebral body wedging. However, with co-occurrence of both anterior and middle column collapse, patients develop a burst fracture, which can be associated with greater pain and instability. Where the vertebral body collapse is asymmetric, patients can develop de novo deformity, which can manifest as de novo scoliosis if the asymmetry is with respect to the sagittal plane. The overarching aims of treatment in metastatic spine disease are palliation—interventions seek to preserve neurological function and restore instability caused by oncologic vertebral destruction [8]. In the case of pathologic fracture with deformity (Fig. 5.1), this intervention may include surgical correction of the deformity. Such interventions are often highly morbid though and are likely best reserved for patients with minimal disseminated disease and good overall functional status [2, 9]. Nevertheless, successful correction of pathologic fracture-associated deformity relies upon appreciation of standard principles for assessing adult degenerative scoliosis, an understanding of the underlying tumor biology and its effect on the adjacent bones, and the relative frailty of the patient.

Biomechanics of Burst Fracture in Metastatic Spine Tumor

There are multiple proposed mechanisms for metastatic spread to the spine, including direct extension, venous hematogenous spread, and arterial hematogenous spread [10]. The most common site for tumor spread is the vertebral body, likely because it is relatively well vascularized and is in direct contact with the valve Batson's venous plexus [1]. Once seeded, the tumor mass begin to grow with resultant destruction of the surrounding cancellous bone.

Multiple cadaveric and finite element analyses have been conducted examining the mechanisms and extent to which progressive tumor infiltration results in spinal column destabilization [11–15]. In one early study by Whealan et al. [16] examined 34 fresh-frozen cadaveric spines divided into three motion segment preparations (eighteen T7-T9 and sixteen L1–3), which were modified with lytic lesions occupying 30% of the vertebral body cross sectional area. They noted that posteriorly located lesions were far better able to tolerate axial compression than vertebrae with lateral or anteriorly positioned defects. However, underlying bone quality appeared to be the most significant predictor of failure load.

Whyne and colleagues [12] used a finite element analysis of the L1 vertebrae to evaluate the impact of tumor size, trabecular bone density, and tumor location on axial load tolerance. They noted that tumor size had the greatest effect on load-bearing capacity, with a tumor occupying 45% of the body leading to a 14-fold increase in vertebral body collapse (as measured by vertebral bulge with axial compression). Low trabecular bone density also caused a significant decrease in load-bearing capacity, as did pedicular involvement. The former has been corroborated by other groups, such as Salvatore et al. [17], who demonstrated that increasing tumor size and poorer baseline bone density work synergistically so that increasing tumor size has a greater effect on decreasing load-bearing capacity in osteoporotic vertebrae.

Whyne et al. [11] employed the same model previously described to demonstrate that in vertebra with greater underlying bone mineral density, fracture occurrence generally followed endplate injury. By contrast, in patients with poor bone mineral density (e.g., osteoporotic patients), burst fracture occurred prior to endplate violation. Such findings may have utility when risk stratifying patients with tumor-affected vertebrae; patients with otherwise good underlying bone mineral density (e.g., younger patients) are likely to be at low risk for burst fracture if imaging demonstrates the endplates of the affected body to be intact. However, they may still be at high risk for compression fracture based on the findings of Taneichi et al., who found 35–40% vertebral body involvement was predictive of impending vertebral body collapse [18].

In another finite element analysis, Tschirhart and colleagues [15] evaluated the relative impact of cortical bone involvement and cephalocaudal location of the affected vertebrae. They noted that central tumor location was associated with the largest increased risk of pathologic burst fracture, whereas transcortical location was associated with decreased risk, with a direct negative correlation of −0.948 between the cross-sectional area of the cortex disruption and burst fracture risk. They also noted that axial loading led to increase in vertebral body bulging at more cephalad segments, suggesting upper thoracic vertebrae are at elevated risk of pathologic burst fracture versus lower levels in the thoracolumbar spine, which may be more prone to compression fractures. The authors also noted that an increased kyphotic angle may predispose the vertebra to fail with a compression as compared to burst morphology. In a contemporaneous analysis using only L1 vertebral body models, the same group [19] demonstrated that tumor ablation (≈30%) followed by injection of a minimum 1–2 mL of polymethylmethacrylate (PMMA) bone cement offers stabilization approaching that expected for an uninvolved vertebra. However, they note that larger PMMA volumes are likely merited for larger tumor sizes following ablation. Posterior localization of the PMMA within the posterior body can help to minimize posterior wall bulging and risk of burst fracture [20]. The authors corroborated these findings in additional finite element [20] and cadaver work [21].

Animal work [22] has demonstrated that lytic tumor invasion is associated with trabecular microdamage. Such damaged regions experience significantly higher stresses than normal vertebra when subjected to the same axial loading. They are closer to their inherent bulk yield, providing a biomechanical underpinning for why these segments are most apt to fail with loading. The progressive microscopic damage accumulated under repeated loading ultimately manifests as a sudden macroscopic fracture when stresses exceed bone strength. In the context of pathologic burst fractures, this suggests a model wherein failure will occur first at the level of the largest lytic lesion. Therefore deformity apex should occur at the most tumor-involved level for lytic lesion, though it may occur at the adjacent vertebra for blastic lesions [23]. Furthermore, eccentric tumor localization allows for asymmetric collapse, as compressive strain distribution is asymmetric in tumor affected vertebrae [24, 25]. Palanca et al. [25] demonstrated this impact of intravertebral tumor location on the pattern of deformation in a strain analysis using 35 cadaveric vertebra from patients with spinal metastases. Stressing of the vertebra to failure showed failure occurred first at the endplate in levels with lytic and mixed tumors [23].

More recently Stadelmann et al. [26] employed microCT (μCT) to correlate microarchitectural and biomechanical properties in 57 cadaveric vertebral bodies with mixed, blastic, or lytic metastases. They noted that blastic lesions required significantly lower amounts of force to undergo plastic deformation in microindentation testing as compared to lytic lesions or non-involved bone, despite having a higher overall bone volume. Micro CT (μCT) of the blastic regions showed thickened, abnormal trabeculae with a preferred orientation, suggesting that the blastic regions, while radiographically "denser," actually have poorer quality bone [27, 28]. Yet macroscopically, their axial compressive strength was greater than that demonstrated by vertebra with lytic or mixed type metastases [26]. By contrast, lytic lesions did not differ appreciably from uninvolved bone with regard to microindentation testing [26]. However, axial compressive strength of vertebrae involved by lytic lesions was appreciably decreased, leading to the conclusion that the impaired load-bearing properties of involved vertebrae is due to rarefaction of the trabecular network in the tumor-involved region. Such findings provide a biomechanical basis for the asymmetric collapse that can result in coronal deformity. Additionally, for corrective surgery, it suggests that pedicle screws may be able to have reasonable purchase in involved segments so long as the screw tract does not include the tumor-affected region. By contrast, given that blastic lesions demonstrated properties more similar to poorly developed cortical bone, they may provide some screw purchase. However, pullout strength is inevitably inferior to that of uninvolved bone and a cortical-pitch screw may be advisable to maximize the purchase of that screw. Cement augmentation ultimately offers the best purchase [29] though it may not be an option for fractured levels as a discontiguous posterior wall can allow for cement leakage into the canal.

Assessment and Preoperative Management

Clinical Assessment

As in any patient presenting with a new spinal mass, patients presenting with pathologic burst fracture and associated deformity require both a thorough clinical and radiographic evaluation. Clinical evaluation should begin with a throughout neurological exam including sensorimotor testing of the upper and lower extremities. Burst fractures are defined by anterior and posterior cortical fracture. Progressive height loss following the fracture can be associated with spinal canal narrowing and neural element compression. Focal deficits on exam and upper motor neuron signs (e.g., Babinski reflex, hyperreflexia, and increased tone) are concerning signs for neural element compression, including metastatic epidural spinal cord compression (MESCC). MESCC merits urgent intervention [2], with groups such as Quraishi et al. [30], Fürstenberg et al. [31], and Chaichana et al. [32] demonstrating that decompression within 48 h of symptom onset is associated with superior long-term neurological outcomes. However, patients need not undergo correction of any associated deformity at the time of decompression, as the goals of the latter are to relieve neural element decompression. Patients with concomitant deformity may be too frail for deformity correction and require optimization prior to considering a deformity correction. Neurological examination should also include assessment for stool or urinary retention. Patients presenting with painful metastases can report concern for incontinence which may be true incontinence or simply increased urgency and inability to make it to the bathroom on time due to mechanical pain with ambulation. To aid in evaluation, patient's reporting symptoms of incontinence should undergo bladder scanning to look for a post-void residual and testing of voluntary rectal tone. Work from the degenerative cauda equina literature [33] suggests that a post-void residual of >200 cc has a high sensitivity (67–88%). A threshold of >500 cc has a marginally higher specificity (67 vs 63%) but a substantially lower sensitivity. Similar work [34] studying the diagnostic accuracy of digital rectal examination shows it to have relatively low sensitivity (23–53%), though testing of voluntary anal squeeze has a higher specificity (up to 96%). Consequently, patients with post-void residuals and a positive anal squeeze are unlikely to have cauda equina and can likely have intervention deferred pending additional workup.

In addition to a sensorimotor exam, patients should be asked about associated pain. Pain should be characterized as mechanical—worse with axial loading/upright posture—or nonmechanical (oncologic). Mechanical pain can indicate underlying instability and such patients can derive significant benefit from surgical stabilization, even in the context of poor expected prognosis [35]. However, such stabilization procedures may seek only to stabilize the affected segment in frail patients or those with poor associated prognoses. More aggressive surgical correction (i.e., correction of significant associated deformity) should likely be relegated to patients with good prognoses and well-controlled disease given the expected healing time for such invasive procedures.

To this end, patients without neurologic concerns requiring urgent decompression should additionally undergo oncologic staging to assess their global disease burden and expected prognoses. Those with newly diagnosed lesions without a known oncologic history should undergo biopsy of the mass if their disease is unifocal to rule out the possibility of a primary vertebral column tumor, which would benefit from *en bloc* resection.

Radiographic Assessment

Radiographic workup for patients with newly diagnosed spinal lesions with associated deformity should include MR, CT, and upright scoliosis films. Upright scoliosis films allow for measurement of the deformity magnitude in the sagittal and coronal planes and allow for characterization of the curve's focality for instrumentation level selection. For those with scoliosis in which deformity correction is being considered, lateral bending films or supine scoliosis films with a bolster can be considered to evaluate for the rigidity of deformity, with Lenke and colleagues having defined <30% curve correction as signifying a stiff deformity [36]. Both supine and lateral bending films have been found to be highly predictive of postoperative Cobb angles in patients undergoing surgery for adult idiopathic scoliosis [37]. An additional benefit of bending films is that they can help to identify the degree to which a patient's coronal imbalance is driven by their primary curve—likely that containing the pathologic fracture in the oncologic population—or by an accompanying fractional curve found at the lumbosacral junction. Coronal imbalance toward the concavity of the fractional curve suggests that the fractional curve is driving the deformity and must be included in the construct, whereas coronal imbalance shifted toward the convexity of the fractional curve suggests it is compensatory [38]. Based on the degenerative literature, it is thought that curves with Cobb angles >30°, >6 mm lateral listhesis, apical rotation greater than 2 [39], or an intercrest line passing through L5 have elevated risk of progression [40, 41]. Here grade 2 is defined by the system of Nash and Moe as the pedicular shadow of the curve concavity having disappeared on posterior-anterior standing radiographs. This corresponds to a rotation of 20–35° in the upper thoracic spine (T2–5), 15–30° in the mid-thoracic spine (T7–10), and 20–35° in the lumbar spine [39].

MR is useful for evaluating the extent of epidural disease and identifying point of neural element compression (oncologic or degenerative) that should be addressed during the operation to correct any underlying deformity. Additionally, for mixed quality lesion, MR may allow for better visualization of the extent of vertebral body involvement. T1-weighted sequences show decreased marrow signal at the fracture site indicating bone edema. T2-weighted and STIR sequences show hyperintense marrow signal at the fractured vertebra as well as adjacent levels, indicating bone edema and hyperemia [42]. The addition of contrast-enhanced sequences is generally recommended, though tumors often show heterogeneous enhancement due to intratumoral necrosis. Though apparent areal bone mineral density evaluated with Hounsfield units likely offers a better assessment of underlying bone quality [43, 44], MR can inform the surgeon of the degree of pedicular and vertebral body involvement. Involved pedicles or levels with significant vertebral body involvement are unlikely to offer good purchase for pedicle screw instrumentation and a priori knowledge of said tumor involvement can help guide level selection.

Computed tomography is also invaluable for preoperative assessment. As mentioned, it allows for assessment of underlying bone quality and provides information about the quality of the bone metastasis, specifically whether it is osteoblastic, osteolytic, or mixed quality. The previously described biomechanical literature has demonstrated that osteolytic lesions have relatively normal trabecular structure but differ from unaffected bone in that there is trabecular rarefaction or greater intertrabecular spacing [26]. Instrumentation at these levels should likely employ cancellous-pitch screws and, if possible, cement augmentation, though such augmentation may displace stresses to the adjacent level. Osteoblastic lesions, by contrast, appear to be histologically more similar to poorly developed cortical bone [26]. Again, cement augmentation significantly improves screw pullout strength [45–47], though maximal gains appear to be achieved with injection of ≈3 mL per pedicle in the lumbar spine [29, 46]. We employed ≈1.5 mL per pedicle in thoracic vertebrae. However, the preoperative CT should be carefully reviewed to identify compromise of the posterior vertebral body cortex (as in a burst fracture), as this is generally considered a contraindication for cement augmentation owing to the risk of cement leakage into the spinal canal. Employing a kyphoplasty technique to create a cavity for cement deposit may allow for cement augmentation and instrumentation of the fractured level; however, this merits thorough discussion with the patient and should only be considered by surgeons with extensive experience with this technique. When employed though, the kyphoplast-style screw augmentation technique offers significantly better pullout properties relative to transpedicular augmentation alone.

In addition to allowing for characterization of bony erosion secondary to tumor involvement and assessment of underlying bone quality, CT is additionally useful to help characterize the rigidity of any associated deformity. While the present chapter focuses on de novo scoliosis following burst fracture, many patients will have a concomitant degenerative de novo scoliosis, as it occurs in approximately 6% of all adults over age 50 [48]. Such degenerative deformity is often characterized by asymmetric disc space collapse [49], facet hypertrophy and anklyosis, and increased ligamentous laxity [40]. Patient with such deformity and a concurrent pathologic burst fracture will likely can have coronal deformity due to both the asymmetric disk space collapse (degenerative process) and asymmetric vertebral body collapse (oncologic-driven deformity). Noting the degree to which the bone-driven and discogenic processes are driving the deformity is valuable for development of the surgical plan. Flexible discogenic deformity can often be corrected with posterior-only osteomies and interbody placement, whereas deformity due to vertebral body collapse will likely require three-column osteotomies and/or corpectomy to restore anterior column height. Last, CT is invaluable for characterizing potential instability of tumor involved vertebra, as it allows for application of the Spinal Instability Neoplastic Score (SINS), which assigns scores based on the degree of posterolateral element involvement, presence and quality of associated pain, lesion quality (lytic/blastic/mixed), extent of vertebral body involvement, cephalocaudal level, and presence of concurrent deformity [50].

Operative Intervention

Percutaneous cement augmentation is the workhorse for the management of most pathologic fracture (see Chap. 7), and there is level 1 evidence that kyphoplasty improves both short- and long-term pain control from pathologic, tumor-related fractures [51]. However, burst fracture (i.e., posterior vertebral body cortical compromise) is a contraindication at many centers. Additionally, where there is concomitant posterolateral involvement and potential instability, patients often see greater improvement with instrumented stabilization [7].

Literature specific to the correction of deformity in the context of pathologic burst fracture is sparse. Consequently, the techniques employed and radiographic goals of deformity correction in this population largely borrow from what is known in the degenerative literature, where it is known that greater deformity correction is in general associated with greater improvements in patient-reported quality-of-life outcomes [52]. Conservatively, curves meriting surgical correction are those at high risk for progression, i.e., those with a coronal Cobb >30° and/or ≥ 6 mm of lateral listhesis. Additionally, patients with serial imaging showing >10° of curve progression or > 3 mm of progressive subluxation are also reasonable surgical candidates [36]. The goals of surgical correction are to reduce lumbopelvic mismatch (lumbar lordosis—pelvic incidence) to less than 10°, pelvic tilt to less than 25°, sagittal vertical axis to less than 5 cm, major curve coronal cobb to less than 30°, and coronal imbalance to less than 3 cm.

Our exact approach varies by the level of the curve apex. However, as recommended by Lenke and colleagues [36] the upper instrumented vertebra (UIV) should be a neutral and stable vertebra, that is a vertebra without significant rotation that is bisected by the central sacral vertical line. However, it is recommended that the UIV not be placed in the thoracic apex (T5/6-T10) and so a more cephalad UIV should be selected if the first stable and neutral vertebra is situated within the region of the apex. This is done to reduce the risk of proximal junctional failure. Selection of the lowest instrumented vertebra (LIV) is variable, but it is again recommended that the level be a neutral and stable vertebra. For scoliosis with lumbar apices, our routine strategy is to extend the fusion distally to the pelvis so as to avoid the risk of distal junctional failure. This in our experience seems to be at higher risk of occurrence in the metastatic spine population owing to the poor bone quality, likely as a combination of age (osteoporosis), tumor burden, and prior chemoradiation. For thoracic curves, an LIV in the lumbar spine can be considered so as to spare additional motion segments [38]. However, if there is a structural fractional curve (i.e., one with the concavity ipsilateral to the patient's trunk shift), the construct should extend caudally into the sacrum/pelvis so as to include the structural curve.

For curves with the pathologic fracture in the thoracic spine, we feel an all-posterior approach can effectively treat the deformity. If there is greater than 50% vertebral body height loss, our strategy is to perform a corpectomy and reconstruct the anterior column with a static or expandable titanium cage. For lumbar lesions, an all-posterior approach can also work given the significant improvement in expandable devices [53] and ability to perform a piecemeal versus *en bloc* corpectomy of the pathologic segment. However, for patients with concurrent sagittal imbalance with multilevel disc space collapse, we consider a combined anterior–posterior approach, assuming the patient has no significant abdominal surgery history and can tolerate the morbidity of a combined procedure. The anterior approach allows for the corpectomy to be performed with relatively minimal risk of neurologic injury while also allowing for concomitant multilevel ALIF to restore sagittal and coronal imbalance driven by disc space collapse. For all approaches, our general preference is to employ cement-augmented pedicle screw constructs due to the superior fatigue and pullout strength of cement augmented screw constructs. We also frequently employ the assistance of plastic surgery for wound closure given the possibility these patients may require future chemoradiation and prior work has suggested plastic surgery assistance can help mitigate some of the increased risk of wound complications seen in this population [54, 55]. This is an approach also favored by many spinal oncologists globally [56]. Last, we also refer patients undergoing these deformity operations for evaluation by an endocrinologist for initiation of antiresorptive therapy (i.e., denosumab, bisphosphonates), if not already initiated by their primary oncology team. These therapies help to reduce the risk of further pathologic fracture and may help reduce postoperative mechanical complications (e.g., proximal junctional kyphosis, hardware pullout, or cut out) by maintaining underlying bone quality [57–62]. Anabolic therapies are generally considered to be contraindicated in this patient population owing to the theoretical increased oncologic risk.

Conclusions

The bony spine is a common site of metastatic disease spread. With progressive tumor involvement, the vertebral body can lose significant biomechanical stability and suffer a burst fracture. With this fracture there can be resultant deformity, which in the case of coronally asymmetric collapse results in scoliosis. While not most patients are not candidates for aggressive deformity correction, those with good prognoses and well-controlled disease can be considered for surgical correction.

Unlike degenerative scoliosis correction, bony resection is almost invariably required as the deformity is secondary to anterior and middle column collapse. We prefer a posterior-only approach, where possible, as it minimizes morbidity relative to circumferential fusion; however, an adjunct anterior approach may be necessary for lumbar lesions with significant collapse. Cement augmentation is highly valuable to improve pedicle screw purchase and reduce the risk of hardware failure. Consideration should also be made to initiate antiresorptive therapy to improve postoperative fusion outcomes and reduce the risks of mechanical complications.

References

1. Pennington Z, Goodwin ML, Westbroek EM, Cottrill E, Ahmed AK, Sciubba DM (2019) Lactate and cancer: spinal metastases and potential therapeutic targets (part 2). Ann Transl Med 7:221
2. Sciubba DM, Pennington Z, Colman MW et al (2021) Spinal metastases 2021: a review of the current state of the art and future directions. Spine J 21:1414–1429
3. Van den Brande R, Cornips MJ et al (2022) Epidemiology of spinal metastases, metastatic epidural spinal cord compression and pathologic vertebral compression fractures in patients with solid tumors: a systematic review. J Bone Oncol 35:100446
4. Pennington Z, Ehresman J, Szerlip NJ, Sciubba DM (2021) Hybrid therapy for metastatic disease. Clin Spine Surg 34:369–376
5. Rothrock R, Pennington Z, Ehresman J, Bilsky MH, Barzilai O, Szerlip NJ, Sciubba DM (2020) Hybrid therapy for spinal metastases. Neurosurg Clin N Am 31:191–200
6. Sahgal A, Myrehaug SD, Siva S et al (2021) Stereotactic body radiotherapy versus conventional external beam radiotherapy in patients with painful spinal metastases: an open-label, multicentre, randomised, controlled, phase 2/3 trial. Lancet Oncol 22:1023–1033
7. Hussain I, Barzilai O, Reiner AS, DiStefano N, McLaughlin L, Ogilvie S, Bilsky M, Laufer I (2018) Patient-reported outcomes after surgical stabilization of spinal tumors: symptom-based validation of the spinal instability neoplastic score (SINS) and surgery. Spine J 18:261–267
8. Kanda Y, Kakutani K, Sakai Y et al (2021) Surgical outcomes and risk factors for poor outcomes in patients with cervical spine metastasis: a prospective study. J Orthop Surg Res 16:423
9. Porras JL, Pennington Z, Hung B, Hersh A, Schilling A, Goodwin CR, Sciubba DM (2021) Radiotherapy and surgical advances in the treatment of metastatic spine tumors: a narrative review. World Neurosurg 151:147–154
10. Shah LM, Salzman KL (2011) Imaging of spinal metastatic disease. Int J Surg Oncol 2011:1–12
11. Whyne CM, Hu SS, Lotz JC (2003) Biomechanically derived guideline equations for burst fracture risk prediction in the metastatically involved spine. J Spinal Disord Tech 16:180–185
12. Whyne CM, Hu SS, Lotz JC (2003) Burst fracture in the metastatically involved spine: development, validation, and parametric analysis of a three-dimensional poroelastic finite-element model. Spine 28:652–660
13. Alkalay RN, Harrigan TP (2016) Mechanical assessment of the effects of metastatic lytic defect on the structural response of human thoracolumbar spine. J Orthop Res 34:1808–1819
14. Tschirhart CE, Nagpurkar A, Whyne CM (2004) Effects of tumor location, shape and surface serration on burst fracture risk in the metastatic spine. J Biomech 37:653–660
15. Tschirhart CE, Finkelstein JA, Whyne CM (2007) Biomechanics of vertebral level, geometry, and transcortical tumors in the metastatic spine. J Biomech 40:46–54
16. Whealan KM, Kwak SD, Tedrow JR, Inoue K, Snyder BD (2000) Noninvasive imaging predicts failure load of the spine with simulated Osteolytic defects*†. J Bone Joint Surg Am 82:1240–1251

17. Salvatore G, Berton A, Giambini H, Ciuffreda M, Florio P, Longo UG, Denaro V, Thoreson A, An K-N (2018) Biomechanical effects of metastasis in the osteoporotic lumbar spine: a finite element analysis. BMC Musculoskelet Disord 19:38
18. Taneichi H, Kaneda K, Takeda N, Abumi K, Satoh S (1997) Risk factors and probability of vertebral body collapse in metastases of the thoracic and lumbar spine. Spine 22:239–245
19. Tschirhart CE, Finkelstein JA, Whyne CM (2006) Optimization of tumor volume reduction and cement augmentation in percutaneous vertebroplasty for prophylactic treatment of spinal metastases. J Spinal Disord Tech 19:584–590
20. Tschirhart CE, Roth SE, Whyne CM (2005) Biomechanical assessment of stability in the metastatic spine following percutaneous vertebroplasty: effects of cement distribution patterns and volume. J Biomech 38:1582–1590
21. Ahn H, Mousavi P, Roth S, Reidy D, Finkelstein J, Whyne C (2006) Stability of the metastatic spine pre and post vertebroplasty. J Spinal Disord Tech 19:178–182
22. Choudhari C, Chan K, Akens MK, Whyne CM (2016) μFE models can represent microdamaged regions of healthy and metastatically involved whole vertebrae identified through histology and contrast enhanced μCT imaging. J Biomech 49:1103–1110
23. Palanca M, Cavazzoni G, Dall'Ara E (2023) The role of bone metastases on the mechanical competence of human vertebrae. Bone 173:116814
24. Costa MC, Eltes PE, Lazary A, Varga PP, Viceconti M, Dall'Ara E (2019) Biomechanical assessment of vertebrae with lytic metastases with subject-specific finite element models. J Mech Behav Biomed Mater 98:268–290
25. Palanca M, Barbanti-Bròdano G, Marras D, Marciante M, Serra M, Gasbarrini A, Dall'Ara E, Cristofolini L (2021) Type, size, and position of metastatic lesions explain the deformation of the vertebrae under complex loading conditions. Bone 151:116028
26. Stadelmann MA, Schenk DE, Maquer G, Lenherr C, Buck FM, Bosshardt DD, Hoppe S, Theumann N, Alkalay RN, Zysset PK (2020) Conventional finite element models estimate the strength of metastatic human vertebrae despite alterations of the bone's tissue and structure. Bone 141:115598
27. Nazarian A, von Stechow D, Zurakowski D, Müller R, Snyder BD (2008) Bone volume fraction explains the variation in strength and stiffness of cancellous bone affected by metastatic cancer and osteoporosis. Calcif Tissue Int 83:368–379
28. Tamada T, Sone T, Jo Y, Imai S, Kajihara Y, Fukunaga M (2005) Three-dimensional trabecular bone architecture of the lumbar spine in bone metastasis from prostate cancer: comparison with degenerative sclerosis. Skeletal Radiol 34:149–155
29. Ehresman J, Pennington Z, Elsamadicy AA et al (2021) Fenestrated pedicle screws for thoracolumbar instrumentation in patients with poor bone quality: case series and systematic review of the literature. Clin Neurol Neurosurg 206:106675
30. Quraishi NA, Rajagopal TS, Manoharan SR, Elsayed S, Edwards KL, Boszczyk BM (2013) Effect of timing of surgery on neurological outcome and survival in metastatic spinal cord compression. Eur Spine J 22:1383–1388
31. Fürstenberg CH, Wiedenhöfer B, Gerner HJ, Putz C (2009) The effect of early surgical treatment on recovery in patients with metastatic compression of the spinal cord. J Bone Joint Surg Br 91:240–244
32. Chaichana KL, Woodworth GF, Sciubba DM, McGirt MJ, Witham TJ, Bydon A, Wolinsky JP, Gokaslan Z (2008) Predictors of ambulatory function after decompressive surgery for metastatic epidural spinal cord compression. Neurosurgery 62:683–692
33. Boktor J, Wong F, Joseph VM, Alshahwani A, Banerjee P, Morris K, Lewis PM, Ahuja S (2023) Predictive value of post-void residual volume as an adjunctive tool in the clinical evaluation of cauda equina syndrome. Bone Joint J 105:487–495
34. Tabrah J, Wilson N, Phillips D, Böhning D (2022) Can digital rectal examination be used to detect cauda equina compression in people presenting with acute cauda equina syndrome? A systematic review and meta-analysis of diagnostic test accuracy studies. Musculoskelet Sci Pract 58:102523

35. Dea N, Versteeg AL, Sahgal A et al (2020) Metastatic spine disease: should patients with short life expectancy be denied surgical care? An international retrospective cohort study. Neurosurgery 87:303–311
36. Silva FE, Lenke LG (2010) Adult degenerative scoliosis: evaluation and management. Neurosurg Focus 28:E1
37. Chan CYW, Tan YWE, Chandren JR, Chandirasegaran S, Chung WH, Chiu CK, Kwan MK (2024) Prediction of postoperative curve correction based on the supine radiographs for adult idiopathic scoliosis patients. Spine J 24:1272–1281
38. Ransom SC, Pennington Z, Brown NJ et al (2024) Assessing the fractional curve for proper management of adult degenerative scoliosis. Neurospine 21:458–473
39. Nash CL, Moe JH (1969) A study of vertebral rotation. J Bone Joint Surg Am 51:223–229
40. Ailon T, Smith JS, Shaffrey CI, Lenke LG, Brodke D, Harrop JS, Fehlings M, Ames CP (2015) Degenerative spinal deformity. Neurosurgery 77:S75–S91
41. Pritchett JW, Bortel DT (1993) Degenerative symptomatic lumbar scoliosis. Spine 18:700–703
42. Shih TT-F, Huang K-M, Li Y-W (1999) Solitary vertebral collapse: distinction between benign and malignant causes using MR patterns. J Magn Reson Imaging 9:635–642
43. Pennington Z, Ehresman J, Lubelski D, Cottrill E, Schilling A, Ahmed AK, Feghali J, Witham TF, Sciubba DM (2021) Assessing underlying bone quality in spine surgery patients: a narrative review of dual-energy X-ray absorptiometry (DXA) and alternatives. Spine J 21:321–331
44. Pennington Z, Mikula AL, Lakomkin N et al (2023) Comparison of Hounsfield units and vertebral bone quality score for the prediction of time to pathologic fracture in mobile spine metastases treated with radiotherapy. J Neurosurg Spine 40:19–27
45. Burval DJ, McLain RF, Milks R, Inceoglu S (2007) Primary pedicle screw augmentation in osteoporotic lumbar vertebrae: biomechanical analysis of pedicle fixation strength. Spine 32:1077–1083
46. Fölsch C, Goost H, Figiel J, Paletta JRJ, Schultz W, Lakemeier S (2012) Correlation of pull-out strength of cement-augmented pedicle screws with CT-volumetric measurement of cement. Biomed Tech Eng 57:473–480
47. Elder BD, Lo S-FL, Holmes C, Goodwin CR, Kosztowski TA, Lina IA, Locke JE, Witham TF (2015) The biomechanics of pedicle screw augmentation with cement. Spine J 15:1432–1445
48. Diebo BG, Shah NV, Boachie-Adjei O, Zhu F, Rothenfluh DA, Paulino CB, Schwab FJ, Lafage V (2019) Adult spinal deformity. Lancet 394:160–172
49. Bao H, Zhu F, Liu Z, Zhu Z, He S, Ding Y, Qiu Y (2014) Coronal curvature and spinal imbalance in degenerative lumbar scoliosis. Spine 39:E1441–E1447
50. Fisher CG, DiPaola CP, Ryken TC et al (2010) A novel classification system for spinal instability in neoplastic disease: an evidence-based approach and expert consensus from the spine oncology study group. Spine 35:E1221–E1229
51. Berenson J, Pflugmacher R, Jarzem P, Zonder J, Schechtman K, Tillman JB, Bastian L, Ashraf T, Vrionis F (2011) Balloon kyphoplasty versus non-surgical fracture management for treatment of painful vertebral body compression fractures in patients with cancer: a multicentre, randomised controlled trial. Lancet Oncol 12:225–235
52. Cawley DT, Takemoto M, Boissiere L et al (2021) The impact of corrective surgery on health-related quality of life subclasses in adult scoliosis: will degree of correction prognosticate degree of improvement? Eur Spine J 30:2033–2039
53. Stinchfield T, Vadapalli S, Pennington Z, Sivagnanam R, Prevost J, Schroeder G, Sciubba DM (2019) Improvement in vertebral endplate engagement following anterior column reconstruction using a novel expandable cage with self-adjusting, multiaxial end cap. J Clin Neurosci 67:249–254
54. Hersh AM, Pennington Z, Schilling AT et al (2021) Plastic surgery wound closure following resection of spinal metastases. Clin Neurol Neurosurg 207:106800
55. Leary OP, Liu DD, Boyajian MK et al (2020) Complex wound closure by plastic surgery following resection of spinal neoplasms minimizes postoperative wound complications in high-risk patients. J Neurosurg Spine 33:77–86

56. Pennington Z, Porras JL, Larry Lo S-F, Sciubba DM (2023) International variability in spinal metastasis treatment: a survey of the AO spine community. Glob Spine J 13:1622–1634
57. Barrionuevo P, Kapoor E, Asi N et al (2019) Efficacy of pharmacological therapies for the prevention of fractures in postmenopausal women: a network meta-analysis. J Clin Endocrinol Metab 104:1623–1630
58. Harris ST, Watts NB, Genant HK et al (1999) Effects of risedronate treatment on vertebral and nonvertebral fractures in women with postmenopausal osteoporosis: a randomized controlled trial. Vertebral efficacy with Risedronate therapy (VERT) study group. JAMA 282:1344–1352
59. Reginster J-Y, Minne HW, Sorensen OH et al (2000) Randomized trial of the effects of risedronate on vertebral fractures in women with established postmenopausal osteoporosis. Osteoporos Int 11:83–91
60. Chesnut CH, Skag A, Christiansen C et al (2004) Effects of oral ibandronate administered daily or intermittently on fracture risk in postmenopausal osteoporosis. J Bone Miner Res 19:1241–1249
61. McClung MR, Zanchetta JR, Høiseth A et al (2013) Denosumab densitometric changes assessed by quantitative computed tomography at the spine and hip in postmenopausal women with osteoporosis. J Clin Densitom 16:250–256
62. Hans D, McDermott M, Huang S, Kim M, Shevroja E, McClung M (2023) Long-term effect of denosumab on bone microarchitecture as assessed by tissue thickness–adjusted trabecular bone score in postmenopausal women with osteoporosis: results from FREEDOM and its open-label extension. Osteoporos Int 34:1075–1084

Chapter 6
De novo Spondylolisthesis from Pathological Posterior Element Disruption

Gabrielle Santangelo, Thomas A. Pieters, Zach Pennington, and Sheng-Fu Larry Lo

Overview of Spondylolisthesis: Classification and Relationship to Global Alignment

Spondylolisthesis—derived from the Greek, *spondylos* (vertebrae) and *olisthesis* (to slip)—was first described in 1782 by an obstetrician, Herbiniaux. It is characterized by the translation of one vertebra over another, usually with the cephalad level anteriorly translated over the caudal level. Spondylolisthesis was first classified in 1932 by Meyerding [1] who identified four grades based on the degree of translation—Grade I (0–25% slip), Grade II (2%–50%), Grade III (50–75%), and Grade IV (75–100%). Spondyloptosis—a slip greater than 100%—was later defined as grade V. Since then, other classification systems have been proposed with that of Wiltse et al. [2] also being popular. The Wiltse system attempts to classify spondylolisthesis into the following five types based on presumed etiology: type I—dysplastic/congenital; type II—isthmic, type III—degenerative, type IV—traumatic, and type V—neoplastic. Type II is further subdivided into type IIA (characterized by pars lysis), type IIB (pars elongation), and type IIC (acute pars fracture). Marchetti and

G. Santangelo
Department of Neurosurgery, University of Rochester, Rochester, NY, USA
e-mail: gabrielle_santangelo@urmc.rochester.edu

T. A. Pieters
Department of Neurosurgery, University of Massachusetts, Worcester, MA, USA

Z. Pennington
Department of Neurologic Surgery, Mayo Clinic, Rochester, MN, USA
e-mail: pennington.zachary@mayo.edu

S.-F. L. Lo (✉)
Department of Neurosurgery, Donald and Barbara Zucker School of Medicine at Hofstra/Northwell, Great Neck, NY, USA
e-mail: larrylo@northwell.edu

D. M. Sciubba (ed.), *Spinal Tumor Associated Deformity*,
https://doi.org/10.1007/978-3-031-87939-5_6

Bartolozzi similarly proposed a classification schema based on presumed etiology, classifying lesions as acquired (traumatic, iatrogenic/post-surgical, pathologic, and degenerative) and developmental, with the latter being subdivided as low- and high-dysplastic [3, 4]. The division based on degree of lumbosacral dysplasia was used to highlight the risk of further slippage.

More recently, attention has been given to how spinopelvic alignment may influence the risk of spondylolisthesis progression [5–10]. The most well-known result of these effort is the classification schema proposed by the Spinal Deformity Study Group (SDSG), which was developed with the aim of guiding clinical and surgical management [5, 11]. The SDSG classification system groups lumbosacral spondylolisthesis into six types. Types 1–3 are low grade (<50% slip) and types 4–6 are high grade (>50% slip) based on the Meyerding classification [1]. Low-grade lesions are further subdivided based on the patient's pelvic incidence (PI)—type 1 (PI<45°), type 2 (PI 45–60°), and type 3 (PI>60°). High-grade lesions are subdivided based on spinopelvic balance. Type 4 lesions have a balanced pelvis, meaning that the combination of sacral slop (SS) and pelvic tilt (PT) places them above the threshold line published by Hresko et al. [10]. Types 5 and 6 have a retroverted pelvis (low SS, high PT), with type 5 having a balanced spine (C7 sagittal plumb line falls at or posterior to the femoral heads) and type 6 having an unbalanced spine (C7 sagittal plumb line falls anterior to the femoral heads) [9].

Other studies have begun to elucidate the relationship between high-grade spondylolisthesis and spinopelvic anatomy, with many noting high pelvic incidence may lead to progression of the slippage [5, 6, 12–15]. Labelle et al. [6] demonstrated that in patients with a spondylolisthesis, the average PI, SS, PT, and LL were significantly greater. While the high PT and high LL can predispose to increased stress at the lumbosacral junction, data are retrospective, and causality has not been established. Nevertheless, the relationship between global alignment and spondylolisthesis should be considered, particularly in the context of a de novo deformity associated with an oncologic process.

Spondylolisthesis in Spine Tumors

Etiology

As primary bone tumors are on the whole uncommon and most metastases localize to the vertebral body [16], pathologic spondylolisthesis in the setting of oncologic disease is relatively uncommon. Where it does occur, the spondylolisthesis is not due to force directly applied by the tumor, but rather due to erosion of the pedicle, facet joints, or isthmus caused by tumor expansion. With the resultant structural incompetence of the posterior elements, the cephalad vertebra can translate over the caudal level, creating a pathologic spondylolisthesis and resultant instability. Involvement of the posterior elements can occur through either localization of the tumor to the posterior elements (as may be seen in primary tumors such as osteoid osteoma), or as is generally the case for metastatic lesions, from extension of a vertebral body lesion into the posterior elements. With the destruction of the posterior elements, most importantly, the pedicles, there is a forward-shearing deformity as forces applied to the cephalad level are no longer resisted by the posterior elements; such instability requires stabilization with instrumented arthrodesis [17].

While an overall less common cause of pathologic spondylolisthesis, primary tumors show a greater propensity to originate in the posterior elements. Primary tumors with known proclivity for the posterior elements include osteochondromas [18–21], osteosarcomas [22, 23], osteoid osteomas and osteoblastoma [24, 25], aneurysmal bone cysts [26, 27], chondrosarcomas [28–32], Ewing sarcoma, and rarely giant cell tumors [33]. The potential that a pathologic spondylolisthesis is associated with a primary tumor should be suspected in young patients with no known oncologic history. Management of these lesions varies from metastases in that surgical resection can be curative and in the case of primary malignancies (i.e., chondrosarcoma, osteosarcoma), resection must be *en bloc* with negative margins to achieve cure.

Metastatic tumors are far more common overall, and management of associated spondylolisthesis should focus on stabilization and neural element decompression. Lesions are most commonly secondary to tumors of the lung, breast, prostate, and kidneys [34, 35] and hematogenous spread through the valveless Batson's plexus cited as a common mechanism for spread to the vertebral body [36–38]. From this point, lesions can directly spread to involve the pedicles and neural arch. It has been shown that metastatic tumors tend to first originate at the posterior vertebral body which increases this likelihood of spread [39]. This spread is thought to be mediated by several immune-mediated factors including TGF-β, RANK/RANKL, IL-1, and IL-6 [40]. Of metastatic spine tumors, hepatocellular carcinoma appears to show the greatest proclivity for the posterior elements. Importantly, HCC lesions are generally osteolytic, which can predispose to a de novo spondylolisthesis [41]. However, ostensibly any pathology can lead to pathologic spondylolisthesis if growth from the vertebral body leads to involvement of the posterior elements [41].

Interestingly, it has been proposed that spinal segments with preexisting spondylolysis have increased vascularization [42], which may predispose them as targets for the hematogenous spread of metastatic disease [43, 44]. Changes in the extracellular matrix at the site of spondylytic defects may also influence the spread of tumor from the vertebral body into the posterior elements [45, 46]. One of note is the increased expression of ligament-associated extracellular matrix structures within the lytic defect, including versican within the fibrocartilaginous enthesis at either end of the defect [42]. Versican has previously been associated with cancer cell self-renewal and also with suppression of cancer cell attachment to extracellular fibronectin, thereby increasing cancer cell motility [47, 48]. It has also been associated with the epithelial-to-mesenchymal transition essential for tumor spread [47, 48] and may also play a role in tumor cell immune system evasion [49].

Classification

At present there is no accepted classification of spondylolisthesis specifically within the oncology population. One study by Cecchinato and Boriani attempted to devise a management algorithm (Fig. 6.1) based on a 27-year experience including 14 patients with tumors and concurrent spondylolysis or spondylolisthesis [50]. Of these, eight patients (57%) had the spondylolisthesis at the level of the tumor or adjacent level, while the remaining six had more than one vertebra separating the slip and the tumor. They grossly divided cases into two types—A and B. Type A cases denoted those with the listhesis/lysis at or adjacent to the tumor-involved level, whereas B cases described those with greater than one level separating the listhesis/lysis and tumor. Within type A they identified three subtypes based on the

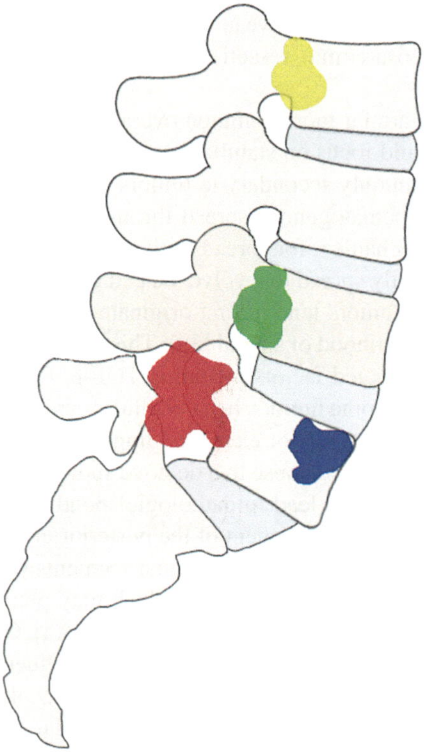

Fig. 6.1 Depiction of Cecchinato et al. classification system. Type A1, seen in red, is when a tumor provokes the spondylolisthesis and treatment should be dictated by the oncologic pathology. Type A2, seen in blue, describes a tumor occurring on a pre-existing spondylolisthesis but the treatment does not require addressing the spondylolisthesis. Type A, seen in green, is when a tumor is found in an adjacent vertebra to a spondylolisthesis in which case extension of fusion to address the underlying misalignment is often required. Finally, type B, seen in yellow, describes any tumor arising at least one or more spinal segment from the spondylolisthesis which does not typically necessitate addressing the slippage

proposed linkage of the tumor and slip. In A1 cases, the tumor is proposed to have caused the slip and the authors argue surgery should be guided by oncologic principles (i.e., *en bloc* resection for primary malignancies) followed by circumferential fusion to stabilize the segment. A2 cases described tumor occurring on a pre-existing spondylolisthesis. Again, they argue oncologic principles should prevail and fusion/stabilization is only necessary where there is overt instability on preoperative evaluation or tumor treatment will result in instability, but the treatment does not require addressing the spondylolisthesis (in the cases of local radiotherapy and limited intralesional excisions). Last, in type A3 lesions the need for instrumentation must be guided jointly by the apparent instability of the listhesis and by any instability that will be generated by oncologic treatment of the tumor; this most commonly involves extending the fusion construct to reduce the spondylolisthesis and stabilize the tumor-affected vertebra. For type B lesions, they note that the surgical plan for the tumor and the listhesis can often be separate, though the degree to which reconstruction following treatment of the tumor will affect sagittal balance and ultimately the listhesis should be considered when developing the operative plan for the tumor. Where there are multiple levels separating the listhesis and tumor they note that the listhesis may reasonably be left alone if low grade and asymptomatic. Interestingly, the authors also note that treatment of patients with longer fusions (over seven levels) that fail to account for overall sagittal balance may lead to poorer functional outcomes irrespective of the oncologic results due to progression of the spondylolisthesis [50]. If such long-segment fusions are stopped adjacent to the spondylolisthesis, they may place increased stresses on this motion segment, increasing the odds of spondylolisthesis progression.

Prior Experiences with Concurrent Tumor and Spondylolisthesis

On the whole the body of literature examining the co-occurrence of tumor and spondylolisthesis is comprised of low-quality evidence, as almost all is derived from case reports and small case series. Klaassen et al. presented one such early description, highlight the case of a 12-year-old boy with a sacral Ewing sarcoma who presented with left-sided weakness and an associated grade II L5 spondylolisthesis with bilateral pars defects [51]. Over 2 weeks, his symptoms worsened, which led to a CT scan demonstrating the tumor involving the left sacral ala with thecal sac impingement; he was treated with chemoradiation, which was accepted oncologic stand of care at the time. His case was most in line with a type A3 lesion in the system of Cecchinato and Boriani [50] and as there was deemed to be no instability, instrumented fusion was not pursued.

A subsequent case reported by Choi and colleagues described a 57-year-old whom who presented with a two-month history of progressive low back pain, right leg radicular pain, and right leg weakness superimposed on a 10-year history of intermittent neurogenic claudication [21]. Imaging demonstrated a grade I L3/4 isthmic spondylolisthesis with an associated exophytic mass of the L3 lamina compressing the thecal sac, which was resected *en bloc* as part of the Gill fragment and shown to be an osteochondroma. The lesion—a type A2 lesion in the system of Cecchinato and Boriani—was treated with concurrent L3-S1 instrumented fusion to address the instability associated with the isthmic spondylolisthesis. The authors posited the fibrous cartilage of the spondylolysis could have been the origin of the diseased cartilage forming the osteochondroma, but note that it is ultimately unclear if the spondylolisthesis predated the tumor [21].

Garneti et al. described a case of cervical spondyloptosis; this description remains the only published case of an aneurysmal bone cyst causing spondyloptosis [27]. The patient, a 11-year-old girl, was initially diagnosed with cervical paralytic scoliosis after presenting with hyperreflexia and an ataxic gait. Imaging ultimately showed a grade III C6/7 anterolisthesis with a collapsed C7 body and an abnormality of the posterior elements at C7. She initially underwent traction to reduce the spondylolisthesis, which was followed by a staged posterior–anterior–posterior approach with gross total resection of the mass and a C6-T1 circumferential fusion. This was followed by 12 weeks in a postoperative halo vest. While the treatment for ABCs do not always involve surgery, given the progressive deformity and neurologic deficit, surgical intervention was deemed to be necessary and a circumferential fusion was performed, in line with the treatment recommended by Cecchinato and Boriani for type A1 lesions [26, 52]. The authors postulated the patient's scoliosis developed as an adaptation to the cervicothoracic junctional dislocation caused by the tumors destruction of the C7 posterior elements.

A similar case was described by Sarmiento and colleagues, though the C4/5 spondylolisthesis (grade 2) was secondary to a rare juxtacortical chondroma. This mass involved the left C5/6 neural foramen and compressed the adjacent thecal sac, causing balance issues and left C6 radicular pain [62]. Imaging also demonstrated kyphotic angulation at the level of the spondylolisthesis with associated mild bowstringing of the cord. This Cecchinato/Boriani type A3 lesion was successfully treated with a C4–6 circumferential fusion to partially reduce the listhesis, and a C4/5-C5/6 decompression to remove the mass. The authors noted the patient was on chronic glucocorticoids and speculated as to whether the spondylolisthesis and associated deformity may have predated the chondroma. Regardless of etiology, because of the anterolisthesis and concurrent kyphotic deformity, the circumferential fusion approach was chosen rather than decompression alone.

A couple of case reports of spondylolisthesis/spondyloptosis in the setting of neurofibromatosis (NF) type 1 have been reported, though scoliosis is the most common deformity and its treatment is outlined in Chap. 2 [53–55]. One report by Cheaney and colleagues described a 26-year-old female who presented with a 12-year history of back and left lower extremity pain refractory to nonoperative management, which was associated with a grade 4 spondylolisthesis. Operative intervention had been previously deferred due to her small, dysmorphic pedicles and significant vertebral body scalloping, which left little fusion surface. Intraoperatively her listhesis progressed to gross spondyloptosis, which was ultimately successfully reduced and treated with a standalone L5/S1 ALIF [56]. Two features highlighted by this case are the often dysmorphic pedicles in patients with NF1, which may affect the choice of instrumentation and level selection, and the presence of dural ectasia, which is relatively common in these patients and can be associated with scalloping of the vertebral bodies [53, 54, 57–60]. Such ectasia must be kept in mind during both instrumentation and decompression as it can increase the risk of dural injury. Such ectasia was also noted in the case reported by Martin-Fuentes and colleagues [61], a 12-year-old girl who had previously undergone multilevel lumbar decompression for cauda equina and subsequently presented with 1-year of progressive low back pain and imaging demonstrating a grade 4 L1/2 spondylolisthesis. The authors opted for an anterior fusion with L2 corpectomy with a plan for a complementary posterior instrumented stage. This was deferred by the parents though and she was instead treated with bracing 1-year postoperatively. This was ultimately associated with a 70° kyphosis above the construct, but her overall sagittal balance was preserved, and she was pain free, so no further intervention was pursued.

Though in the above cases, workup of the patient's pain led to diagnosis of the spondylolisthesis and associated mass, pre-existing spondylolisthesis and associated pain may delay diagnosis of the underlying tumor. This is true for both lesions of the vertebral body, and in rare cases, intramedullary tumors [63]. Pain in the context of tumor and concurrent spondylolisthesis may be due to either tumor progression or progression of the spondylolisthesis [17, 44, 63].

Evaluation and Treatment of Spondylolisthesis

A patient with spondylolisthesis often will present with back pain, leg pain, or a combination of both [64–66]. In the context of a known primary cancer, any acute onset of this symptomatology should prompt spinal imaging to look for the presence of metastatic disease to the vertebral column. While non-pathologic spondylolisthesis pain may be relieved with recumbency, pathologic spondylolisthesis will likely have both mechanical and oncologic components. The latter is unlikely to be relieved with recumbency. In patients with pathologic spondylolisthesis evaluation should include a complete neurologic exam with motor and sensory testing, along with visual inspection for deformity, and palpation of the spine, which can reveal a step-off at the spinous process above the listhesis or midline tenderness [67]. A Phalen-Dickson sign (knee-flexed, hip-flexed gait) can be observed as well as compensatory hyperlordosis above the spondylolisthesis. Sensorimotor deficits on exam may be from neural element compression by the tumor, or compression in either the lateral recess or affected foramen secondary to the spondylolisthesis. In cases where the lesion is associated with pedicular lysis, the exiting nerve root is more likely to be affected, as in other cases of isthmic spondylolisthesis. With a higher-grade spondylolisthesis, a global deformity may be noted [68–70].

Imaging should include full-length standing radiographs that visualize the spine from the cranium to the femoral heads to assess global alignment. Ideally extension of the film to include the knees and look for compensatory mechanisms is also preferable [50, 71]. Flexion/extension view of the spine region involved by the spondylolisthesis can also be useful to assess the mobility of the listhesis and need for a stabilization procedure [67]. Advanced neuraxial imaging including CT to assess the underlying bone quality and MR to assess the epidural disease burden are also warranted [26].

The aggressiveness of the surgical correction is dictated by the patient's symptomatology, the patient's ability to tolerate an aggressive deformity correction, and the underlying bone quality, which is key in determining whether the patient's spine will support such a correction. Borrowing from the SDSG classification system, it is recommended that patients with high-grade slips (types 4–6) undergo reduction and realignment. In types 5 and 6, wherein the pelvis is unbalanced, reduction should also be attempted so as to try and restore global balance [5, 8]. This is based on data suggesting that global spinal alignment and spinopelvic parameters are associated with superior pain relief and improved quality of life, though long-term follow-up is wanting [5, 10, 72, 73]. Other retrospective studies examining spinopelvic parameters in the context of high-grade spondylolisthesis have suggested that in patients with an unbalanced pelvis, reduction may be beneficial [10]. Overall, there is a paucity of quality studies examining the influence of spinopelvic parameters on the outcomes of surgical treatment of spondylolisthesis though, which may explain the lack of consensus on which patients benefit from treatment.

Ultimately, the patient's overall fitness for surgery, oncologic disease burden, and presenting clinical picture must be considered when outlining the goals of surgery and developing an individualized surgical plan. Independent of the plan for correction of the underlying spondylolisthesis, surgery must also be designed to achieve the appropriate oncologic goals, as highlighted by Cecchinato and Boriani [50]. A surgery that corrects the listhesis, but which violates oncologic principles (e.g., curettage of a primary bony spine malignancy) is ultimately determinantal to the patient's overall outcome. In most described cases, the listhesis is observed in the context of a benign lesion or metastatic disease, in which case greater emphasis may be placed on successful correction. If the listhesis is itself asymptomatic, it may be left out of the surgical plan unless the construct proposed as part of the plan for tumor resection will involve the listhesed segment or the construct will place the listhesis at an adjacent segment. In such case it becomes a stress riser and would likely benefit from inclusion in the proposed construct. If the spondylolisthesis is to be addressed, surgical principles will be the same as described in the degenerative or isthmic literature [74–79]. Of course, given the relationship to global spine alignment, a longer construct may be necessary in the case of higher-grade spondylolisthesis to address the misalignments to improve the functional outcomes and effectively alleviate pain [71].

Conclusion

De novo spondylolisthesis, though rare, can be seen in a variety of spine tumors where the neoplastic process involves the posterior elements. Spondylolisthesis can also be seen adjacent to a nascent oncologic process, in which case the surgeon must consider whether operative management should seek to address both the deformity and the tumor, or only the neoplastic process. It is also important to recognize that with improvements in oncologic treatments, patient prognoses are improving and many who would've previously succumbed to their cancer now survive long enough for their degenerative disease to become symptomatic. Given this, if evaluation of the patient's oncologic disease burden, fitness for surgery, and clinical symptoms favors concurrent treatment of the spondylolisthesis, the construct should incorporate the principles used in the management of degenerative and isthmic spondylolisthesis. Lastly, especially in cases where the spondylolisthesis occurs with a surgically curable lesion, the patient's overall spinal alignment must be considered in the surgical plan so as to avoid creating new or worsening preexisting deformity.

References

1. Meyerding HW (1932) Spondyloptosis. Surg Gynecol Obstet 54:371–377
2. Wiltse LL, Newman PH, Macnab I (1976) Classification of spondylolisis and spondylolisthesis. Clin Orthop Relat Res:23–29
3. Marchetti P, Bartolozzi P (1997) Classification of spondylolisthesis as a guideline for treatment. In: Bridwell KH, DeWald RL (eds) Textbook of spinal surgery, 2nd edn. Lippincott Williams & Wilkins, Inc, pp 1211–1254
4. Batra S, Garg B (2021) Classification of spondylolisthesis: current concepts. Indian Spine J 4:10
5. Labelle H, Mac-Thiong J-M, Roussouly P (2011) Spino-pelvic sagittal balance of spondylolisthesis: a review and classification. Eur Spine J 20:641–646
6. Labelle H, Roussouly P, Berthonnaud É, Transfeldt E, O'Brien M, Chopin D, Hresko T, Dimnet J (2004) Spondylolisthesis, pelvic incidence, and spinopelvic balance. Spine 29:2049–2054
7. Hanson DS, Bridwell KH, Rhee JM, Lenke LG (2002) Correlation of pelvic incidence with low- and high-grade isthmic spondylolisthesis. Spine 27:2026–2029
8. Mac-Thiong J-M, Duong L, Parent S, Hresko MT, Dimar JR, Weidenbaum M, Labelle H (2012) Reliability of the spinal deformity study group classification of lumbosacral spondylolisthesis. Spine 37:E95–E102
9. Duval-Beaupère G, Schmidt C, Cosson P (1992) A barycentremetric study of the sagittal shape of spine and pelvis: the conditions required for an economic standing position. Ann Biomed Eng 20:451–462
10. Hresko MT, Labelle H, Roussouly P, Berthonnaud E (2007) Classification of high-grade spondylolistheses based on pelvic version and spine balance: possible rationale for reduction. Spine 32:2208–2213
11. Camino Willhuber G, Kido G (2020) Classifications in brief: the spinal deformity study group classification of lumbosacral spondylolisthesis. Clin Orthop Relat Res 478:681–684
12. Boulay C, Tardieu C, Hecquet J, Benaim C, Mouilleseaux B, Marty C, Prat-Pradal D, Legaye J, Duval-Beaupère G, Pélissier J (2006) Sagittal alignment of spine and pelvis regulated by pelvic incidence: standard values and prediction of lordosis. Eur Spine J 15:415–422

13. Schwab FJ, Lafage V, Farcy J-P, Bridwell KH, Glassman S, Shainline MR (2008) Predicting outcome and complications in the surgical treatment of adult scoliosis. Spine 33:2243–2247
14. Lafage V, Schwab F, Skalli W, Hawkinson N, Gagey P-M, Ondra S, Farcy J-P (2008) Standing balance and sagittal plane spinal deformity: analysis of spinopelvic and gravity line parameter. Spine 33:1572–1578
15. Lafage V, Schwab F, Patel A, Hawkinson N, Farcy J-P (2009) Pelvic tilt and truncal inclination: two key radiographic parameters in the setting of adults with spinal deformity. Spine 34:E599–E606
16. Sciubba DM, Pennington Z, Colman MW et al (2021) Spinal metastases 2021: a review of the current state of the art and future directions. Spine J 21:1414–1429
17. Harrington KD (1993) Metastatic tumors of the spine: diagnosis and treatment. J Am Acad Orthop Surg 1:76–86
18. Sakai D, Mochida J, Toh E, Nomura T (2002) Spinal osteochondromas in middle-aged to elderly patients. Spine 27:E503–E506
19. Gille O, Pointillart V, Vital J-M (2005) Course of spinal solitary osteochondromas. Spine 30:E13–E19
20. Gaetani P, Tancioni F, Merlo P, Villani L, Spanu G, Baena RR et al (1996) Spinal chondroma of the lumbar tract: case report. Surg Neurol 46:534–539
21. Choi BK, Han IH, Cho WH, Cha SH (2010) Lumbar osteochondroma arising from spondylolytic L3 lamina. J Korean Neurosurg Soc 47:313
22. Ilaslan H, Sundaram M, Unni KK, Shives TC (2004) Primary vertebral osteosarcoma: imaging findings. Radiology 230:697–702
23. Hassankhani EG (2009) Solitary lower lumbar osteochondroma (spinous process of L3 involvement): a case report. Cases J 2:9359
24. Kransdorf MJ, Stull MA, Gilkey FW, Moser RP (1991) Osteoid osteoma. Radiographics 11:671–696
25. Jackson RP, Reckling FW, Mantz FA (1977) Osteoid osteoma and osteoblastoma. Similar histologic lesions with different natural histories. Clin Orthop Relat Res 128:303–313
26. Boriani S, De Iure F, Campanacci L, Gasbarrini A, Bandiera S, Biagini R, Bertoni F, Picci P (2001) Aneurysmal bone cyst of the mobile spine: report on 41 cases. Spine 26:27–35
27. Garneti N, Dunn D, El Gamal E, Williams DA, Nelson IW, Sandemon DR (2003) Cervical spondyloptosis caused by an aneurysmal bone cyst. Spine 28:E68–E70
28. Hirsh LF, Thanki A, Spector HB (1984) Primary spinal chondrosarcoma with eighteen-year follow-up: case report and literature review. Neurosurgery 14:747–749
29. Quiriny M, Gebhart M (2008) Chondrosarcoma of the spine: a report of three cases and literature review. Acta Orthop Belg 74:885–890
30. Katonis P, Alpantaki K, Michail K, Lianoudakis S, Christoforakis Z, Tzanakakis G, Karantanas A (2011) Spinal chondrosarcoma: a review. Sarcoma 2011:1–10
31. Pennington Z, Ehresman J, Pittman PD, Ahmed AK, Lubelski D, McCarthy EF, Goodwin CR, Sciubba DM (2021) Chondrosarcoma of the spine: a narrative review. Spine J 21:2078–2096
32. Vaidya M, Shenoy A, Goel N (2019) Chondrosarcoma of the dorsal spine – a rare case. J Craniovertebr Junction Spine 10:250
33. Kumar A, Nehete L, Chaturvedi J, Hussain N (2018) Large giant cell tumor at dorsal spine with spinal instability. J Spinal Surg 5:174–177
34. Sohn S, Kim J, Chung CK, Lee NR, Park E, Chang U-K, Sohn MJ, Kim SH (2016) A nationwide epidemiological study of newly diagnosed spine metastasis in the adult Korean population. Spine J 16:937–945
35. Wright E, Ricciardi F, Arts M et al (2018) Metastatic spine tumor epidemiology: comparison of trends in surgery across two decades and three continents. World Neurosurg 114:e809–e817
36. Kumar N, Tan WLB, Wei W, Vellayappan BA (2020) An overview of the tumors affecting the spine – inside to out. Neuro-Oncol Pract 7:i10–i17

37. Yuh WTC, Quets JP, Lee HJ, Simonson TM, Michalson LS, Nguyen PT, Sato Y, Mayr NA, Berbaum KS (1996) Anatomic distribution of metastases in the vertebral body and modes of hematogenous spread. Spine 21:2243–2250
38. Pennington Z, Goodwin ML, Westbroek EM, Cottrill E, Ahmed AK, Sciubba DM (2019) Lactate and cancer: spinal metastases and potential therapeutic targets (part 2). Ann Transl Med 7:221
39. Guo M, Kolberg KL, Smith EC et al (2018) Predominance of spinal metastases involving the posterior vertebral body. World Neurosurg 119:e991–e996
40. Roodman GD (2004) Mechanisms of bone metastasis. N Engl J Med 350:1655–1664
41. An C, Lee YH, Kim S, Cho HW, Suh J-S, Song H-T (2013) Characteristic MRI findings of spinal metastases from various primary cancers: retrospective study of pathologically-confirmed cases. J Korean Soc Magn Reson Med 17:8–18
42. Boszczyk BM, Boszczyk AA, Boos W, Korge A, Mayer HM, Putz R, Benjamin M, Milz S (2006) An immunohistochemical study of the tissue bridging adult spondylolytic defects – the presence and significance of fibrocartilaginous entheses. Eur Spine J 15:965–971
43. Nordström D, Santavirta S, Seitsalo S, Hukkanen M, Polak JM, Nordsletten L, Konttinen YT (1994) Symptomatic lumbar spondylolysis. Spine 19:2752–2758
44. Galasso O, Gasparini G, Mariconda M, Signorelli F (2013) Isolate metastasis of listhetic vertebra. J Back Musculoskelet Rehabil 26:255–259
45. Zheng Y, Chow S-O, Boernert K et al (2014) Direct crosstalk between cancer and osteoblast lineage cells fuels metastatic growth in bone via auto-amplification of IL-6 and RANKL signaling pathways. J Bone Miner Res 29:1938–1949
46. Bendre M, Gaddy D, Nicholas RW, Suva LJ (2003) Breast cancer metastasis to bone: bone: it is not all about PTHrP. Clin Orthop Relat Res 415:S39–S45
47. Karagiorgou Z, Fountas PN, Manou D, Knutsen E, Theocharis AD (2022) Proteoglycans determine the dynamic landscape of EMT and cancer cell stemness. Cancers (Basel) 14:5328
48. Du WW, Yang W, Yee AJ (2013) Roles of versican in cancer biology – tumorigenesis, progression and metastasis. Histol Histopathol 28:701–713
49. Hirani P, Gauthier V, Allen CE, Wight TN, Pearce OMT (2021) Targeting versican as a potential immunotherapeutic strategy in the treatment of cancer. Front Oncol 11:712807
50. Cecchinato R, Boriani S (2018) Spondylolisthesis and tumors: a treatment algorithm. Eur Spine J 27:206–212
51. Klaassen MA, Hoffman G (1987) Ewing sarcoma presenting as spondylolisthesis. Report of a case. J Bone Joint Surg Am 69:1089–1092
52. Turker RJ, Mardjetko S, Lubicky J (1998) Aneurysmal bone cysts of the spine: excision and stabilization. J Pediatr Orthop 18:209–213
53. Wong-Chung J, Gillepsie R (1991) Lumbosacral spondyloptosis with neurofibromatosis: case report. Spine 16:986–987
54. Rockower S, McKay D, Nason S (1982) Dislocation of the spine in neurofibromatosis. A report of two cases. J Bone Joint Surg Am 64:1240–1242
55. Hanna BG, Pill SG, Drummond DS (2002) Irreducible thoracic spondyloptosis in a child with neurofibromatosis: a rationale for treatment. Spine 27:E342–E347
56. Cheaney B, Krause KL, Jung E, Than KD (2023) Treatment of L5-S1 spondyloptosis with stand-alone anterior lumbar interbody fusion in a patient with neurofibromatosis. Br J Neurosurg 37:512–517
57. Modi HN, Srinivasalu S, Suh SW, Yang JH (2009) Grade 4 spondylolisthesis of the L5 vertebra associated with dural ectasia in neurofibromatosis. Singapore Med J 50:e287–e292
58. Gioia G, Mandelli D, Capaccioni B, Sartori A (1998) Postlaminectomy cervical dislocation in von recklinghausen's disease. Spine 23:273–276
59. Stone JW, Bridwell KH, Shackelford GD, Abramson CL (1987) Dural ectasia associated with spontaneous dislocation of the upper part of the thoracic spine in neurofibromatosis. A case report and review of the literature. J Bone Joint Surg Am 69:1079–1083

60. Toyoda K, Taguchi T, Kaneko K, Kato Y, Imajo Y, Imagama T (2005) High-grade L5 spondylolisthesis associated with dural ectasia in neurofibromatosis. J Orthop Sci 10:233–236
61. Martín-Fuentes AM, Pretell-Mazzini J, Curto de la Mano A, Viña-Fernández R (2013) High-grade spondyloretrolisthesis in a 12-year-old girl with neurofibromatosis type 1. J Pediatr Orthop B 22:110–116
62. Sarmiento JM, Medina O, Do AS-MS, Farber S, Chu RM (2019) Resection of cervical juxtacortical chondroma and circumferential spinal stabilization for kyphotic deformity. Cureus 11:e4523
63. Yoon SH, Kim K-J, Chung SK, Kim H-J, Choe G, Chung SB, Jin YJ (2010) Inflammatory myofibroblastic tumor in the intradural extramedullary space of the lumbar spine with spondylolisthesis: case report and review of the literature. Eur Spine J 19:153–157
64. DeWald CJ, Vartabedian JE, Rodts MF, Hammerberg KW (2005) Evaluation and management of high-grade spondylolisthesis in adults. Spine 30:S49–S59
65. Tanguay F, Labelle H, Wang Z, Joncas J, de Guise JA, Mac-Thiong J-M (2012) Clinical significance of lumbosacral kyphosis in adolescent spondylolisthesis. Spine 37:304–308
66. Fredrickson BE, Baker D, McHolick WJ, Yuan HA, Lubicky JP (1984) The natural history of spondylolysis and spondylolisthesis. J Bone Joint Surg Am 66:699–707
67. Kasliwal MK, Smith JS, Kanter A, Chen C-J, Mummaneni PV, Hart RA, Shaffrey CI (2013) Management of high-grade spondylolisthesis. Neurosurg Clin N Am 24:275–291
68. Lenke LG, Bridwell KH (2003) Evaluation and surgical treatment of high-grade isthmic dysplastic spondylolisthesis. Instr Course Lect 52:525–532
69. Lamartina C, Zavatsky JM, Petruzzi M, Specchia N (2009) Novel concepts in the evaluation and treatment of high-dysplastic spondylolisthesis. Eur Spine J 18:133–142
70. Li Y, Hresko TM (2012) Radiographic analysis of spondylolisthesis and sagittal spinopelvic deformity. J Am Acad Orthop Surg 20:194–205
71. Berjano P, Cecchinato R, Pun A, Boriani S (2020) Revision surgery for tumors of the thoracic and lumbar spine: causes, prevention, and treatment strategy. Eur Spine J 29:66–77
72. Schwab F, Patel A, Ungar B, Farcy J-P, Lafage V (2010) Adult spinal deformity-postoperative standing imbalance: how much can you tolerate? An overview of key parameters in assessing alignment and planning corrective surgery. Spine 35:2224–2231
73. Videbaek TS, Bünger CE, Henriksen M, Neils E, Christensen FB (2011) Sagittal spinal balance after lumbar spinal fusion: the impact of anterior column support results from a randomized clinical trial with an eight- to thirteen-year radiographic follow-up. Spine 36:183–191
74. Alfieri A, Gazzeri R, Prell J, Röllinghoff M (2013) The current management of lumbar spondylolisthesis. J Neurosurg Sci 57:103–113
75. Steiger F, Becker H-J, Standaert CJ, Balague F, Vader J-P, Porchet F, Mannion AF (2014) Surgery in lumbar degenerative spondylolisthesis: indications, outcomes and complications. A systematic review. Eur Spine J 23:945–973
76. Mannion AF, Pittet V, Steiger F, Vader J-P, Becker H-J, Porchet F (2014) Development of appropriateness criteria for the surgical treatment of symptomatic lumbar degenerative spondylolisthesis (LDS). Eur Spine J 23:1903–1917
77. Jacobs WCH, Vreeling A, De Kleuver M (2006) Fusion for low-grade adult isthmic spondylolisthesis: a systematic review of the literature. Eur Spine J 15:391–402
78. Kalichman L, Hunter DJ (2008) Diagnosis and conservative management of degenerative lumbar spondylolisthesis. Eur Spine J 17:327–335
79. Schulte TL, Ringel F, Quante M, Eicker SO, Muche-Borowski C, Kothe R (2016) Surgery for adult spondylolisthesis: a systematic review of the evidence. Eur Spine J 25:2359–2367

Chapter 7
Interventional Image-Guided Deformity-Correcting Options for Pathological Fractures

Aladine A. Elsamadicy, Benjamin C. Reeves, Stephanie M. Robert, Igor Latich, Luis Kolb, Maxwell Laurans, and Ehud Mendel

Introduction

Vertebral compression fractures (VCFs) occur when the loads subjected to the vertebra exceed its inherent load-bearing capacity. While multiple etiologies can weaken the underlying cancellous bone and increase the fracture risk (e.g., infection and osteoporosis), where the underlying pathology is tumor, the fracture is described as a pathologic fracture [1–4]. The vertebral bodies are most commonly affected by pathologic fracture in patients with cancer as they are the most common site of metastasis within the spine and are responsible for the majority of axial load bearing [5]. Pathologic VCFs are defined by collapse of the anterior vertebral body and are the most common pathologic fracture, with approximately 1.5 million new cases reported in the United States (US) each year [3, 6]. These fractures most commonly arise with minimal or no associated trauma and are initially asymptomatic in two-thirds of cases. However, VCFs predispose to additional pathologic fractures and with progressive height loss they can cause kyphotic deformation of the spinal column [3, 7]. In one-third of patients who are symptomatic at presentation, the chief complaint is progressive pain, though in some cases, this may be accompanied by neurological deficits from spinal cord or nerve root compression [8, 9]. Irrespective

A. A. Elsamadicy (✉) · S. M. Robert · M. Laurans · E. Mendel
Department of Neurosurgery, Yale University School of Medicine, New Haven, CT, USA
e-mail: aladine.elsamadicy@yale.edu; maxwell.laurans@yale.edu; ehud.mendel@yale.edu

B. C. Reeves · L. Kolb
Department of Neurosurgery, Barrow Neurological Institute, Phoenix, AZ, USA
e-mail: benjamin.reeves@barrowbrainandspine.com; luis.kolb@yale.edu

I. Latich
Department of Radiology and Biomedical Imaging, Yale University School of Medicine, New Haven, CT, USA
e-mail: igor.latich@yale.edu

D. M. Sciubba (ed.), *Spinal Tumor Associated Deformity*,
https://doi.org/10.1007/978-3-031-87939-5_7

of presentation, pathologic vertebral fractures are associated with an increased overall morbidity and mortality [9, 10].

Treatment for pathologic fractures of the spine can range from noninvasive immobilization with bracing to open instrumented fusion depending on the fracture severity and location, degree of associated deformity, symptoms, and overall medical fitness of the patients for surgical intervention. Historically, open surgical stabilization predominated as the gold-standard for invasive intervention. While there is still a role for an open approach in select cases, minimally invasive image-guided techniques have emerged an effective alternative for the management of most VCFs [11]. Percutaneous vertebroplasty and balloon kyphoplasty are the oldest such techniques and are nearly universally accepted minimally invasive alternative to surgery for patients with minimal associated deformity [12–16]. Recent advancements in the technological and procedural design of classic percutaneous VCF stabilization have been associated with improved pain control, reduced disability, and fewer reduced complications [5, 12–16]. Examples of these developments include pairing of traditional cement-based kyphoplasty with radiofrequency ablation or implantation of a device that may improve the load-bearing capacity of the treated vertebra (e.g., OsseoFix®, SpineJack®, and Kiva system) [5].

Herein, we outline the presentation and complications of pathologic spine fractures and highlight minimally invasive, image-guided procedures to stabilize affected segments and correct underlying deformity.

Presentation of Patients with VCF

Pathologic fractures of the spine often present without obvious precipitating trauma; they may occur during trivial events such as lifting a light object, coughing, or even turning over in bed. For many, VCFs are asymptomatic, but in patients who develop symptoms, the most common presentation is acutely progressive axial pain that increases with upright posture and improves with recumbency [3, 17–19]. Neurological deficits are infrequent but may occur if the fracture also involves the middle column with resultant bony retropulsion into the spinal canal (i.e., burst fracture) [3]. If left untreated, a single VCF increases the load imposed on adjacent spinal levels, greatly increasing the risk of subsequent fracture and progressive spinal degeneration [20].

Pathologic Fractures in Spine Metastases

Spine metastases are reported to affect 14%, 8%, and 6% of patients with breast, lung, and prostate cancer, respectively [21]. Other common pathologies include multiple myeloma (MM) and lymphoma; MM affects the spine in 24% of cases [21, 22] and lymphoma has been reported to involve the spine in 5–6% of cases [23, 24].

Primary pathology is largely independent of clinical presentation. Most patients present with focal back pain due to pathologic spine fracture. With progressive vertebral collapse, the patient can develop a kyphotic deformity that places increased strain on the paraspinal musculature and restricts expansion of the thoracic cavity in severe cases [25, 26]. In such event patients have impaired ambulation tolerance and poor pulmonary function, elevating the risk for atelectasis, pneumonia, and decreased exercise tolerance [18, 19, 27–29].

Unlike osteoporotic VCF, where spontaneous resolution of the fracture is often observed, pathologic fractures show a dispensation for progressive height loss and worsened associated deformity [30]. However, patients with metastatic disease are commonly frail, with many comorbidities and a limited life-expectancy, which has been conventionally used as a reason to avoid surgical intervention [30, 31]. Because of this, initial management in neurologically intact patients has been external stabilization (bracing), often with concurrent radiation therapy, unless there is evidence of gross instability [30, 32]. Radiotherapy is associated with sufficient pain control in 60–70% of patients [33], but carries the downside of further weakening of vertebral bone and elevating the risk of VCFs [30, 34, 35]. Particularly in the setting of stereotactic body radiation therapy (SBRT), higher occurrences of VCF have been identified with reported rates ranging between 15% and 40% [36–38]. Adjacent level VCFs are also relatively common following radiotherapy with Lockney et al. observing adjacent-level VCF in 10.8% of cases after SBRT [39]. Pathologic fractures can also be the initial presentation of primary lesions, such as giant cell tumor, for which surgery can be curative. As such, in patients with pathological fracture and no oncologic history, biopsy is crucial to obtain tissue diagnosis and guide therapy [30].

Vertebral Body Augmentation Modalities

Considerations and Contraindications

The primary goal of vertebral body augmentation is pain reduction so as to allow patients to comfortably return to normal daily activities. Conservative management with oral analgesics and noninvasive intervention has conventionally been first line, but more recently validity of this approach has been called into question due to the life-threatening risks of prolonged immobilization in frail or elderly patients (e.g., atelectasis, pneumonia, and pressure sores) [40–42]. Given that open surgery can carry significant risks and be poorly tolerated by frail patients [30], percutaneous, image-guided augmentation procedure are increasingly favored for patients presenting with pathologic fracture without associated instability or mild instability, with or with mild concomitant deformity.

Not all patients are candidates for percutaneous augmentation though. Absolute contraindications to include active local infections (e.g., osteomyelitis, discitis, and epidural abscess) and at many centers compromise of the posterior vertebral body cortex and the presence of retropulsed tumor are considered absolute indications [32, 43]. The latter imposes a potential risk of inducing spinal cord compression following percutaneous intervention [43]. Relative contraindications (Fig. 7.1) include the presence of osteoblastic lesions, three column involvement (evidence of gross instability), and vertebrae plana (complete vertebral body collapse). Other potential contraindications to vertebral body cement augmentation are severe vertebral body collapse (>70% height loss), pedicle fractures, or need for vertebroplasty of more than three levels in a single procedure.

Vertebroplasty

First introduced in 1984 [44], percutaneous vertebroplasty uses image-guidance to transpedicularly insert a needle into the fractured body, through which polymethylmethacrylate (PMMA) cement is delivered. After the cement hardens it results in a significant increase in vertebral body stiffness and crush strength [45], though the amount of cement required depends upon the underlying cement composition and vertebral body size [46]. Percutaneous vertebroplasty is widely employed for VCF secondary to both osteoporosis [47] and neoplastic processes [48]. They are employed commonly in patients with mild-to-moderate deformity in which conservative management cannot control pain and there are no neurological defects

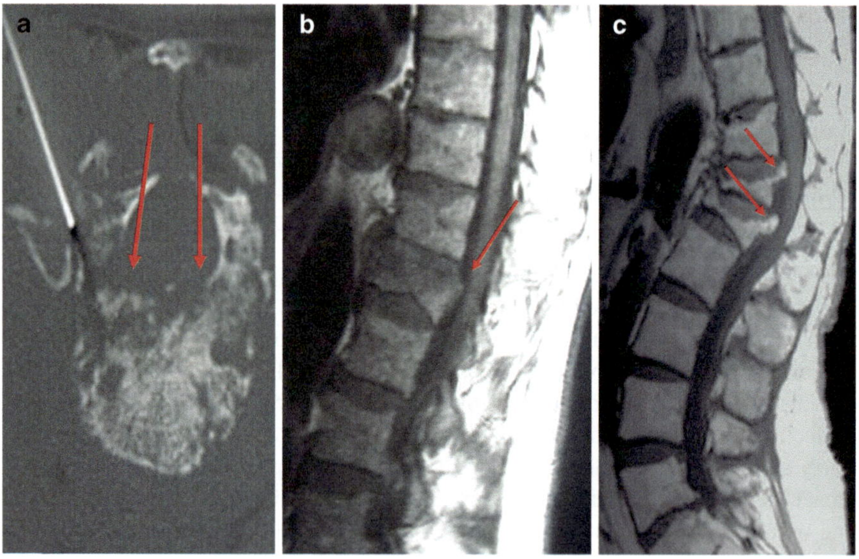

Fig. 7.1 Relative contraindications for vertebroplasty include (**a**) absent margins; (**b**) posterior wall integrity compromise; and (**c**) moderate to severe retropulsion of the posterior vertebral body cortex into the spinal canal with severe collapse

(Fig. 7.2). In general, unilateral percutaneous vertebroplasty is preferred over bilateral, as it is associated with similar outcomes, shorter procedure times, and reduced radiation exposure [49, 50]. Biomechanical testing has also suggested similar stabilizing effects in vertebra subjected to axial loading following unipedicular and bipedicular vertebroplasty [45]. It is noted that when a unilateral approach is employed though, efforts should be made to have a midline cement fill within the vertebral body.

Much of the highest quality data for vertebroplasty comes from the management of patients with osteoporotic VCFs. In one early randomized controlled trial comparing vertebroplasty and sham for osteoporosis-related VCF, Kallmes et al. found no additive benefit of vertebroplasty in the control of pain or functional recovery [51]. Similarly, the randomized, double-blind placebo-controlled study of

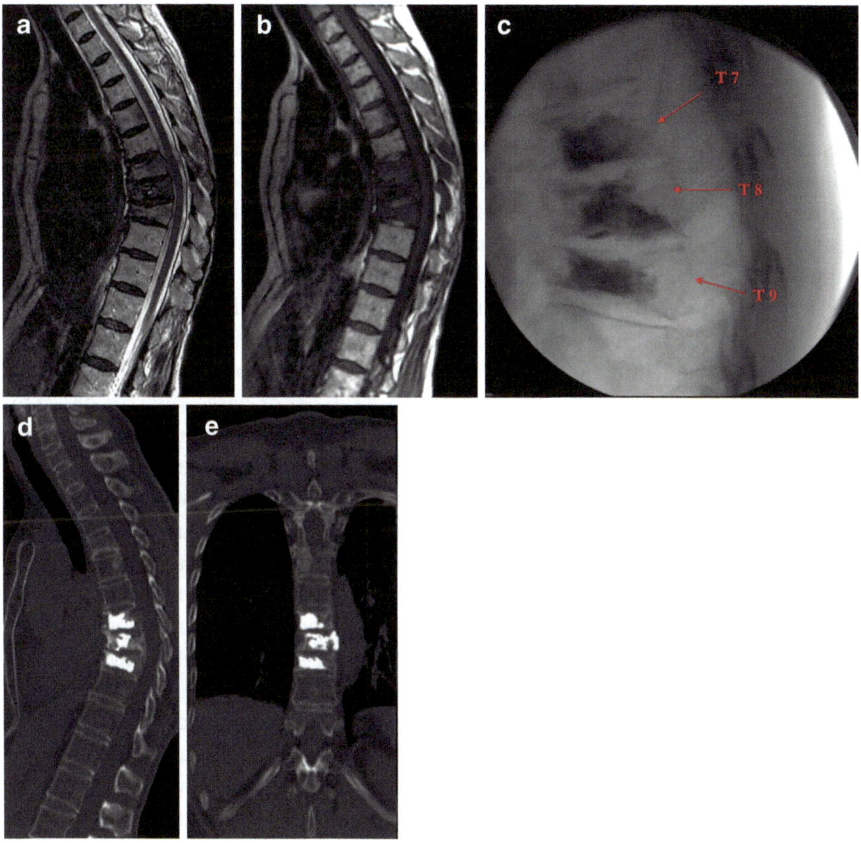

Fig. 7.2 A 56-year-old female patient presenting with mid-thoracic mechanical back pain. Sagittal (**a**) T2; (**b**) T1 pre-contrast demonstrating T7-T9 pathological vertebral body pathological fractures secondary to metastatic lesions. The patient subsequently underwent 3-level vertebroplasty (**c**) intraoperative lateral film—the arrows indicating the vertebral body levels; post-vertebroplasty CT (**d**) sagittal and (**e**) axial

Buchbinder et al. comparing vertebroplasty to sham operation found patients in both groups had similar reductions in overall pain, and similar improvements in physical function, quality of life, and perceived recovery at 6 months post-intervention [52]. However, more recent cohort data has suggested improved pain relief with vertebroplasty relative to nonoperative management. One prospective study by Yang et al. examined 544 patients with at least one osteoporotic VCF and found vertebroplasty to be associated with lower pain and disability index scores at 1-week and 1-, 3-, and 6-month follow-ups, allowing for earlier return to daily activities [53]. Thillainadesan et al. likewise showed sustained efficacy of vertebroplasty up to 29 months in a small prospective cohort of patients treated for osteoporotic fractures [54]. In patients with neoplastic-related VCF, previous studies have shown shorter hospitalizations, better vertebral body height restoration, and better pain reduction relative to conventional minimally invasive spine surgery [55, 56].

While closed vertebroplasties are more common, for patients requiring operative intervention for severe deformity or neural element decompression, open vertebroplasty can be performed (Fig. 7.3). In a study of 68 patients with thoracolumbar vertebral metastases who were undergoing vertebroplasty (routine or bone filling mesh pocket vertebroplasty) combined with pedicle screw fixation, Zhu et al. demonstrated a significant reduction in pain, with commensurate improvements in neural function, and spinal stability [57]. However, with the introduction of fenestrated pedicle screw fixation [58], the need for open vertebroplasty has been reduced as the cement may be placed through a fenestrated screw into the vertebral body, thereby supplementing the screw strength (Fig. 7.4) [59].

Despite perceived benefits, vertebroplasty is not without risks (Fig. 7.5). Complications include neuraxial anesthesia, new adjacent and non-adjacent vertebral fractures, and infection [60]. The most common complication, however, is cement leakage, which has been reported in 41–62% of cases [59, 61–63]. This leakage is most common in patients with highly morselized fractures and fractures with significant height loss, where there is often radiological evidence of intravertebral clefts or cortical disruption that allow for leakage of cement out of the vertebral body. This complication is less common in modern practice due to advances in technique, but is still seen at a nontrivial rate, though most cases are asymptomatic [61, 62]. CT is the most sensitive method for detection (82% sensitivity) and may identify embolization events not seen during intraprocedural fluoroscopic monitoring [64]. The vast majority of embolization events are asymptomatic [59], but cement leakage into the canal should be suspected in those with new onset neurological symptoms (e.g., radicular pain, bowel/bladder incontinence, weakness, and numbness) following cement injection. Cement augmentation also increases the risk of adjacent-level vertebral fractures by placing a rigid cement-augmented vertebral body adjacent to a nonaugmented level with an undoubtedly lower yield strength. Such fractures have been reported to occur in up to 19.9% of cases [65]. Other complications of vertebroplasty include arterial and venous particle embolization, which can lead to cement pulmonary emboli, intraprocedural pedicle fracture, epidural hematoma [66], and access site hematomas. The latter complications

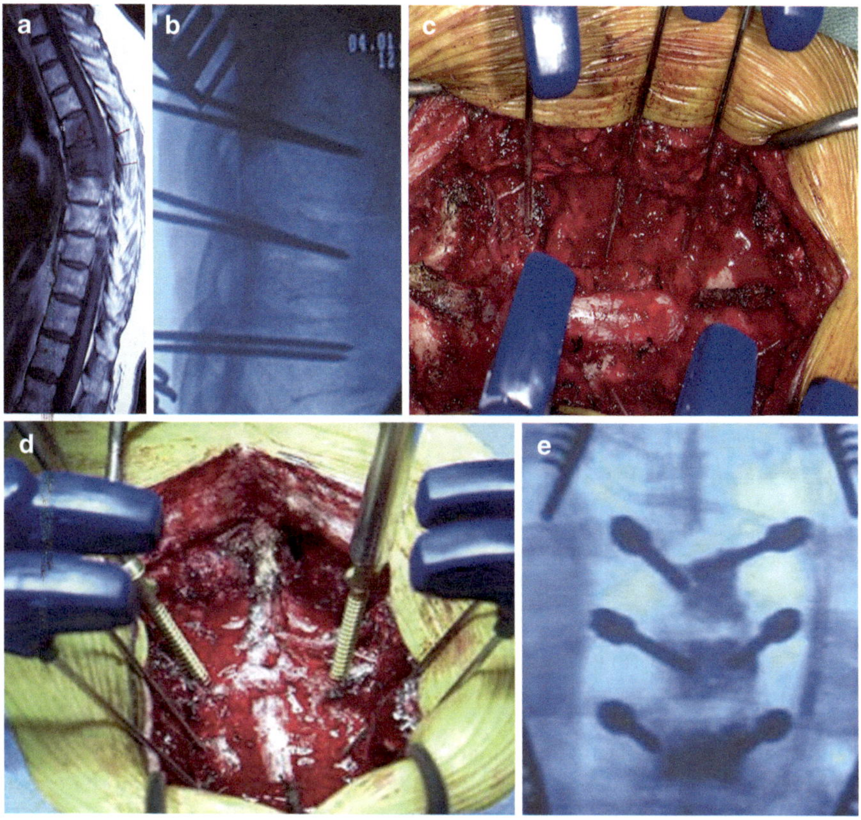

Fig. 7.3 A 63-year-old male presenting with intractable mechanical back pain. (**a**) Sagittal pre-contrast MRI demonstrating osseous lesions at T5 and T6 vertebral bodies with dorsal epidural spinal cord compression. Plan for open multi-level vertebroplasties with pedicle screw placement. Intraoperative (**b**) lateral films demonstrating canulated pedicle needle insertion; (**c**) operative field view of the multi-level canulated pedicle needles; (**d**) insertion of pedicle screw after cement inserted; (**e**) postoperative anterior–posterior film of pedicle screws inserted into the vertebroplasty cement at each vertebral body level

are generally seen in patients on chronic anticoagulation, which for many proceduralists is a contraindication to cement augmentation.

Balloon Kyphoplasty

Kyphoplasty is similar to vertebroplasty with the exception that prior cement injection, a balloon is passed through the cannula into the vertebral body and expanded (Fig. 7.6). The objective of this is to restore vertebral body height and create a repository of the PMMA cement so as to potentially decrease the risk of cement

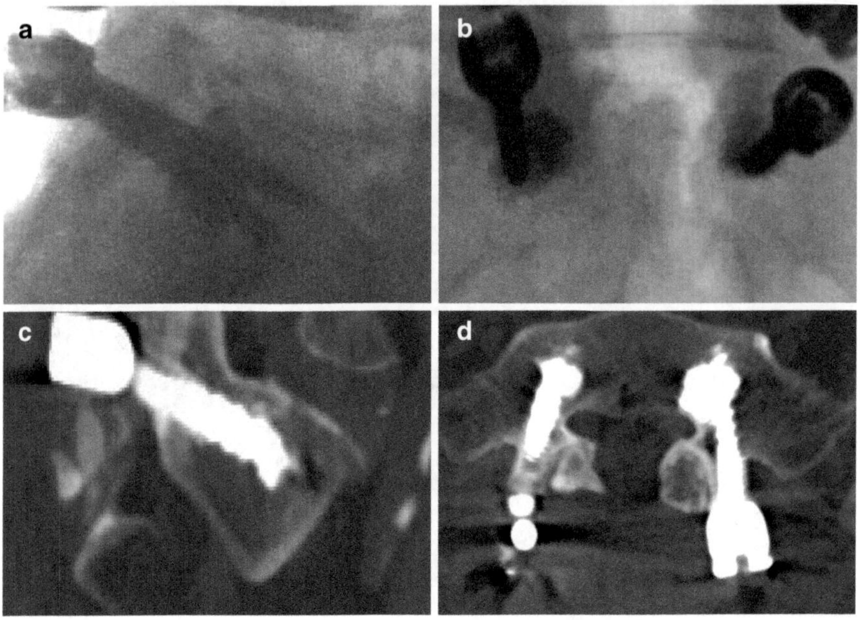

Fig. 7.4 (**a**) Lateral and (**b**) PA film; (**c**) lateral and (**d**) axial CT of S1 fenestrated pedicle screws placement

extravasation. Kyphoplasty has similar indications to vertebroplasty, and unilateral, rather than bilateral, injection typically yields comparable outcomes, shorter operation times, lower radiation dose, and less injected cement [50].

As with vertebroplasty, the best evidence for the efficacy of kyphoplasty is from the osteoporotic/fragility fracture literature. In one randomized control trial of 300 patients, Boonen et al. found that patients who underwent kyphoplasty had improved pain and motor function at 24-month follow-up, without an increase in additional fractures [67]. Cohort series have similarly suggest good outcomes, but have also suggested kyphoplasty may offer superior vertebral height restoration, making it a better option for patients with fracture-associated deformity [68, 69]. Furthermore, a randomized control trial comparing vertebroplasty and kyphoplasty for patients with osteoporotic VCFs showed kyphoplasty to have a lower rate of cement leakages and offer both superior pain control and greater improvements in functional status [70, 71]. Similar results were reported in a subsequently performed meta-analysis [70, 71].

Berenson and colleagues also demonstrated the utility of kyphoplasty for patients with pathologic fracture in the CAFÉ trial, randomizing 131 patients with 1–3 painful VCFs to kyphoplasty or nonoperative management. Patients treated with kyphoplasty had significantly better pain and disability scores at 1 month; they also had significantly fewer reduced activity days and days in which they were bed bound [72].

Common complications following kyphoplasty are similar to those of percutaneous vertebroplasty; however, cement leakage is less common (18 vs 55%) [73]. It

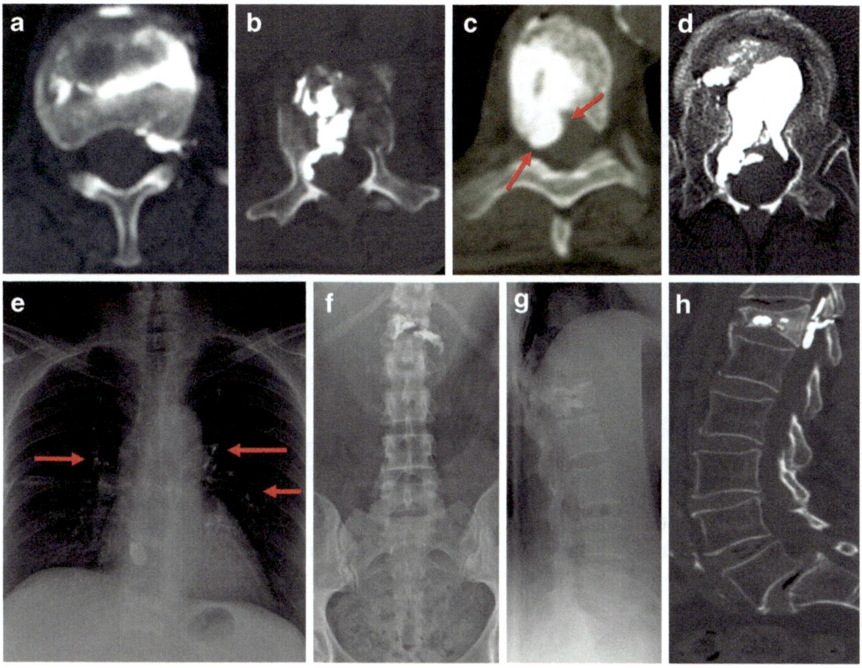

Fig. 7.5 Complications of vertebroplasties include (**a**–**d**) axial CT of cement leakage posteriorly into the spinal canal. (**e**) Posterior–anterior [PA] chest film demonstrating particle embolization to bilateral lungs—arrows demonstrating the cement particles. (**f**) PA lumbar film demonstrating lateral leakage of cement and (**g**) lateral film demonstrating leakage through the inferior endplate. (**h**) Sagittal lumbar CT demonstrating cement leakage into the spinal canal with intact posterior well

has been hypothesized that initial vertebral body expansion using the balloon reduces cement leakage by creating a cavity into which cement can be injected under a lower pressure [74]. As with vertebroplasty, it has been reported that kyphoplasty can increase the risk of adjacent level fracture, though meta-analyses have reached contradictory conclusion regarding this risk [75, 76]. Last, kyphoplasty is associated with greater radiation exposure for both patient and proceduralist [77].

Mechanical Reinforcement

Kiva System

The Kiva system is a vertebral augmentation technique that supplements cement augmentation with a cylindrical polyetheretherketone (PEEK) implant. This technique uses transpedicular access like conventional cement augmentation, but prior to cement injection the PEEK implant is passed down a guidewire into the vertebral

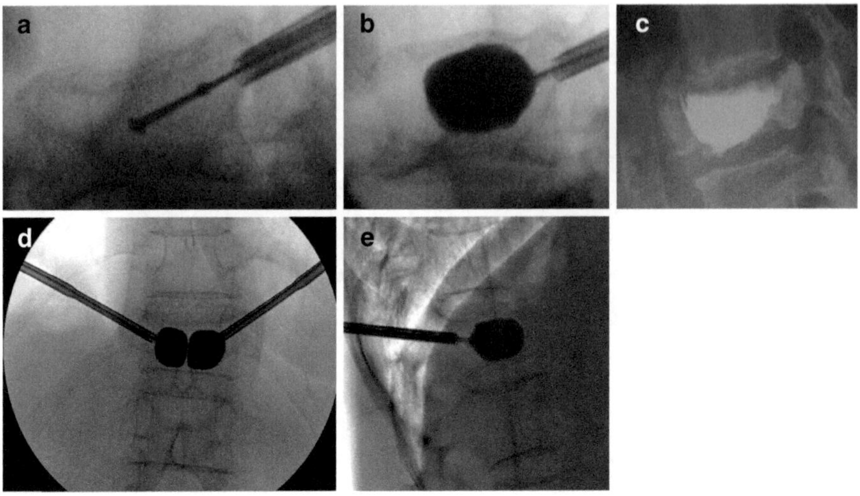

Fig. 7.6 (**a**) Lateral film demonstrating unilateral pedicle insertion into vertebral body of balloon kyphoplasty; (**b**) inflation of balloon. (**c**) Post-cement insertion into balloon occupying space in the vertebral body. (**d**) PA film and (**e**) lateral film demonstrating bilateral pedicle insertion into vertebral body of balloon kyphoplasty

body tool where it coils into its cylindrical shape. Once the desired vertebral height has been achieved, the wire is removed and cement is injected into the implant [60].

In a pilot study of 57 patients with osteoporotic VCFs by Olivarez et al., the authors found that the Kiva system resulted in a 66% and 63% decrease in pain and functional impairment at 12 months following the procedure [78]. A subsequent study by Otten et al. compared Kiva to balloon kyphoplasty for osteoporotic VCF and noted superior improvements in back pain for those treated with the Kiva system though vertebral height restoration and improvements in disability were similar between groups [79]. Korovessis et al. [80] randomized 168 patients with osteoporotic VCF to KIVA or kyphoplasty and noted similar improvements in vertebral height, disability scores, and pain scores, though they suggested Kiva may be superior for restoring kyphotic angulation as compared to conventional kyphoplasty. They did report lower rates of cement extravasation though, which was also observed in the subsequent Kiva Safety and Effectiveness Trial (KAST) [81]. However, as with the prior studies, the KAST trial demonstrated Kiva to be non-inferior to balloon kyphoplasty with regard to improvements in pain and function at 12-month follow-up. Overall, the data appear to suggest equipoise between Kiva and conventional kyphoplasty, with the main benefits of Kiva being lower rates of cement leakage [80, 81] and potentially lower rates of new fractures when compared to balloon kyphoplasty [78, 79].

OsseoFix® System

The OsseoFix® system, which became available in 2009, is a percutaneous stabilization method available for both osteoporotic and cancer-related VCFs [82]. In this procedure, a titanium cage is placed transpedicularly into the anterior third of the vertebral body and then filled with cement. In a prospective study of 32 patients with osteoporotic VCFs treated with OsseoFix®, Ender et al. reported significant improvements in patient disability and pain, as well as a reduction in overall kyphosis at 12 months [83]. A follow-up study, which included both patients with osteoporotic and tumorous VCFs, demonstrated similar results [84]. The main advantage of the OsseoFix® system is that it requires significantly less bone cement than traditional kyphoplasty and may lower rates of cement leakage, as there have been no reports of symptomatic cement leak to date [83].

SpineJack® System

The SpineJack® system is third widely available vertebral augmentation system designed to improve upon conventional kyphoplasty. Like the OsseoFix® device, the SpineJack® device is made of titanium and is placed into the vertebral body via a transpedicular approach prior to augmentation with polymethylmethacrylate cement. The device can be distracted after placement to facilitate vertebral body height restoration and is designed to support the surrounding bone [85]. Similar to OsseoFix®, SpineJack® also shares the benefit of needing less cement than balloon-assisted procedures. In studies that directly compare its performance to conventional augmentation procedures, SpineJack® has been found to maintain vertebral height, correct kyphosis, and limit refractures better than traditional kyphoplasty for osteoporotic and trauma-induced VCFs [86–88]. In a prospective, consecutive, multicenter observational registry study of 103 patients with 108 traumatic VCF, Noriega et al. reported no adverse events with no need for removal and a 1-year adjacent fracture rate of 2.9% [89]. The subsequent multicenter randomized controlled SAKOS trial [90] compared SpineJack® and balloon kyphoplasty for osteoporotic VCF and found the SpineJack® device to offer superior vertebral height restoration at 6 and 12 months. Patients treated with SpineJack® also achieved the primary composite outcome, where the composite outcome was defined as improvement in fracture-related pain with maintenance or improvement in functional status and without device-related adverse events or surgical reintervention.

Radiofrequency Kyphoplasty

Radiofrequency kyphoplasty (RFK) was developed in 2009 for the treatment of VCF due to a variety of underlying disease processes. In RFK, an articulating osteotome creates channels within the cancellous bone of the affected vertebrae and then the vertebral body is filled with ultrahigh viscosity cement [91]. The artificial channels allow for improved integration of the cement within the cancellous bone, further reinforcing stability [91]. RFK has been used in patients with painful aggressive primary and metastatic spine tumors and in patients with VCFs due to osteoporosis that fail conservative management. In one prospective study comparing 80 patients with osteoporotic VCF treated with RFK or balloon kyphoplasty, RFK required less cement and offered greater reduction in the kyphotic deformity while producing similar reductions in pain at 12 months [92]. In another prospective single-armed study of patients who underwent RFK for myeloma-related VCFs, Ali et al. showed that at 12-month follow up, patients demonstrated a marked reduction in pain, disability, and angle of kyphosis [93]. However, all three outcome measures gradually worsened between 12- and 24-month follow-up, and 10% of patients experienced new fractures [93]. To date, no large, randomized control trials have been completed; thus, further studies are needed to validate the findings described above.

Radiofrequency Ablation

Radiofrequency ablation (RFA) is a fluoroscopy- or computer tomography (CT)-guided interventional technique that uses electrical energy to heat tissue to roughly 90 °C and cause tumor necrosis [94–97]. Both bipolar and monopolar configurations use a generator to produce a rapidly alternating current that is transferred between an cathode and an anode [16]. The small cross-sectional area of the needle tip allows for a high-energy flux that excites ions in the tissue it contacts, resulting in extensive heating and cell death [16, 98]. Of note, the current transmitted through the RFA needle tip is not visible with standard imaging and thus, utilization of this technique requires extensive knowledge of the lesion anatomy [16, 98]. However, there has been increased use of cone beam CT which allows for a more precise localization of ablation probes.

The role of RFA in bony spine disease is primarily palliative pain control, though it can help with local control in metastatic disease and some aggressive primary tumors [94–97]. While some studies have suggested isolated RFA to have similar efficacy when compared to traditional kyphoplasty for pathologic VCFs [99], it is common practice to pair RFA with cement augmentation (Fig. 7.7). RFA allows for lesional ablation and may enable cement to be injected at lower pressure. In one prospective, single-institution study of 12 patients with malignant VCFs treated with RFA and vertebroplasty, Song et al. found that 92% of patients reported good or excellent pain relief [100]. In another single-institution, prospective study of 30 patients with vertebral body metastases, Sayed et al. found combined RFA and vertebroplasty was associated with significantly improved pain and quality of life at 3 days, 1 week, and 1 and 2 months following the procedure [101]. Subsequent studies by Ragheb et al. [102] and Wang et al. [103] similarly endorsed good results. Ragheb et al. [102] similarly noted good improvements in pain up to 6 months post-procedurally but also noted lower rates of local tumor recurrence relative to historic

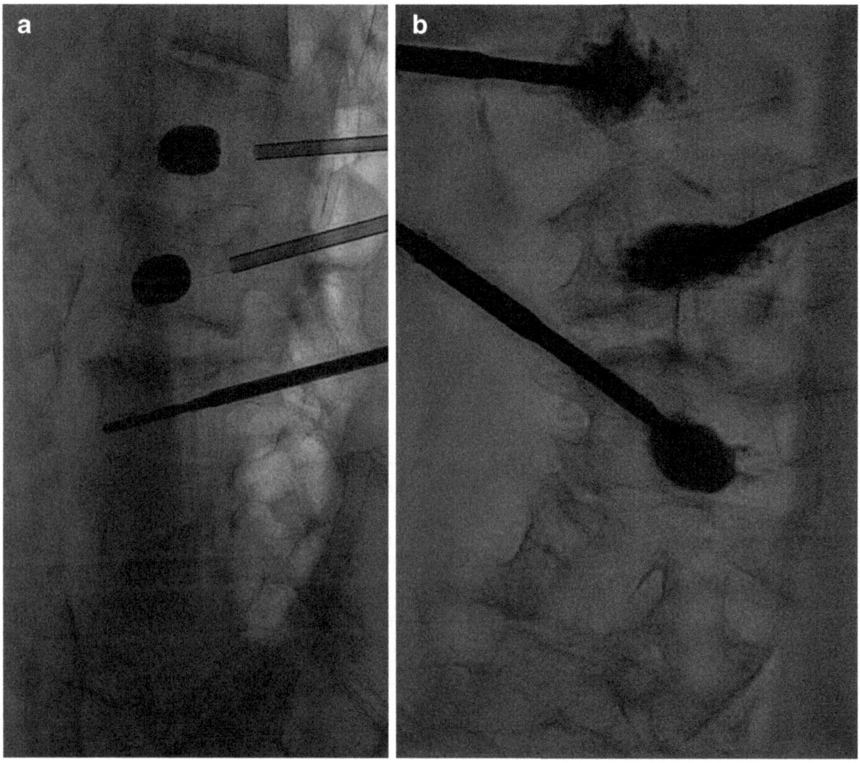

Fig. 7.7 (**a**) Lateral and (**b**) PA films demonstrating radio-frequency ablation followed by osteoplasty and cement augmentation

literature values, suggesting the addition of RFA may improve local tumor control. Last, Wang et al. compared RFA and vertebroplasty to vertebroplasty alone and noted patients in the combined group had better pain outcomes at 6 months and lower rates of cement leak [103]. Additional investigation is merited and cryoablation may serve a similar function to RFA when paired with cement augmentation [32, 104–106].

Conclusion

Given the frailty of many patients with metastatic disease, alternatives to surgical intervention are often preferred. Cement augmentation with vertebroplasty and kyphoplasty are effective options for stabilization of vertebral body metastases with mild-to-moderate associated stability. Augmentation of these approaches with additional device implantation (e.g., OsseoFix®, SpineJack®, and Kiva system) may help improve the load-bearing properties of affected vertebra while offering similar to improved deformity correction and lower rates of cement leakage. Additionally, RFA and cryoablation may be combined with augmentation procedures to decrease cement leakage and improve local control. Prior to pursuing any of these interventions the fracture must be carefully assayed for evidence of posterior cortex compromise, active infection, or complete vertebral collapse, all of which are absolute or relative contraindications to cement augmentation. None of these interventions can supplant surgery for severe deformity, but they appear to be good, minimally invasive options for select patients.

References

1. Montagu A, Speirs A, Baldock J, Corbett J, Gosney M (2012) A review of vertebroplasty for osteoporotic and malignant vertebral compression fractures. Age Ageing 41:450–455
2. Tobert DG, Schwab JH (2019) Pathologic vertebral fractures: diagnosis, treatment, complications, and controversies through case-based learning. Instr Course Lect 68:585–591
3. Alexandru D, So W (2012) Evaluation and management of vertebral compression fractures. Perm J 16:46–51
4. Robinson Y, Heyde CE, Försth P, Olerud C (2011) Kyphoplasty in osteoporotic vertebral compression fractures – guidelines and technical considerations. J Orthop Surg Res 6:43
5. Imamudeen N, Basheer A, Iqbal AM, Manjila N, Haroon NN, Manjila S (2022) Management of osteoporosis and spinal fractures: contemporary guidelines and evolving paradigms. Clin Med Res 20:95–106
6. Barr JD, Barr MS, Lemley TJ, McCann RM (2000) Percutaneous vertebroplasty for pain relief and spinal stabilization. Spine (Phila Pa 1976) 25:923–928
7. Lindsay R (2001) Risk of new vertebral fracture in the year following a fracture. JAMA 285:320
8. Yeung Y-K, Ho S-T (2017) Delayed neurological deficits after osteoporotic vertebral fractures: clinical outcomes after surgery. Asian Spine J 11:981–988
9. Hoyt D, Urits I, Orhurhu V, Orhurhu MS, Callan J, Powell J, Manchikanti L, Kaye AD, Kaye RJ, Viswanath O (2020) Current concepts in the management of vertebral compression fractures. Curr Pain Headache Rep 24:16
10. Lau E, Ong K, Kurtz S, Schmier J, Edidin A (2008) Mortality following the diagnosis of a vertebral compression fracture in the medicare population. J Bone Joint Surg Am 90:1479–1486
11. Health Quality Ontario (2016) Vertebral augmentation involving vertebroplasty or kyphoplasty for cancer-related vertebral compression fractures: a systematic review. Ont Health Technol Assess Ser 16:1–202
12. Clark W, Bird P, Gonski P, Diamond TH, Smerdely P, McNeil HP, Schlaphoff G, Bryant C, Barnes E, Gebski V (2016) Safety and efficacy of vertebroplasty for acute painful osteoporotic fractures (VAPOUR): a multicentre, randomised, double-blind, placebo-controlled trial. Lancet 388:1408–1416
13. Firanescu CE, de Vries J, Lodder P et al (2018) Vertebroplasty versus sham procedure for painful acute osteoporotic vertebral compression fractures (VERTOS IV): randomised sham controlled clinical trial. BMJ 361:k1551
14. Solberg J, Copenhaver D, Fishman SM (2016) Medial branch nerve block and ablation as a novel approach to pain related to vertebral compression fracture. Curr Opin Anaesthesiol 29:596–599
15. Dassa M, Roux C, Tselikas L et al (2020) Image-guided percutaneous fixation with internal cemented screws of impending femoral neck pathologic fractures in patients with metastatic cancer: safety, efficacy, and durability. Radiology 297:721–729

16. Ahmed O, Feinberg N, Lea WB (2019) Interventional techniques for the ablation and augmentation of extraspinal lytic bone metastases. Semin Intervent Radiol 36:221–228
17. Lad SP, Patil CG, Lad EM, Boakye M (2007) Trends in pathological vertebral fractures in the United States: 1993 to 2004. J Neurosurg Spine 7:305–310
18. Meunier P, Delmas P, Eastell R, McClung M, Papapoulos S, Rizzoli R, Seeman E, Wasnich R (1999) Diagnosis and management of osteoporosis in postmenopausal women: clinical guidelines. Clin Ther 21:1025–1044
19. Lindsay R, Burge RT, Strauss DM (2005) One year outcomes and costs following a vertebral fracture. Osteoporos Int 16:78–85
20. Ross PD, Genant HK, Davis JW, Miller PD, Wasnich RD (1993) Predicting vertebral fracture incidence from prevalent fractures and bone density among non-black, osteoporotic women. Osteoporos Int 3:120–126
21. Saad F, Lipton A, Cook R, Chen Y-M, Smith M, Coleman R (2007) Pathologic fractures correlate with reduced survival in patients with malignant bone disease. Cancer 110:1860–1867
22. Eseonu KC, Panchmatia JR, Streetly MJ, Grauer JN, Fakouri B (2023) The role of vertebral augmentation procedures in the management of vertebral compression fractures secondary to multiple myeloma. Hematol Oncol 41:323–334
23. Hashi S, Goodwin CR, Ahmed AK, Sciubba DM (2018) Management of extranodal lymphoma of the spine: a study of 30 patients. CNS Oncol 7:CNS11
24. Uehara M, Takahashi J, Hirabayashi H, Kitahara J, Kamijyo T, Ebara S, Kato H (2013) Hodgkin's disease of the thoracic vertebrae. Spine J 13:e59–e63
25. Kim DH, Vaccaro AR (2006) Osteoporotic compression fractures of the spine; current options and considerations for treatment. Spine J 6:479–487
26. Truumees E, Hilibrand A, Vaccaro AR (2004) Percutaneous vertebral augmentation. Spine J 4:218–229
27. Theodorou DJ, Theodorou SJ, Duncan TD, Garfin SR, Wong WH (2002) Percutaneous balloon kyphoplasty for the correction of spinal deformity in painful vertebral body compression fractures. Clin Imaging 26:1–5
28. Vaccaro AR, Kim DH, Brodke DS, Harris M, Chapman JR, Schildhauer T, Routt ML, Sasso RC (2004) Diagnosis and management of thoracolumbar spine fractures. Instr Course Lect 53:359–373
29. Wu SS, Lachmann E, Nagler W (2003) Current medical, rehabilitation, and surgical management of vertebral compression fractures. J Women's Heal 12:17–26
30. Aghayev K, Papanastassiou ID, Vrionis F (2011) Role of vertebral augmentation procedures in the management of vertebral compression fractures in cancer patients. Curr Opin Support Palliat Care 5:222–226
31. Pennington Z, Ehresman J, Cottrill E, Lubelski D, Lehner K, Feghali J, Ahmed AK, Schilling A, Sciubba DM (2021) To operate, or not to operate? Narrative review of the role of survival predictors in patient selection for operative management of patients with metastatic spine disease. J Neurosurg Spine 34:135–149
32. Sciubba DM, Pennington Z, Colman MW et al (2021) Spinal metastases 2021: a review of the current state of the art and future directions. Spine J 21:1414–1429
33. Foro Arnalot P, Fontanals AV, Galcerán JC et al (2008) Randomized clinical trial with two palliative radiotherapy regimens in painful bone metastases: 30Gy in 10 fractions compared with 8Gy in single fraction. Radiother Oncol 89:150–155
34. Mikula AL, Pennington Z, Lakomkin N et al (2022) Independent predictors of vertebral compression fracture following radiation for metastatic spine disease. J Neurosurg Spine 37:617–623
35. Pennington Z, Mikula AL, Lakomkin N et al (2023) Comparison of Hounsfield units and vertebral bone quality score for the prediction of time to pathologic fracture in mobile spine metastases treated with radiotherapy. J Neurosurg Spine 40:19–27

36. Kowalchuk RO, Johnson-Tesch BA, Marion JT et al (2022) Development and assessment of a predictive score for vertebral compression fracture after stereotactic body radiation therapy for spinal metastases. JAMA Oncol 8:412
37. Sahgal A, Atenafu EG, Chao S et al (2013) Vertebral compression fracture after spine stereotactic body radiotherapy: a multi-institutional analysis with a focus on radiation dose and the spinal instability neoplastic score. J Clin Oncol 31:3426–3431
38. Tseng C-L, Soliman H, Myrehaug S et al (2018) Imaging-based outcomes for 24 Gy in 2 daily fractions for patients with de novo spinal metastases treated with spine stereotactic body radiation therapy (SBRT). Int J Radiat Oncol 102:499–507
39. Lockney DT, Hopkins B, Lockney NA et al (2019) Adjacent level fracture incidence in single fraction high dose spinal radiosurgery. Ann Transl Med 7:211–211
40. Lyles KW, Gold DT, Shipp KM, Pieper CF, Martinez S, Mulhausen PL (1993) Association of osteoporotic vertebral compression fractures with impaired functional status. Am J Med 94:595–601
41. Lyritis GP, Mayasis B, Tsakalakos N, Lambropoulos A, Gazi S, Karachalios T, Tsekoura M, Yiatzides A (1989) The natural history of the osteoporotic vertebral fracture. Clin Rheumatol 8:66–69
42. Phillips FM, Pfeifer BA, Lieberman IH, Kerr EJ, Choi IS, Pazianos AG (2003) Minimally invasive treatments of osteoporotic vertebral compression fractures: vertebroplasty and kyphoplasty. Instr Course Lect 52:559–567
43. Shaibani A, Ali S, Bhatt H (2007) Vertebroplasty and kyphoplasty for the palliation of pain. Semin Intervent Radiol 24:409–418
44. Galibert P, Deramond H, Rosat P, Le Gars D (1987) Preliminary note on the treatment of vertebral angioma by percutaneous acrylic vertebroplasty. Neurochirurgie 33:166–168
45. Tohmeh AG, Mathis JM, Fenton DC, Levine AM, Belkoff SM (1999) Biomechanical efficacy of unipedicular versus bipedicular vertebroplasty for the management of osteoporotic compression fractures. Spine (Phila Pa 1976) 24:1772–1776
46. Belkoff SM, Mathis JM, Jasper LE, Deramond H (2001) The biomechanics of vertebroplasty. The effect of cement volume on mechanical behavior. Spine (Phila Pa 1976) 26:1537–1541
47. Buchbinder R, Johnston RV, Rischin KJ, Homik J, Jones CA, Golmohammadi K, Kallmes DF (2018) Percutaneous vertebroplasty for osteoporotic vertebral compression fracture. Cochrane Database Syst Rev 2018:CD006349
48. Lieberman I, Reinhardt MK (2003) Vertebroplasty and kyphoplasty for osteolytic vertebral collapse. Clin Orthop Relat Res 415:S176–S186
49. Chen Y-C, Zhang L, Li E-N, Ding L-X, Zhang G-A, Hou Y, Yuan W (2019) Unilateral versus bilateral percutaneous vertebroplasty for osteoporotic vertebral compression fractures in elderly patients. Medicine (Baltimore) 98:e14317
50. Yin P, Ji Q, Wang Y, Liu Y, Wu Y, Yu Y, Hai Y, Su Q (2019) Percutaneous kyphoplasty for osteoporotic vertebral compression fractures via unilateral versus bilateral approach: a meta-analysis. J Clin Neurosci 59:146–154
51. Kallmes DF, Comstock BA, Heagerty PJ et al (2009) A randomized trial of vertebroplasty for osteoporotic spinal fractures. N Engl J Med 361:569–579
52. Buchbinder R, Osborne RH, Ebeling PR, Wark JD, Mitchell P, Wriedt C, Graves S, Staples MP, Murphy B (2009) A randomized trial of vertebroplasty for painful osteoporotic vertebral fractures. N Engl J Med 361:557–568
53. Yang W, Song J, Liang M, Cui H, Chen H, Yang J (2019) Functional outcomes and new vertebral fractures in percutaneous vertebroplasty and conservative treatment of acute symptomatic osteoporotic vertebral compression fractures. World Neurosurg 131:e346–e352
54. Thillainadesan J, Schlaphoff G, Gibson K, Hassett G, McNeil H (2010) Long-term outcomes of vertebroplasty for osteoporotic compression fractures. J Med Imaging Radiat Oncol 54:307–314
55. Reinas R, Kitumba D, Pereira L, Alves O (2021) Minimally invasive surgery for spinal fractures due to multiple myeloma. J Craniovertebr Junction Spine 12:117–122

56. Ramazanoglu AF, Sarikaya C, Etli MU, Yaltirik CK, Onen MR, Naderi S (2022) Results of percutaneous cervical vertebroplasty using an anterolateral approach for cervical spine tumors. Acta Orthop Traumatol Turc 56:268–271
57. Zhu Q, Qiao Y, Li T et al (2022) Study on the clinical efficacy of bone-filled mesh vertebroplasty combined with posterior screw and rod internal fixation in the treatment of thoracolumbar metastases: a retrospective cohort study. Ann Palliat Med 11:1401–1409
58. Waits C, Burton D, McIff T (2009) Cement augmentation of pedicle screw fixation using novel cannulated cement insertion device. Spine (Phila Pa 1976) 34:E478–E483
59. Ehresman J, Pennington Z, Elsamadicy AA et al (2021) Fenestrated pedicle screws for thoracolumbar instrumentation in patients with poor bone quality: case series and systematic review of the literature. Clin Neurol Neurosurg 206:106675
60. Long Y, Yi W, Yang D (2020) Advances in vertebral augmentation systems for osteoporotic vertebral compression fractures. Pain Res Manag 2020:1–9
61. Nieuwenhuijse MJ, Van Erkel AR, Dijkstra PDS (2011) Cement leakage in percutaneous vertebroplasty for osteoporotic vertebral compression fractures: identification of risk factors. Spine J 11:839–848
62. Bula P, Lein T, Straßberger C, Bonnaire F (2010) Ballonkyphoplastie zur Behandlung osteoporotischer Wirbelfrakturen: Indikationen – Behandlungsstrategie – Komplikationen. Z Orthop Unfall 148:646–656
63. Martín-Fernández M, López-Herradón A, Piñera AR, Tomé-Bermejo F, Duart JM, Vlad MD, Rodríguez-Arguisjuela MG, Alvarez-Galovich L (2017) Potential risks of using cement-augmented screws for spinal fusion in patients with low bone quality. Spine J 17:1192–1199
64. Martin DJ, Rad AE, Kallmes DF (2012) Prevalence of extravertebral cement leakage after vertebroplasty: procedural documentation versus CT detection. Acta Radiol 53:569–572
65. Trout AT, Kallmes DF, Kaufmann TJ (2006) New fractures after vertebroplasty: adjacent fractures occur significantly sooner. Am J Neuroradiol 27:217–223
66. Zou P, Gong H-L, Wei J-M, Wei D-M, Qian L-X, Liu P, Hao D-J, Yang J-S, Zhao Y-T (2020) Spinal epidural hematoma after percutaneous kyphoplasty: case report and literature review. J Pain Res 13:2799–2804
67. Boonen S, Van Meirhaeghe J, Bastian L, Cummings SR, Ranstam J, Tillman JB, Eastell R, Talmadge K, Wardlaw D (2011) Balloon kyphoplasty for the treatment of acute vertebral compression fractures: 2-year results from a randomized trial. J Bone Miner Res 26:1627–1637
68. Zhu J, Zhang K, Luo K, Qiu Z, Yang S, Cui F, Weng X, Jiang G (2019) Mineralized collagen modified Polymethyl methacrylate bone cement for osteoporotic compression vertebral fracture at 1-year follow-up. Spine (Phila Pa 1976) 44:827–838
69. Voggenreiter G (2005) Balloon kyphoplasty is effective in deformity correction of osteoporotic vertebral compression fractures. Spine (Phila Pa 1976) 30:2806–2812
70. Dohm M, Black CM, Dacre A, Tillman JB, Fueredi G (2014) A randomized trial comparing balloon kyphoplasty and vertebroplasty for vertebral compression fractures due to osteoporosis. Am J Neuroradiol 35:2227–2236
71. Liang L, Chen X, Jiang W, Li X, Chen J, Wu L, Zhu Y (2016) Balloon kyphoplasty or percutaneous vertebroplasty for osteoporotic vertebral compression fracture? An updated systematic review and meta-analysis. Ann Saudi Med 36:165–174
72. Berenson J, Pflugmacher R, Jarzem P, Zonder J, Schechtman K, Tillman JB, Bastian L, Ashraf T, Vrionis F (2011) Balloon kyphoplasty versus non-surgical fracture management for treatment of painful vertebral body compression fractures in patients with cancer: a multicentre, randomised controlled trial. Lancet Oncol 12:225–235
73. Zhan Y, Jiang J, Liao H, Tan H, Yang K (2017) Risk factors for cement leakage after vertebroplasty or kyphoplasty: a meta-analysis of published evidence. World Neurosurg 101:633–642
74. Peh WCG, Gilula LA, Peck DD (2002) Percutaneous vertebroplasty for severe osteoporotic vertebral body compression fractures. Radiology 223:121–126

75. Zhang H, Xu C, Zhang T, Gao Z, Zhang T (2017) Does percutaneous vertebroplasty or balloon kyphoplasty for osteoporotic vertebral compression fractures increase the incidence of new vertebral fractures? A meta-analysis. Pain Physician 20:E13–E28
76. Zhu R-S, Kan S-L, Ning G-Z, Chen L-X, Cao Z-G, Jiang Z-H, Zhang X-L, Hu W (2019) Which is the best treatment of osteoporotic vertebral compression fractures: balloon kyphoplasty, percutaneous vertebroplasty, or non-surgical treatment? A Bayesian network meta-analysis. Osteoporos Int 30:287–298
77. Kopparapu S, Lubelski D, Pennington Z, Khan M, Theodore N, Sciubba D (2021) Comparison of operator and patient radiation exposure during fluoroscopy-guided vertebroplasty and kyphoplasty: a systematic review and meta-analysis. J Neurosurg Spine 35:117–126
78. Rosales Olivarez LM, Dipp JM, Escamilla RF, Bajares G, Perez A, Stubbs HA, Block JE (2011) Vertebral augmentation treatment of painful osteoporotic compression fractures with the kiva VCF treatment system. SAS J 5:114–119
79. Otten LA, Bornemnn R, Jansen TR, Kabir K, Pennekamp PH, Wirtz DC, Stuwe B, Pflugmacher R (2013) Comparison of balloon kyphoplasty with the new kiva® VCF system for the treatment of vertebral compression fractures. Pain Physician 16:E505–E512
80. Korovessis P, Vardakastanis K, Repantis T, Vitsas V (2013) Balloon kyphoplasty versus kiva vertebral augmentation – comparison of 2 techniques for osteoporotic vertebral body fractures. Spine (Phila Pa 1976) 38:292–299
81. Tutton SM, Pflugmacher R, Davidian M, Beall DP, Facchini FR, Garfin SR (2015) KAST study: the kiva system as a vertebral augmentation treatment-a safety and effectiveness trial: a randomized, noninferiority trial comparing the kiva system with balloon kyphoplasty in treatment of osteoporotic vertebral compression fractures. Spine (Phila Pa 1976) 40:865–875
82. Vanni D, Galzio R, Kazakova A, Pantalone A, Grillea G, Bartolo M, Salini V, Magliani V (2016) Third-generation percutaneous vertebral augmentation systems. J Spine Surg 2:13–20
83. Ender SA, Wetterau E, Ender M, Kühn J-P, Merk HR, Kayser R (2013) Percutaneous stabilization system Osseofix® for treatment of osteoporotic vertebral compression fractures – clinical and radiological results after 12 months. PLoS One 8:e65119
84. Ender SA, Gradl G, Ender M, Langner S, Merk HR, Kayser R (2013) Osseofix® system for percutaneous stabilization of osteoporotic and tumorous vertebral compression fractures – clinical and radiological results after 12 months. RöFo 186:380–387
85. Vanni D, Pantalone A, Bigossi F, Pineto F, Lucantoni D, Salini V (2012) New perspective for third generation percutaneous vertebral augmentation procedures: preliminary results at 12 months. J Craniovertebr Junction Spine 3:47
86. Noriega DC, Rodríguez-Monsalve F, Ramajo R, Sánchez-Lite I, Toribio B, Ardura F (2019) Long-term safety and clinical performance of kyphoplasty and SpineJack® procedures in the treatment of osteoporotic vertebral compression fractures: a pilot, monocentric, investigator-initiated study. Osteoporos Int 30:637–645
87. Krüger A, Baroud G, Noriega D, Figiel J, Dorschel C, Ruchholtz S, Oberkircher L (2013) Height restoration and maintenance after treating unstable osteoporotic vertebral compression fractures by cement augmentation is dependent on the cement volume used. Clin Biomech 28:725–730
88. Lin J-H, Wang S-H, Lin E-Y, Chiang Y-H (2016) Better height restoration, greater kyphosis correction, and fewer refractures of cemented vertebrae by using an intravertebral reduction device: a 1-year follow-up study. World Neurosurg 90:391–396
89. Noriega D, Maestretti G, Renaud C et al (2015) Clinical performance and safety of 108 SpineJack implantations: 1-year results of a prospective multicentre single-arm registry study. Biomed Res Int 2015:1–10
90. Noriega D, Marcia S, Theumann N et al (2019) A prospective, international, randomized, noninferiority study comparing an implantable titanium vertebral augmentation device versus balloon kyphoplasty in the reduction of vertebral compression fractures (SAKOS study). Spine J 19:1782–1795

91. Hegazy R, El-Mowafi H, Hadhood M, Hannout Y, Allam Y, Silbermann J (2019) The outcome of radiofrequency kyphoplasty in the treatment of vertebral compression fractures in osteoporotic patients. Asian Spine J 13:459–467
92. Petersen A, Hartwig E, Koch EMW, Wollny M (2016) Clinical comparison of postoperative results of balloon kyphoplasty (BKP) versus radiofrequency-targeted vertebral augmentation (RF-TVA): a prospective clinical study. Eur J Orthop Surg Traumatol 26:67–75
93. Ali T, Bornemann R, Roessler PP, Sander K, Wirtz DC, Pflugmacher R, Frey SP (2016) Mid-term outcomes after radiofrequency-targeted vertebral augmentation in the treatment of myeloma associated vertebral fractures. Technol Health Care 24:745–751
94. Goetz MP, Callstrom MR, Charboneau JW et al (2004) Percutaneous image-guided radiofrequency ablation of painful metastases involving bone: a multicenter study. J Clin Oncol 22:300–306
95. Callstrom MR, Charboneau JW, Goetz MP et al (2002) Painful metastases involving bone: feasibility of percutaneous CT- and US-guided radio-frequency ablation. Radiology 224:87–97
96. Carrafiello G, Laganà D, Ianniello A, Nicotera P, Fontana F, Dizonno M, Cuffari S, Fugazzola C (2009) Radiofrequency thermal ablation for pain control in patients with single painful bone metastasis from hepatocellular carcinoma. Eur J Radiol 71:363–368
97. Dupuy DE, Liu D, Hartfeil D, Hanna L, Blume JD, Ahrar K, Lopez R, Safran H, DiPetrillo T (2010) Percutaneous radiofrequency ablation of painful osseous metastases. Cancer 116:989–997
98. Guenette JP, Lopez MJ, Kim E, Dupuy DE (2013) Solitary painful osseous metastases: correlation of imaging features with pain palliation after radiofrequency ablation – a multicenter American college of radiology imaging network study. Radiology 268:907–915
99. Jain S, Kinch L, Rana M, Anitescu M (2020) Comparison of post-operative pain scores and opioid use between kyphoplasty and radiofrequency ablation (RFA) systems combined with cement augmentation. Skeletal Radiol 49:1789–1794
100. Song H-M, Gu Y-F, Li Y-D, Wu C-G, Sun Z-K, He C-J (2014) Interventional tumor removal: a new technique for malignant spinal tumor and malignant vertebral compression fractures without epidural involvement. Acta Radiol 55:976–984
101. Sayed D, Jacobs D, Sowder T, Haines D, Orr W (2019) Spinal radiofrequency ablation combined with cement augmentation for painful spinal vertebral metastasis: a single-center prospective study. Pain Physician 22:E441–E449
102. Ragheb A, Vanood A, Fahim DK (2022) The addition of radiofrequency tumor ablation to kyphoplasty may reduce the rate of local recurrence in spinal metastases secondary to breast cancer. World Neurosurg 161:e500–e507
103. Wang F, Gu J, Xu C, Li G, Lv P (2022) The combination of radiofrequency ablation and vertebroplasty shows advantages over single vertebroplasty in treating vertebral neoplastic lesions. Skeletal Radiol 51:565–571
104. Sagoo NS, Haider AS, Ozair A et al (2022) Percutaneous image-guided cryoablation of spinal metastases: a systematic review. J Clin Neurosci 96:120–126
105. Moses ZB, Lee TC, Huang KT, Guenette JP, Chi JH (2020) MRI-guided cryoablation for metastatic spine disease: intermediate-term clinical outcomes in 14 consecutive patients. J Neurosurg Spine 32:676–681
106. Hadzipasic M, Giantini-Larsen AM, Tatsui CE, Shin JH (2020) Emerging percutaneous ablative and radiosurgical techniques for treatment of spinal metastases. Neurosurg Clin N Am 31:141–150

Chapter 8
Pathological Fractures Following High-Dose Radiation

Grace X. Xiong and Joseph H. Schwab

Introduction

The bony spine is one of the most common sites for metastatic disease, being affected in up to 70% of cancer patients on post-mortem studies [1]. Significant advances in palliative therapies have allowed for significant symptomatic relief, and the advent of focused radiation modalities such as stereotactic body radiation therapy (SBRT) have allowed for improved local control relative to conventional external beam radiation therapy (EBRT) [2–5]. Nonetheless, complications of radiation therapy persist, and some, notably vertebral column fractures (VCF), may be more frequent in patients treated with these focused modalities. Post-radiotherapy fractures can range from incidental asymptomatic fractures with minimal height loss to highly symptoms fractures that cause functional decline and increased narcotic usage [6]. The goal of this chapter is to cover pathophysiology, risk factors, initial evaluation, and a summary of possible treatment options for pathologic vertebral fractures following high-dose radiation.

G. X. Xiong
Department of Orthopaedic Surgery, Stanford University, Redwood City, CA, USA
e-mail: gxiong@stanford.edu

J. H. Schwab (✉)
Department of Orthopaedic Surgery, Cedars Sinai Medical Center, Los Angeles, CA, USA
e-mail: Joseph.schwab@cshs.org

D. M. Sciubba (ed.), *Spinal Tumor Associated Deformity*,
https://doi.org/10.1007/978-3-031-87939-5_8

Pathophysiology

Radiation therapy has well-described deleterious impacts on bone health. In particular, hematopoietic stem cells are sensitive to radiation effects even more so than mesenchymal stem cells (MSCs) [7], resulting in fat marrow replacement and increased intramedullary adiposity [7, 8]. In vitro work has suggested that one of the possible effects of radiation on bone may be altering MSC differentiation away from the osteoblast lineage and toward an adipocyte [9] or osteoclast lineage [10], resulting in fatty marrow replacement. Additionally, osteoblasts appear to be far more radiation susceptible to radiation than MSCs [9, 11], which are relatively radiation resistant [7, 12]. This results in bone changes primarily derived from osteoblast impedance more so than upregulation of resorption [9]. Prior studies in mouse models have demonstrated cellular changes start as early as 2 weeks following radiation [9, 13], mediated by downregulation of growth factors and changes in mineral/matrix ratios and collagen crosslink ratios. These changes include reduced trabecular thickness and volume [14] and increased trabecular spacing [15]. Radiotherapy appears to affect both cancellous bone and all components of cortical bone, from the periosteum through the endosteal region [16]. Such morphological changes lead to worsening of the load-bearing properties of irradiated vertebra with Emerzian et al. showing fractionated radiotherapy (30Gy delivered in 10 fractions) to reduce bone strength by 28% when subjected to axial loading. Decreases in bone strength were proportional to changes in bone mass. Mouse models have also demonstrated deleterious effects on regions adjoining the irradiated tissue, but which are not in the treatment field proper. Specifically, Zou et al. noted decreases in contralateral limb trabecular volume and increases in cortical porosity in a rat model of lower extremity radiotherapy [9].

Mouse models and in vitro studies have additionally provided some insights regarding how the aforementioned changes in underlying bone microarchitecture may be prevented. One such intervention is cyclical loading. Govey and colleagues [17] demonstrated this in a murine model of bone marrow transplant. Mice were treated with 600 + 475 cGy split dose of whole body and then subjected to cyclical mechanical loading of the tibia 5 days per week for a 3-week regimen. Comparison of the tibial microarchitecture using micro-CT (μCT) showed significantly greater decreases in trabecular bone volume and trabecular connectivity relative to mice who were irradiated and not loaded. Additionally, mice undergoing loading showed increased trabecular thickness and tissue mineral density relative to baseline, consistent with the known principles of Wolff's law—bone will adapt to mechanical loading [18]. However, the effectiveness of such loading protocols has yet to be tested in the clinical sphere to any significant extent. An additional potentially protective mechanism is through the use of pulsed electromagnetic fields. Again using a rodent hindlimb radiation model, Yan and colleagues [19] demonstrated that application of a 15 Hz, 2mT pulsed electrical magnetic field was able to stimulate expression of osteogenic genes and proteins in irradiated osteoblasts. More importantly, histologic staining of irradiated femora in rats that had been treated with the pulsed electromagnetic fields showed significant improvements in trabecular thickness, trabecular number, and bone volume fraction along with a significant decrease in trabecular spacing. Biomechanical testing was not done, but the initial results are promising. Externally applied pulsed electromagnetic field devices have been clinically approved and suggested to have some efficacy for improving fusion rates in the degenerative population, though the overall quality of evidence is weak [20]. Given the noninvasive nature of these devices though, further investigation in the oncology population is merited.

Risk Factors for Pathologic Fracture

Vertebral column fractures (VCF) in the setting of radiation therapy have described incidence rates that vary based on methods of radiation therapy. Vertebral column fractures in the setting of stereotactic body radiation therapy (SBRT) was initially described in 2009 by collaborators at Memorial Sloan Kettering Cancer Center [6]. They described a 38% VCF rate in a series of 61 patients (71 lesions) who received a single fraction SBRT with doses ranging from 18 to 24 Gy. This early series noted that the occurrence of VCF was independently predicted by lytic [vs mixed/sclerotic] bone quality and the lesion occupying >40% of the vertebral body. These data concord with both earlier and subsequent cadaveric data [21–27]. For example, Stadelmann and colleagues [21] tested 11 cadaver spines from patients with known primary tumors and found that lytic lesions deformed at significantly lower pressures than mixed or blastic lesions in an axial loading model of compression fracture. MicroCT of the lytic lesions also demonstrated more expansive degradation of the trabecular bone network, providing an explanation for the decreased loading capacity. Alkalay et al. [27] similarly found blastic lesions to have greater axial compression tolerances. They also found that volumetric bone mineral density estimates derived from μCT also predicted failure strength in blastic and mixed-type lesions. Tschirhart and colleagues employed a finite element model to demonstrate that tumor location likely influences failure mode [22], with tumors situated posteriorly within the vertebral body having increased risk of pathologic burst fracture. Using a similar model they also suggested larger tumor size is associated with greater fracture risk [23]. These findings were echoed by Ebihara and colleagues [24] in an ovine model using fresh thoracic spine preparations. Consistent with the findings of Rose et al. [6] regarding SBRT, Ebihara and colleagues noted lesions occupying 40% of the vertebral cross-sectional area were associated with a 25% decrease in failure load.

Incidence rates for conventional external beam therapy (EBRT) have been reported to be lower than rates for SBRT—5% versus 11–39% for SBRT with further increases in SBRT regimens employed dose per fraction above 19 Gy [28, 29]. One study [30] conducted a direct comparison between EBRT and SBRT in 90 propensity-matched patients (45 in each group) and found significantly higher 5-year rates of VCF (22.2%) compared with EBRT (6.7%).

Several large-scale pooled studies have examined risk factors for VCF following radiotherapy. One multi-institutional study of 252 patients treated with SBRT (410 treated levels) saw a 14% overall VCF rate of which 47% were new fractures and 53% were progressions of existing fractures [29]. The authors noted that independent risk factors for VCF were dose per fraction, pre-existing VCF, lytic tumor quality (vs blastic/mixed), and the presence of pre-existing spinal deformity. Another multi-institutional pooled study of 541 patients (594 treated tumors) observed new VCF in only 3% of patients and progressive VCF in 2.7% using a median dose of 20 Gy delivered in one fraction [31]. Independent risk factors for VCF again included pre-existing VCF; other factors were the presence of a solitary metastasis and a prescribed radiation dose of 38.4 Gy or more. A sub-analysis focusing only on new VCF found the only independent risk factors were the presence of a solitary metastasis and lack of MRI for target delineation. Finally, Mantel et al. published the results of a multinational European phase II SBRT trial of 56 patients (61 lesions). VCF occurred in 34.4% VCF rate, of which 18.0% were new and 16.4% progressive VCF [32]. It is important to note that only three patients were symptomatic in this cohort. Multivariable analysis demonstrated that the relative amount of vertebral body involvement, the osteolytic volume, and pre-existing VCF were predictive of subsequent VCF. In these studies, it appears that in general pre-existing VCF, higher radiation doses, and larger or lytic lesions are associated with new or progressive fracture risk.

More recent studies have focused on developing predictive scores and algorithms for pre-procedural risk stratification. One study from the Mayo Clinic [33] developed a predictive score for VCF following SBRT using a cohort of 331 patients (464 treatments) treated with either single fraction (16–24Gy) or multifraction SBRT (median 30 Gy). Using a 70%/15%/15% training/validation/testing protocol they devised a scoring algorithm allocating one point each to: gross tumor volume greater than 10 cc, lumbar location, epidural extension, and a SINS greater than 6. Analysis identified three patient tiers: low risk (0–1 points), intermediate risk (2 points), and high risk (3–4 points) with distinct cumulative hazard of new VCF. "High-risk" patients had a 2-year cumulative risk of 35% compared to only 7% in the low-risk group. Other studies have focused on radiomic parameters, such as those of Ehresman et al. [34] and Gui et al. [35] with the later developing a combined radiomic and clinical model predicting VCF after SBRT that outperformed either the SINS or clinical criteria alone.

Although uncommon, several studies have also described the risk of VCF in the setting of re-irradiation for tumor progression or recurrence. Two studies analyzed VCF risk in patients previously treated with conventional EBRT who subsequently underwent SBRT for progression/recurrence. The first, a multinational, multicenter study by Hashmi and colleagues, examined 215 patients (247 lesions) and observed a VCF rate of 4.5% [36]. A subsequent study by Detsky et al. similarly noted a 4% risk of new or progressive VCF in their study of 43 patients treated at 83 levels [37]. Florez et al. examined the reverse treatment paradigm—salvage EBRT following SBRT in 54 patients and observed a 9.3% VCF rate [38]. However, given the small sample sizes, the data are insufficient to determine if EBRT as salvage therapy following initial SBRT increases fracture risk relative to the reverse paradigm. To date, there has been one study examining repeat SBRT after prior SBRT. This study, published by Thibault et al., observed no episodes of VCF in this cohort of 40 patients treated at 56 levels with median follow-up 6.8 months [39]. Further study in this area is needed to elucidate further risk factors and methods of prevention in the setting of re-irradiation.

Clinical Presentation and Evaluation

Vertebral column fractures may be identified either incidentally (e.g., as part of repeat staging for a patient with a history of cancer), or as part of evaluation for a newly symptomatic patient, often with a known history of cancer. Patients in the latter group often present with an acute increase in back pain, which may be superimposed on a history of chronic oncologic back pain stemming for metastatic spine involvement. The increased pain often develops a mechanical component, which may even precede the occurrence of a radiographically detectable fracture. All patients presenting with new onset back pain and imaging showing a vertebral body lesion should undergo thorough neurological examination in addition to being interviewed about their presenting symptoms and medical history. The neurological exam should include a thorough sensorimotor exam and interrogation of bowel/bladder function, including rectal tone examination in a patient with complaints of new urinary or fecal incontinence. Patients with focal neurological deficits may have lesions with associated neural element compression that require surgical intervention to preserve function (Fig. 8.1). Radiographic workup should include upright radiographs (as tolerated), MRI with and without contrast of the affected region, and non-contrast CT of the affected region to assess underlying bone quality. For patients with new oncologic disease or those with a known history of cancer without recent staging, new radiographic staging should be performed, which is often performed with a whole-body PET/CT, but in the semi-urgent setting may be performed with a CT chest/abdomen/pelvis. In evaluating the lesion for radiotherapy, a thorough assessment of the epidural disease burden associated with the potential target lesion should be performed, as Bilsky grade 2/3 epidural disease [40] is considered a contraindication to radiotherapy at many center. In lesions that are to be considered for irradiation, radiation oncology should be engaged early to weigh in on the feasibility of radiation treatment and to provide recommendations about imaging for radiotherapy planning [41–43].

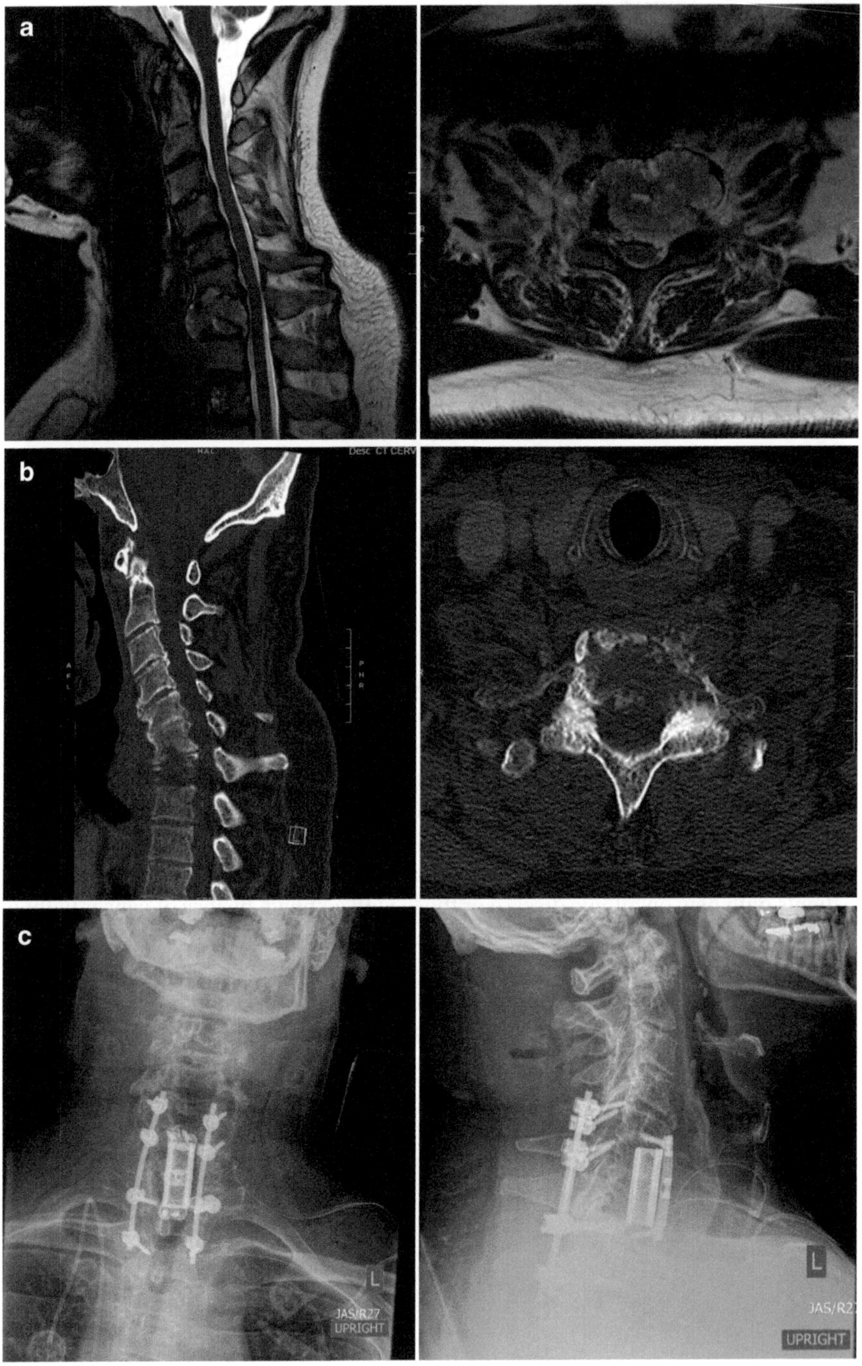

Fig. 8.1 A 51-year-old male with metastatic intrahepatic cholangiocarcinoma with metastases to the C7 vertebral body (panel **a**). The patient underwent radiation therapy with 30 Gy over 10 fractions to the C4-T3 region. Ten weeks following irradiation the patient noted progressive pain and radiculopathy to the left upper extremity with lytic destruction and possible spinal instability at the C7 segment (panel **b**). The patient was subsequently treated with a C6-C7 anterior cervical corpectomy, fusion, and C5-T2 posterior spinal instrumented fusion

Prevention and Treatment of Pathologic Fracture

Pathologic Fracture Prevention

In many cases, it is impossible to prevent pathologic fracture given that biomechanical data have found fracture risk to be proportional to tumor size and underlying lesion quality, which are inherently fixed characteristics [21–27]. However, several mechanisms have been proposed to mitigate the risk. Bisphosphonates have been proposed for the prevention of radiation-associated fracture with promising results in animal models [44–46]. Clinical results have been more mixed though. In one recent clinical study by Patel et al. [47], the authors examined the influence of anti-resorptive medication on post-radiotherapy VCF risk. They noted that while antiresorptive therapy prior to SBRT was associated with reduced fracture incidence, neither bisphosphonate dose nor duration predicted the occurrence of VCF. By contrast, a contemporary study by Te Velde et al. looked at VCF risk in 127 patients with multiple myeloma and found bisphosphonate use to be associated with a more than two-fold hazard reduction [48]. Ozdemir et al. [49] likewise noted bisphosphonate use >6 months to be a significant independent predictor of reduced VCF risk. Other anti-resorptive medications such as denosumab have also shown promise in fracture prevention in cancer patients [50], though there is at present no strong evidence suggesting a protective effect in radiated patients. In fact, the aforementioned study of Patel et al. [47] failed to see a significant association between denosumab dose or duration of use and post-radiotherapy VCF risk. Anabolic agents such as parathyroid hormone analogs have shown promise in animal models [51], but their use is limited in the oncology population due to the risk, however small, of primary bone cancers in the setting of prior malignancy [52].

Literature suggests that the use of fractionated versus single-fraction SBRT dosing may help to mitigate risk of VCF [53]. One multi-institutional study by Redmond et al. demonstrated a dose-dependent relationship between dose and VCF risk. Specifically, per fraction doses ≥24Gy (HR 5.25) and 20–23Gy (HR 4.91) were associated with significantly increased risk of post-radiotherapy VCF [54]. These results were subsequently supported by a systematic review published by Faruqi et al. [53] that found the extant literature to support higher per fraction dose as a risk factor for VCF, in addition to greater tumor involvement, lytic lesion quality, baseline vertebral compression fracture, advanced age, and baseline deformity. The results were heterogeneous though and so only a range of hazard ratios were reported, making it unclear if there is a specific threshold above which VCF risk increases substantially. It has also been reported that SBRT hypofractionation may mitigate the risk of other radiotherapy complications such as pain flares and radiation-associated myelopathy.

Post-radiotherapy Pathologic Fracture Management

Treatment of VCF varies according to symptomatology and the potential for instability at the fractured level. In cases of symptomatic VCF causing significant functional limitations or pain without spinal instability, vertebroplasty or balloon kyphoplasty can offer significant pain relief (see Chap. 7). Although more commonly used in the treatment of symptomatic osteoporotic vertebral compression fractures, vertebral augmentation procedures have gained popularity since being described in the early 2000s for pathologic VCF [55]. Balloon kyphoplasty may offer benefits over vertebroplasty with regard to restoration of height and correction of kyphosis in comparison to vertebroplasty [56]. In the CAFE trial, a multinational randomized-controlled trial, 134 patients were randomized to either kyphoplasty or non-surgical management. The trial found a significant reduction in pain for patients managed with kyphoplasty compared with non-surgical management at 7 days [57].

There is no definitive metric for determining underlying instability with 100% fidelity. However, the Spine Instability Neoplastic Score (SINS) is a commonly employed clinical tool that has become widely adopted and was designed by the Spine Oncology Study Group to help predict tumor-related spinal instability. In brief, patients are graded along six parameters—tumor lesion quality (e.g., lytic), presence and quality of associated pain, lesion location/spinal level, radiographic alignment, extent of vertebral body involvement/collapse, and extent of posterolateral element involvement. Scores are assigned to each parameter and summed to give an aggregate score (0–18) based on which the lesion is classified into one of three groups: stable (score 0–6), potentially unstable (score 7–12), and unstable (score 13–18) [58]. Notably, part of the composite score includes an assessment of radiological collapse, enabling it to capture an interval instability imparted by post-radiotherapy VCF.

Several studies have assessed the utility of the SINS specifically in the setting of pathologic VCF after radiation therapy. One study by Virk and colleagues [59] analyzed 323 patients treated with 24Gy single-fraction stereotactic radiosurgery (SRS), noting a 5-year cumulative incidence of symptomatic VCF of 7.2% [59]. Though no multivariable analysis was performed, univariate linear regression showed a moderate, significant correlation between higher SINS and time to post-radiotherapy VCF ($R^2 = 0.4$, $p < 0.001$). Several other studies [32–34, 60] have also found increased SINS to predict VCF risk following SBRT, including those by Kowalchuk et al. [33], Ehresman et al. [34], Mantel et al. [32], and Pennington et al. [60]. Some portions of the SINS score appear to be more impactful in predicting postradiotherapy VCF risk though. Cunha et al. [61] published one of the earlier such studies, examining 90 patients treated at 167 segments with SBRT. Nineteen patients (11%) experienced new or progressive fracture and multivariable analysis showed fraction dose ≥20Gy, lytic vs mixed lesion quality (SINS component), and de novo deformity at the fracture level (SINS component) all predicted increased fracture risk. In a subsequent, expanded multicenter cohort of 252 patients (410 levels), Sahgal et al. performed a similar analysis [29]. Fractures occurred in 13.9%

of treated levels and on multivariable analysis and fraction dose (≥24Gy or 20–23Gy vs <20Gy), and three SINS components predicted VCF risk. Again, lytic bone lesion type and the presence of deformity at baseline predicted VCF risk, as did more extensive vertebral body involvement. The same author group evaluated fracture risk within 116 patients with renal cell carcinoma from the multi-institutional cohort (187 levels). Higher fraction dose, baseline malalignment (SINS component), and baseline extent of vertebral body involvement (SINS component) predicted increased fracture risk.

For patients who require decompressive surgery or surgical stabilization, the exact selection of surgical approaches and techniques vary and are outside the scope of this chapter. In general, surgery in the setting of VCF shows good, durable, symptomatic relief [62], though improvements appear best for patients with SINS scores ≥10 at presentation [63]. For those undergoing surgery and adjuvant radiotherapy, the latter is typically administered 1–2 weeks after surgical stabilization to avoid wound complications [64], although recent studies have suggested that close interval SBRT followed by surgery may have good results without increased risk of wound complications [65].

Conclusion

Significant advancements have been made in radiation therapy, including the ability of SBRT to provide improved local control relative to conventional EBRT while reducing off-target toxicities. SBRT, however, may be accompanied by an increased risk of vertebral column fractures owing to its toxic effect on the vertebral bone, with resultant reduction in vertebral body strength. A subset of patients who suffer post-radiotherapy VCF will experience pain and associated functional decline. Studies have attempted to elucidate various risk factors for VCF, with greater lesion size, lytic versus blastic or mixed bone quality, and poorer underlying bone quality having noted associations with VCF risk. Preventative measures to avoid VCF following radiotherapy may include anti-resorptive therapies such as bisphosphonates or denosumab, though the available evidence is of limited quality. Prophylactic cement augmentation may also be considered for patients who are symptomatic at the time of presentation. Cement augmentation is similarly the treatment of choice for VCF without overt instability, and balloon kyphoplasty may offer superior pain palliation relative to vertebroplasty. However, some lesions will require stabilization and so it is essential to assay both epidural disease burden and the underlying instability associated with the metastasis being targeted. The Spine Instability Neoplastic Score is clinically focused too that can aid with assessing spinal instability and identify patients who may benefit from surgical stabilization.

References

1. Coleman RE (2006) Clinical features of metastatic bone disease and risk of skeletal morbidity. Clin Cancer Res 12:6243s–6249s
2. Myrehaug S, Sahgal A, Hayashi M et al (2017) Reirradiation spine stereotactic body radiation therapy for spinal metastases: systematic review. J Neurosurg Spine 27:428–435
3. Schaub SK, Tseng YD, Chang EL et al (2019) Strategies to mitigate toxicities from stereotactic body radiation therapy for spine metastases. Neurosurgery 85:729–740
4. Zeng KL, Tseng C-L, Soliman H, Weiss Y, Sahgal A, Myrehaug S (2019) Stereotactic body radiotherapy (SBRT) for oligometastatic spine metastases: an overview. Front Oncol 9:337
5. Zeng KL, Myrehaug S, Soliman H et al (2022) Mature local control and reirradiation rates comparing spine stereotactic body radiation therapy with conventional palliative external beam radiation therapy. Int J Radiat Oncol Biol Phys 114:293–300
6. Rose PS, Laufer I, Boland PJ, Hanover A, Bilsky MH, Yamada J, Lis E (2009) Risk of fracture after single fraction image-guided intensity-modulated radiation therapy to spinal metastases. J Clin Oncol 27:5075–5079
7. Green DE, Rubin CT (2014) Consequences of irradiation on bone and marrow phenotypes, and its relation to disruption of hematopoietic precursors. Bone 63:87–94
8. Mitchell MJ, Logan PM (1998) Radiation-induced changes in bone. Radiographics 18:1125–1136
9. Zou Q, Hong W, Zhou Y, Ding Q, Wang J, Jin W, Gao J, Hua G, Xu X (2016) Bone marrow stem cell dysfunction in radiation-induced abscopal bone loss. J Orthop Surg Res 11:3
10. Lima F, Swift JM, Greene ES, Allen MR, Cunningham DA, Braby LA, Bloomfield SA (2017) Exposure to low-dose X-ray radiation alters bone progenitor cells and bone microarchitecture. Radiat Res 188:433–442
11. Chandra A, Lin T, Tribble MB et al (2014) PTH1–34 alleviates radiotherapy-induced local bone loss by improving osteoblast and osteocyte survival. Bone 67:33–40
12. Oliver L, Hue E, Séry Q, Lafargue A, Pecqueur C, Paris F, Vallette FM (2013) Differentiation-related response to DNA breaks in human mesenchymal stem cells. Stem Cells 31:800–807
13. Mandair GS, Oest ME, Mann KA, Morris MD, Damron TA, Kohn DH (2020) Radiation-induced changes to bone composition extend beyond periosteal bone. Bone Rep 12:100262
14. Green DE, Adler BJ, Chan ME, Rubin CT (2012) Devastation of adult stem cell pools by irradiation precedes collapse of trabecular bone quality and quantity. J Bone Miner Res 27:749–759
15. Sakyi MY, Miller BJ, Coleman MC, Rodman SN, Brouillette MJ, Johnson JE, Fredericks DC, Goetz JE (2023) Effects of radiotherapy upon bone structure-strength relationships vary with sex and fractionation of dosing. Iowa Orthop J 43:77–86
16. Thio QCBS, van Wulfften Palthe ODR, Bramer JAM, DeLaney TF, Bredella MA, Dempster DW, Zhou H, Hornicek FJ, Chen Y-LE, Schwab JH (2023) Pilot study: short term impact of radiation therapy on bone mineral density and bone metabolism. Calcif Tissue Int 113:640–650
17. Govey PM, Zhang Y, Donahue HJ (2016) Mechanical loading attenuates radiation-induced bone loss in bone marrow transplanted mice. PLoS One 11:e0167673
18. Wolff J (1893) Das Gesetz der Transformation der Knochen. DMW Dtsch Medizinische Wochenschrift 19:1222–1224
19. Yan Z, Wang D, Cai J, Shen L, Jiang M, Liu X, Huang J, Zhang Y, Luo E, Jing D (2022) High-specificity protection against radiation-induced bone loss by a pulsed electromagnetic field. Sci Adv 8:eabq0222
20. Cottrill E, Pennington Z, Ahmed AKK, Lubelski D, Goodwin ML, Perdomo-Pantoja A, Westbroek EM, Theodore N, Witham T, Sciubba D (2020) The effect of electrical stimulation therapies on spinal fusion: a cross-disciplinary systematic review and meta-analysis of the preclinical and clinical data. J Neurosurg Spine 32:106–126
21. Stadelmann MA, Schenk DE, Maquer G, Lenherr C, Buck FM, Bosshardt DD, Hoppe S, Theumann N, Alkalay RN, Zysset PK (2020) Conventional finite element models estimate the

strength of metastatic human vertebrae despite alterations of the bone's tissue and structure. Bone 141:115598
22. Tschirhart CE, Nagpurkar A, Whyne CM (2004) Effects of tumor location, shape and surface serration on burst fracture risk in the metastatic spine. J Biomech 37:653–660
23. Whyne CM, Hu SS, Lotz JC (2001) Parametric finite element analysis of verterbral bodies affected by tumors. J Biomech 34:1317–1324
24. Ebihara H, Ito M, Abumi K, Taneichi H, Kotani Y, Minami A, Kaneda K (2004) A biomechanical analysis of metastatic vertebral collapse of the thoracic spine: a sheep model study. Spine (Phila Pa 1976) 29:994–999
25. Roth SE, Mousavi P, Finkelstein J, Chow E, Kreder H, Whyne CM (2004) Metastatic burst fracture risk prediction using biomechanically based equations. Clin Orthop Relat Res 419:83–90
26. Whyne CM, Hu SS, Lotz JC (2003) Biomechanically derived guideline equations for burst fracture risk prediction in the Metastatically involved spine. J Spinal Disord Tech 16:180–185
27. Alkalay RN, Groff MW, Stadelmann MA, Buck FM, Hoppe S, Theumann N, Mektar U, Davis RB, Hackney DB (2022) Improved estimates of strength and stiffness in pathologic vertebrae with bone metastases using CT-derived bone density compared with radiographic bone lesion quality classification. J Neurosurg Spine 36:113–124
28. Rich SE, Chow R, Raman S, Liang Zeng K, Lutz S, Lam H, Silva MF, Chow E (2018) Update of the systematic review of palliative radiation therapy fractionation for bone metastases. Radiother Oncol 126:547–557
29. Sahgal A, Atenafu EG, Chao S et al (2013) Vertebral compression fracture after spine stereotactic body radiotherapy: a multi-institutional analysis with a focus on radiation dose and the spinal instability neoplastic score. J Clin Oncol 31:3426–3431
30. Vargas E, Susko MS, Mummaneni PV, Braunstein SE, Chou D (2020) Vertebral body fracture rates after stereotactic body radiation therapy compared with external-beam radiation therapy for metastatic spine tumors. J Neurosurg Spine 33:870–876
31. Jawad MS, Fahim DK, Gerszten PC et al (2016) Vertebral compression fractures after stereotactic body radiation therapy: a large, multi-institutional, multinational evaluation. J Neurosurg Spine 24:928–936
32. Mantel F, Sweeney RA, Klement RJ, Hawkins MA, Belderbos J, Ahmed M, Toussaint A, Polat B, Flentje M, Guckenberger M (2019) Risk factors for vertebral compression fracture after spine stereotactic body radiation therapy: long-term results of a prospective phase 2 study. Radiother Oncol 141:62–66
33. Kowalchuk RO, Johnson-Tesch BA, Marion JT et al (2022) Development and assessment of a predictive score for vertebral compression fracture after stereotactic body radiation therapy for spinal metastases. JAMA Oncol 8:412
34. Ehresman J, Schilling A, Pennington Z et al (2020) A novel MRI-based score assessing trabecular bone quality to predict vertebral compression fractures in patients with spinal metastasis. J Neurosurg Spine 32:499–506
35. Gui C, Chen X, Sheikh K, Mathews L, Lo S-FL, Lee J, Khan MA, Sciubba DM, Redmond KJ (2022) Radiomic modeling to predict risk of vertebral compression fracture after stereotactic body radiation therapy for spinal metastases. J Neurosurg Spine 36:294–302
36. Hashmi A, Guckenberger M, Kersh R et al (2016) Re-irradiation stereotactic body radiotherapy for spinal metastases: a multi-institutional outcome analysis. J Neurosurg Spine 25:646–653
37. Detsky JS, Nguyen TK, Lee Y, Atenafu E, Maralani P, Husain Z, Tseng C-L, Myrehaug S, Soliman H, Sahgal A (2020) Mature imaging-based outcomes supporting local control for complex reirradiation salvage spine stereotactic body radiotherapy. Neurosurgery 87:816–822
38. Florez MA, De B, Chapman BV et al (2023) Safety and efficacy of salvage conventional re-irradiation following stereotactic radiosurgery for spine metastases. Radiat Oncol J 41:12–22
39. Thibault I, Campbell M, Tseng C-L, Atenafu EG, Letourneau D, Yu E, Cho BCJ, Lee YK, Fehlings MG, Sahgal A (2015) Salvage stereotactic body radiotherapy (SBRT) following in-field failure of initial SBRT for spinal metastases. Int J Radiat Oncol Biol Phys 93:353–360

40. Bilsky MH, Laufer I, Fourney DR, Groff M, Schmidt MH, Varga PP, Vrionis FD, Yamada Y, Gerszten PC, Kuklo TR (2010) Reliability analysis of the epidural spinal cord compression scale. J Neurosurg Spine 13:324–328
41. Sciubba DM, Pennington Z, Colman MW et al (2021) Spinal metastases 2021: a review of the current state of the art and future directions. Spine J 21:1414–1429
42. Rothrock R, Pennington Z, Ehresman J, Bilsky MH, Barzilai O, Szerlip NJ, Sciubba DM (2020) Hybrid therapy for spinal metastases. Neurosurg Clin N Am 31:191–200
43. Pennington Z, Ehresman J, Szerlip NJ, Sciubba DM (2021) Hybrid therapy for metastatic disease. Clin Spine Surg 34:369–376
44. Arrington SA, Fisher ER, Willick GE, Mann KA, Allen MJ (2010) Anabolic and Antiresorptive drugs improve trabecular microarchitecture and reduce fracture risk following radiation therapy. Calcif Tissue Int 87:263–272
45. Keenawinna L, Oest ME, Mann KA, Spadaro J, Damron TA (2013) Zoledronic acid prevents loss of trabecular bone after focal irradiation in mice. Radiat Res 180:89–99
46. Willey JS, Livingston EW, Robbins ME, Bourland JD, Tirado-Lee L, Smith-Sielicki H, Bateman TA (2010) Risedronate prevents early radiation-induced osteoporosis in mice at multiple skeletal locations. Bone 46:101–111
47. Patel PP, Esposito EP, Zhu J et al (2024) Antiresorptive medications prior to stereotactic body radiotherapy for spinal metastasis are associated with reduced incidence of vertebral body compression fracture. Glob Spine J 14:1778–1785
48. te Velde JP, Zijlstra H, Lans A, Patel CG, Raje N, Delawi D, Kempen DHR, Verlaan J-J, van Royen BJ, Schwab JH (2024) Fracture rate after conventional external beam radiation therapy to the spine in multiple myeloma patients. Spine J 24:137–145
49. Ozdemir Y, Torun N, Guler OC, Yildirim BA, Besen AA, Yetisken AG, Onal HC, Topkan E (2019) Local control and vertebral compression fractures following stereotactic body radiotherapy for spine metastases. J Bone Oncol 15:100218
50. Açil Y, Gierloff M, Behrens C, Möller B, Gassling V, Niehoff P, Wiltfang J, Simon M (2013) Effects of Zoledronate on irradiated bone in vivo: analysis of the collagen types I, V and their cross-links Lysylpyridinoline, Hydroxylysylpyridinoline and Hydroxyproline. Calcif Tissue Int 92:251–260
51. Chandra A, Lan S, Zhu J, Lin T, Zhang X, Siclari VA, Altman AR, Cengel KA, Liu XS, Qin L (2013) PTH prevents the adverse effects of focal radiation on bone architecture in young rats. Bone 55:449–457
52. Oest ME, Mann KA, Zimmerman ND, Damron TA (2016) Parathyroid hormone (1–34) transiently protects against radiation-induced bone fragility. Calcif Tissue Int 98:619–630
53. Faruqi S, Tseng C-L, Whyne C et al (2018) Vertebral compression fracture after spine stereotactic body radiation therapy: a review of the pathophysiology and risk factors. Neurosurgery 83:314–322
54. Redmond KJ, Sahgal A, Foote M et al (2015) Single versus multiple session stereotactic body radiotherapy for spinal metastasis: the risk–benefit ratio. Future Oncol 11:2405–2415
55. Fourney DR, Schomer DF, Nader R, Chlan-Fourney J, Suki D, Ahrar K, Rhines LD, Gokaslan ZL (2003) Percutaneous vertebroplasty and kyphoplasty for painful vertebral body fractures in cancer patients. J Neurosurg Spine 98:21–30
56. Eseonu KC, Panchmatia JR, Streetly MJ, Grauer JN, Fakouri B (2023) The role of vertebral augmentation procedures in the management of vertebral compression fractures secondary to multiple myeloma. Hematol Oncol 41:323–334
57. Berenson J, Pflugmacher R, Jarzem P, Zonder J, Schechtman K, Tillman JB, Bastian L, Ashraf T, Vrionis F (2011) Balloon kyphoplasty versus non-surgical fracture management for treatment of painful vertebral body compression fractures in patients with cancer: a multicentre, randomised controlled trial. Lancet Oncol 12:225–235
58. Fisher CG, Schouten R, Versteeg AL et al (2014) Reliability of the Spinal Instability Neoplastic Score (SINS) among radiation oncologists: an assessment of instability secondary to spinal metastases. Radiat Oncol 9:69

59. Virk MS, Han JE, Reiner AS, McLaughlin LA, Sciubba DM, Lis E, Yamada Y, Bilsky M, Laufer I (2017) Frequency of symptomatic vertebral body compression fractures requiring intervention following single-fraction stereotactic radiosurgery for spinal metastases. Neurosurg Focus 42:E8
60. Pennington Z, Mikula AL, Lakomkin N et al (2023) Comparison of Hounsfield units and vertebral bone quality score for the prediction of time to pathologic fracture in mobile spine metastases treated with radiotherapy. J Neurosurg Spine 40:19–27
61. Cunha MVR, Al-Omair A, Atenafu EG et al (2012) Vertebral compression fracture (VCF) after spine stereotactic body radiation therapy (SBRT): analysis of predictive factors. Int J Radiat Oncol 84:e343–e349
62. Moussazadeh N, Rubin DG, McLaughlin L, Lis E, Bilsky MH, Laufer I (2015) Short-segment percutaneous pedicle screw fixation with cement augmentation for tumor-induced spinal instability. Spine J 15:1609–1617
63. Hussain I, Barzilai O, Reiner AS, McLaughlin L, DiStefano NM, Ogilvie S, Versteeg AL, Fisher CG, Bilsky MH, Laufer I (2019) Spinal instability neoplastic score component validation using patient-reported outcomes. J Neurosurg Spine 30:432–438
64. Itshayek E, Yamada J, Bilsky M, Schmidt M, Shaffrey C, Gerszten P, Polly D, Gokaslan Z, Varga PP, Fisher CG (2010) Timing of surgery and radiotherapy in the management of metastatic spine disease: a systematic review. Int J Oncol 36:533–544
65. Azad TD, Varshneya K, Herrick DB et al (2021) Timing of adjuvant radiation therapy and risk of wound-related complications among patients with spinal metastatic disease. Glob Spine J 11:44–49

Chapter 9
Post-Laminectomy Kyphosis Following Intradural Tumor Resection

Zach Pennington, Daniel M. Sciubba, and Benjamin D. Elder

Overview and Epidemiology of Intradural Tumors

Based on the latest data from the Central Brain Tumor Registry of the United States [1], tumors of the spinal cord, nerve roots, and meninges affect 4058 persons per year. Peak incidence is from the sixth to ninth decades of life, with roughly equal sex distributions [2]. Pathology varies by anatomic compartment, but, of intradural tumors, ependymomas and astrocytomas represent the bulk of intramedullary lesions (IMSCT), whereas meningiomas and schwannomas represent the bulk of extramedullary lesions (EMSCT) [3–7]. Surgical resection is considered standard of care for both intramedullary and extramedullary lesions; in the case of ependymomas, meningiomas, and schwannomas, resection is often curative.

Unlike tumors of the vertebral body, lesions of the intradural space are seldom destabilizing in and of themselves. However, the intraoperative bone removal, coupled with neuromuscular dysfunction of the paraspinal musculature from spinal cord dysfunction from the tumor itself, can create subsequent instability that must be considered. Though the optimal surgical approach is dependent upon lesion location, for most lesions, a posterior approach with laminectomy or laminoplasty is performed to access the thecal sac. For lesions with ventrolateral or ventral positions, as occurs in some meningiomas, a more oblique approach angle may be required, up to and including removal of the facet joint or proximal rib (in the case

Z. Pennington (✉) · B. D. Elder
Department of Neurologic Surgery, Mayo Clinic, Rochester, MN, USA
e-mail: pennington.zachary@mayo.edu; elder.benjamin@mayo.edu

D. M. Sciubba
Department of Neurosurgery, Zucker School of Medicine at Hofstra, Long Island Jewish Medical Center and North Shore University Hospital, Northwell Health, Great Neck, NY, USA
e-mail: dsciubba1@northwell.edu

D. M. Sciubba (ed.), *Spinal Tumor Associated Deformity*,
https://doi.org/10.1007/978-3-031-87939-5_9

of thoracic lesions). Disruption of the posterior tension band can result in disequilibrium between the kyphosing moments placed on the spine by the ventrally positioned viscera and the opposing lordotic moments imparted by the paraspinal musculature. Such mismatch may result in progressive postlaminectomy kyphosis. As a delayed outcome of surgery [8–10], postlaminectomy kyphosis may not be appreciated for years after the index surgery. In this chapter, we provide a brief overview of spinal biomechanics, describe risk factors for postlaminectomy kyphosis, and identify potential strategies for preventing this outcome.

Overview of Spinal Biomechanics and the Posterior Tension Band

The spine can be divided into bony load-bearing elements and tension-bearing musculoligamentous elements, which control the movement of the spinal units (vertebrae) along three linear axes (compression–distraction, anterior–posterior translation, and lateral translation) and three rotational axes (flexion–extension, axial rotation, and lateral bending). Regarding surgery for intradural pathologies, rotation about a horizontally oriented axis through the instantaneous axis of rotation (IAR) is of chief importance. Additionally, the tension-bearing musculoligamentous ligaments along with the posterior bony elements (spinous processes, laminae) to which they attach are of greatest importance for controlling this motion (flexion–extension). The ligaments and muscles comprise the posterior ligamentous complex (PLC), and they are responsible for maintaining extensor forces applied by the paraspinal muscles to the spinal column. The major ligaments opposing flexion are the ligamentum flavum (yellow ligament), interspinous ligament, capsular ligaments, and supraspinous ligament. The latter is absent in the cervical spine, in which occipitocervical flexion is partially opposed by the nuchal ligament that runs from the external occipital protuberance to the spinous process of C7 [11].

Some of the seminal work on spinal biomechanics was performed by White and Punjabi [12–16] in the 1970s and 1980s. Among their experiments were those looking at the impact of ligament transection on flexion–extension stability of the mobile spine. The first of their series of experiments [14–16] examined flexion–extension deformation of cervical functional spine units (motion segments)—two vertebrae constructs denuded of muscle and overlying soft tissue but with preservation of the ligaments linking the two bodies. In this study, they found that kyphosis under flexion loads increased serially with transection of the interspinous ligament, yellow ligament, facet capsule, and ultimately violation of the facet joint. However, critical instability (failure) only resulted following transection of the posterior longitudinal ligament. A more recent study by Hartman and colleagues [17] reported similar results using C6–7 motion segments, which were tested in flexion–extension, lateral bending, and axial rotation movements following resection of the: (1) supraspinous and interspinous ligaments, (2) ligamentum flavum, (3) facet capsules, and (4) facets. They noted that range of motion in flexion increased by approximately 2° (17.8%) after resection of the supraspinous and interspinous ligaments and by 1.7° (12.7%) after resection of the ligamentum flavum. The increased range of motion following supraspinous and interspinous ligament resection was statistically significant, as was the reduction in end-range moment following ligament flavum resection—a measure of resistance to flexion. In fact, the authors noted the ligamentum flavum to provide 32.8% of the resistance to flexion in the intact spine. The contribution of the facet capsule was also found to be significant, providing 14.3% of the resistance to flexion. Histological studies by others have suggested that the resistance to flexion offered by the supraspinous and interspinous ligaments likely decreases with age [18, 19] secondary to a decrease in oxytalan elastic fibers [19]. Finite element analysis has similarly suggested that exclusion of the interspinous ligament results in excessive flexion instability [20].

Following the examination of cervical spine ligaments, Panjabi, Hausfeld, and White examined the impact of posterior element ligamentous structures in the thoracic spine. Again using fresh-frozen cadaveric spines, ligaments were serially transected in two-vertebrae functional spine units that were then subjected to loads constituting 11, 21, 32, and 43 percent of the body weight of the cadaveric specimen [13]. As compared to the cervical spine, transection of the supraspinous, interspinous, and capsular ligaments, along with facet joint disruption, only resulted in a small increase in rotation/kyphosis with application of kyphosing forces. By contrast, severing of the PLL and violation of the posterior annulus were both highly destabilizing and also allowed for significant horizontal translation. The authors acknowledged that their results did not account for the stability offered by the paraspinal musculature or by the rib cage, both of which resist flexion movement. Nevertheless, they suggested that the thoracic, or at least the mid-thoracic spine, should be relatively resistant to deformation by kyphosing forces even with compromise of the supraspinous, interspinous, and yellow ligaments, as occurs in laminectomy. Similar results may not hold true at the thoracolumbar junction, however, as cadaveric work by Li et al [21] using thoracolumbar models of compression fracture has found that the ligamentum flavum and supraspinous ligament both contribute significantly to flexion resistance. At the junctional T12-L1 segment, supraspinous ligament transection resulted in a 0.84° (11.7%) increase in flexional movement and ligamentum flavum transection resulted in a 1.26° (15.3%) increase in flexional movement. At the L1–2 segment, supraspinous ligament and ligamentum flavum transection resulted in only minor increases in the range of motion relative to the destabilized segment (injury model with intact ligaments).

Shortly thereafter, Posner et al. published a similar study examining the flexional resistance ability of lumbar functional spine units derived from fresh-frozen cadavers [12]. As in the Panjabi et al. study, ligaments were divided serially in posterior-to-anterior direction and after each transection were subjected to progressively greater loads. As compared to the earlier study, transection of the ligamentum flavum resulted in a substantial decrease in resistance to flexion forces when the segment was loaded at maximum physiological loads. Additionally, violation of the facet joint was again highly destabilizing, to the point that flexion forces caused significantly increased segmental kyphosis even in the absence of preloading forces. Heuer and colleagues [22] subsequently identified a lesser contribution from the posterior ligaments. They found that while resection of the supraspinous ligament, interspinous ligament, and ligamentum flavum also resulted in significant increases in flexion, it was only with removal of the vertebral arch that flexion range of motion increased significantly.

These data suggest the integrity of the posterior ligamentous complex, especially the posterolateral complex, is more important for maintenance of posture in lumbar pathologies than for thoracic pathologies. As aforementioned, this may in part be due to the presence of the rib cage in the thoracic spine but may also be due to differences in the position of the IAR in the thoracic [vs lumbar] vertebrae and the relative orientation of the spinous processes [23]. The more anteriorly positioned IAR in the thoracic motion segments offers the capsular ligaments and posterior longitudinal ligament a greater lever arm upon which to act to prevent kyphosis of the functional spine unit. Additionally, the more horizontally oriented spinous processes of the lumbar spine create a longer moment arm for the supraspinous ligament. Consequently, compromise of the supraspinous ligament would be expected to have a greater impact on lumbar spine stability. Animal studies have similarly suggested this principle, such as the work by Gillespie and Dickey [24], which showed using a porcine model that the supraspinous and interspinous ligaments provided significant flexion resistance—14% and 10.5%, respectively. The interaction of these two ligaments in flexion was also significant. The ligamentum flavum contributed a further 24.7% suggesting that resection of these posterior ligaments may result in destabilization of the spine in flexion.

In aggregate, the above results demonstrate that the contributions of the ligamentum flavum, supraspinous ligament, and interspinous ligament to flexion resistance are significant in the cervical and lumbar spine. However, in the thoracic spine, their contribution is less, likely due to the stabilizing effect of the rib cage. In light of this, resection of these ligaments may account for the biomechanical basis for postlaminectomy kyphosis. Additionally, there is evidence to suggest that the relative contributions to flexion resistance vary with the degree of flexion present [18]; therefore, baseline posture may dictate the degree to which laminectomy [versus laminoplasty] destabilizes the spine in flexion.

Previous Examinations of Postlaminectomy Kyphosis and Risk Factors for the Condition

Studies in Tumor Populations

Given that all posterior approaches to the spine involve soft tissue dissection and at least some disruption of the posterior tension band, undergoing surgical resection is the precipitating event for all postlaminectomy kyphosis, though there is likely some contribution for spinal cord dysfunction and resultant damage to the neuromuscular control of the paraspinal musculature. Nevertheless, only a minority of patients suffer this complication, and previous examinations have suggested laminectomy length and the strategy for posterior element removal as the chief risk factors. In their series of 164 pediatric patients (mean age 8.6 ± 5 years) who underwent laminectomy or laminoplasty for resection of intramedullary spinal cord tumors, McGirt et al [25] reported postoperative progressive spinal deformity requiring fusion occurred in 44 patients (26.8%). Postoperative deformity was scoliosis in 14 patients, kyphosis in 15, and a mixed kyphoscoliosis in the remaining 14. Patients who underwent laminectomy had a significantly higher rate of progressive deformity (30%) compared to those treated with laminoplasty (5%), a difference that remained significant (odds ratio 0.13; $p = 0.05$) on multivariable analysis. For their closure, the authors both replaced the lamina using titanium microplates and sutured the paraspinal musculature to the interspinous ligaments and laminae to help reconstruct the posterior tension band. Their findings echoed those of Yeh et al [26] and Sciubba et al. [27] Yeh et al. had observed progressive deformity requiring fusion in 5 of 27 pediatric patients (mean age 5.6 years) who underwent laminectomy or laminoplasty for IMSCT. They noted risk factors for subsequent deformity requiring fusion were laminectomy across the thoracolumbar junction, increasing number of laminectomy levels, and the use of laminectomy versus laminoplasty. Sciubba et al [27] focused their cohort specifically on adult patients treated for cervical IMSCT. They found that length of the laminectomized segment was a strong predictor of subsequent deformity, with 33% of patients undergoing ≥3-level laminectomy requiring subsequent fusion (at a median of 25.2 months) as compared to 5% of those undergoing ≤2-level laminectomy. Interestingly, soft-tissue dissection at the craniocervical or cervicothoracic junction predicted subsequent kyphosis requiring fixation.

These same authors also published a grading scale to evaluate the relative risk of developing progressive deformity postoperatively [28]. The grading scale was based on a previous evaluation of independent predictors for progressive spinal deformity requiring fusion in a cohort of 161 patients, of whom 27% required operation for deformity [29]. Patients were scored from a grade of I-V based on four factors: number of prior operations (index versus revision operation), preoperative scoliosis (defined by Cobb angle >10°), crossing of the thoracolumbar junction with the laminectomy, and age (<13 vs ≥ 13 years of age). There was a stepwise increase in deformity risk with increasing number of risk factors; patients with all four risk factors suffered postlaminectomy progressive deformity in 75% of cases [27].

In a subsequent series of 238 patients, McGirt et al [9] compared rates of progressive kyphosis following laminectomy and laminoplasty. As compared to their prior series, this chapter examined predominately adult patients (88%; mean age 46 ± 20 years) and included both intramedullary (57%) and extramedullary lesions (43%). Progressive deformity occurred in 11% of patients at a mean of 14 months postoperatively. Six patients developed cervical lordosis, two developed cervical kyphosis, four developed progressive thoracic kyphosis and 14 experienced progression of their preoperative coronal deformity. Interestingly, only five patients required surgical management of their deformity (i.e., instrumented fusion). In contrast to the prior studies, rates of deformity were similar in both the laminoplasty and laminectomy cohorts; however, they did note that laminoplasty trended toward lower rates of incisional cerebrospinal fluid leak.

In line with this, Hersh et al [30] performed a study of 66 pediatric patients (age < 21 years) treated with laminectomy (29%) or laminoplasty (71%) for IMSCT, predominately of the cervicothoracic region (92%). They noted postoperative deformity in 81.8% of patients, with similarly high rates in the laminoplasty (83%) and laminectomy groups (79%). The most common deformity was progressive kyphosis (61%). Only a minority of patients required instrumented fusion (15%), which was performed at a median 31.9 months following the initial resection. Though a multivariable analysis was not performed, they suggested that decompression length was the highest predictor of progressive postoperative deformity, in line with the similar findings of Sciubba [27].

Though none of these studies found age to be a significant risk factor for progressive deformity, only Sciubba et al [27] explicitly looked at this association, finding one to exist, though the correlation was statistically insignificant. Yet, in aggregate, the studies do appear to indicate a trend toward higher rates of deformity requiring operative revision in the pediatric population, suggesting that younger age may be a risk factor for progressive postoperative deformity.

Other Clinical Work

The importance of sagittal alignment for predicting progressive deformity—"deformity begets deformity"—has become increasingly recognized over the past decade. In accordance with this, clinical work from nononcologic populations has begun to document the role of sagittal alignment in outcomes following laminoplasty. In their series of 53 patients treated with open-door or French-door laminoplasty for cervical spondylotic myelopathy, Kim et al [31] found the postoperative progressive kyphotic deformity was independently predicted by increased T1 slope (more forward sloping T1), decreased baseline C2–7 range of motion (stiffer subaxial spine), and decreased C2–7 extension at baseline (weak extensor musculature). Interestingly, regional cervical spine balance as measured by C2–7 sagittal vertical axis was not predictive of kyphosis on either univariable or multivariable analysis. The authors concluded that a spine with a weak posterior tension band at baseline was apt to suffer kyphosis especially if observed in conjunction with a high T1 slope, likely because strong extensors are necessary to maintain proper alignment in this scenario and provide compensatory cervical hyperlordosis for the thoracolumbar deformity resulting in the high T1 slope. This corroborated the findings of an earlier study by Passias and colleagues, who noted that fatty infiltration of the paraspinal muscles following posterior cervical fusion was associated with worse overall sagittal imbalance at 1-year follow-up. Work supporting this in the lumbar literature is more abundant. Muellner et al [32, 33] and Elysee et al [34] both demonstrated that paraspinal muscle cross-sectional area was negatively associated with pelvic tilt, while extent of fatty infiltration was positively correlated with pelvic tilt and sagittal imbalance. This suggests a weakened or atrophic posterior tension band may place the patient at risk for positive sagittal imbalance.

Fatty infiltration and paraspinal muscle atrophy are known side effects of surgery, thought to occur secondary to muscle ischemia in the setting of prolonged retraction as well as simply cauterization during the surgical exposure [35, 36]. In one study, atrophy following posterior cervical spine surgery was found to approach a 6% rate following laminoplasty, as compared to 13% following laminectomy [37]. However, the authors acknowledged that the extent of postlaminectomy atrophy was likely related to the extent of exposure, with an increasingly lateral exposure in the case of posterior cervical fusion having been previously correlated with more extensive postoperative atrophy in a series by Sangala and colleagues [38].

In addition to limiting exposure, it has been suggested that such muscular atrophy may be preventable with repeated release of retractors during surgery. Reasonable quality evidence supporting the association of continued retraction with muscle fiber atrophy has been provided using several animal models of lumbar fusion [18, 19]. No similar human studies exist that directly vary length or extent of retractor use with postoperative cross-sectional area. Nevertheless, work by Styf and Willén [39], Taylor et al. [40], and Mukai et al [41] has provided reasonable evidence suggesting that the increased intramuscular pressures thought to contribute to postoperative atrophy are also observed in human subjects undergoing spine surgery.

Biomechanical Work: Cadaveric Studies and Finite Element Analyses

From a biomechanical study, previous cadaveric work has been performed examining the relative destabilization caused by laminoplasty and laminectomy. Nowinski et al [42] studied loading and motion properties of nine fresh-frozen cervical spine preparations with normal confirmed bone density that had been denuded of all non-ligamentous soft tissue. Specimens underwent C3–6 open-door laminoplasty followed by laminectomy with staged facetectomies, ranging from 25 to 75% of the facet joint. Comparison between laminoplasty and the intact spine showed no significant difference, but the range of motion was significantly increased after laminectomy with 25% facetectomy in flexion/extension. Laminoplasty also had a marginally increased range of motion for axial torsion relative to the intact specimen, but laminectomy significantly increased instability relative to either laminoplasty or the intact state. These results conflicted with earlier work by Zdeblick and colleagues [43], who noted that laminectomy alone did not result in a significant increase in segmental mobility. They noted significant hypermobility only after removal of ≥50% of the facet.

Other cadaveric studies by Subramaniam et al [44] and Kode et al [45] both found laminectomy to be more destabilizing than laminoplasty. The former evaluated the range of motion in seven fresh-frozen C2-T1 cervical spine preparations denuded of all musculoligamentous attachments. Spines were tested intact under three conditions: (1) a stenosis-stimulating condition with attached hemispheric wooden beads, (2) stenosis following laminoplasty, and (3) stenosis following laminectomy. While laminoplasty was not associated with a significant change in flexion–extension range of motion relative to the intact preparation, laminectomy resulted in a 12 ± 9% increase in flexion ROM and a 17 ± 13% increase in extension ROM. Kode and colleagues [45] examined range of motion across the subaxial cervical spine of C2-T1 in fresh-frozen cadaveric preparations in lateral bending, flexion/extension, and axial rotation following progressively larger bony removal—two-level open-door laminoplasty, four-level open-door laminoplasty, and then four-level laminectomy [45]. The authors found that both the two-level and four-level laminoplasty resulted in no appreciable increase in the range of motion relative to intact specimens. By contrast, four-level laminectomy was associated with a significant increase in ROM across all tested conditions.

A later finite element analysis by Kode and colleagues [46] supported the notion of laminectomy as a more destabilizing procedure. Using a C2-T1 model of the cervical spine with the five major ligaments—anterior longitudinal ligament (ALL), posterior longitudinal ligament (PLL), ligamentum flavum, interspinous ligament, and capsular ligaments—the authors compared the range of motion between patients treated with C3–6 laminectomy and either C3–6 open door or French door/double-door laminoplasty. While the range of motion for lateral bending and axial rotation was comparable between groups, flexion ROM was significantly increased in the laminectomy group. Additionally, annular stresses exerted on the intervertebral disks were appreciably elevated in the laminoplasty group under flexion.

More recently, Xu et al [47] reported the results of a finite element analysis evaluating the range of motion in C2-T1 cervicothoracic models with regard to flexion–extension, lateral bending, and axial rotation following three distinct laminoplasty procedures. They found that the optimal method for laminoplasty reconstruction employed tension band replacement (TBR) plates at the cephalad and caudad levels and traditional miniplates at the intervening segment. This construct had similar lateral bending and axial rotation relative to the other modalities but had lower flexional movement that a construct comprised solely of tension band replacement plates and lower extension ROM relative to both the all-TBR and all-miniplate constructs. It also reduced the von Mises stresses on plates in the middle of the construct.

Strategies for Prevention

As one of the primary drivers for progressive postlaminectomy deformity appears to be disruption of the posterior tension band, strategies to prevent the occurrence of progressive postoperative deformity focus on minimizing its disruption. For many authors, this involves laminoplasty as opposed to laminectomy. Such a strategy was advocated by Hersh et al [30] and McGirt and colleagues [25] in their studies examining pediatric populations. In their series, McGirt et al. described the closure of their laminoplasty, including reattachment of the paraspinal musculature to the interspinous ligaments and laminae with suture to explicitly reconstruct the posterior tension band.

As atrophy of the cervical paraspinal musculature also appears to play a strong role in postoperative progressive deformity, some groups have made attempts to preserve the musculature as a means of preserving biomechanical function. Kim et al. previously described a "myoarchitectonic spinolaminoplasty" as a muscle-sparing alternative to the conventional open-door and French-door/double door laminoplasty techniques. The authors described using sharp dissection and bipolar cautery to divide the nuchal ligament at three levels—at the insertion of the trapezius, at the insertion of the splenius capitis, and at the insertion of the semispinalis capitis. Furthermore, monopolar cautery was avoided to minimize soft tissue injury, and the spinous process was split in the midline, leaving the attachments of the splenius capitis and semispinalis cervicis intact (cortical plates). Grooves were cut at the spinolaminar junction bilaterally to release the spinous process, followed by cutting of a central groove in the base of the spinous process, between the attachments of the multifidus. As with the conventional double-door technique, gutters were formed at the lateral aspect of the laminae bilaterally, and the laminae were fractured dorsally and then secured to a hydroxyapatite implant placed between them, to which the cortical plates were attached using nonabsorbable suture. The authors noted this technique was associated with both a significantly lower increase in the range of motion from the native state and a smaller decrease in lordosis from baseline, supporting its potential utility for preventing progressive postoperative deformity. Postoperative cross-sectional imaging additionally found no significant decrease in the cross-sectional area of any of the major paraspinal muscle groups, as compared to the conventional laminoplasty group, in which there was significant atrophy of the semispinalis capitis, semispinalis cervicis, and multifidus at 1 year postoperatively. The myoarchitectonic spinolaminoplasty group additionally experienced less gapping of the splenius capitis postoperatively, potentially resulting in improved cosmetic outcomes. Despite these advantages, it is unclear whether the exposure offered by such a technique is adequate to provide the visualization necessary for intradural surgery. Additionally, the eschewing of monopolar electrocautery increases the difficulty of maintaining hemostasis. Rundown from inadequately coagulated muscle can obfuscate the surgical field and complicate resection. Similar concerns arise for muscle-sparing variations of open-door laminoplasty, such as that of Shiraishi [48] and Hosono et al. [49] Open-door laminoplasty in general does not offer sufficient visualization of the thecal sac to allow for intradural tumor resection.

In adults and some pediatric patients, instrumented fusion can be a preferred alternative to laminoplasty, especially for patients undergoing resection of lesions with long craniocaudal extents. However, in growing pediatric patients, this approach can be suboptimal as continued expansion of the anterior column can result in a crankshaft deformity. This is characterized by progressive rotational deformity resulting from the spreading apart of vertebral bodies that are fixed posteriorly by rigid instrumentation, which forces growth to occur predominately in the axial plan [30, 50]. This was originally described by Dubousset in 1973 based on observations of progressive deformity in skeletally immature patients who had undergone rigid instrumentation for their deformity [50]. The crankshaft phenomenon has been most well-described in this group [51], in whom younger skeletal age appears to be the strongest independent predictor [51]. However, similar principles guide growth in the cervical spine, and it seems logical that such a complication could occur following posterior cervical fusion. Yet, the relatively low rates of cervical fusion performed in pediatric patients limit the ability to evaluate this phenomenon.

Case Examples

Case 1

A 16-year-old otherwise healthy male with past medical history significant for von Hippel-Lindau syndrome presented with left upper extremity weakness and sensory loss and was found to be myelopathic in the lower extremities. On MRI, he had an avidly contrast-enhancing nodule with an expansive associated syrinx extending from the level of C4 cranially to T11 caudally (Fig. 9.1). The patient was taken to the operating room and underwent a C6–7 osteoplastic laminotomy and gross total resection of the lesion, which was subsequently demonstrated to be a hemangioblastoma on pathologic examination. At 3-month follow-up, the patient had complete resolution of his preoperative sensory and motor symptoms. Imaging demonstrated gross total resection of the lesion with recurrence and significant improvement in his syrinx (Fig. 9.2). However, upright cervical radiographs demonstrated early focal kyphosis at the C6-T1 level, across the laminoplasty site. The patient denied mechanical neck or arm pain and is currently being followed with serial imaging.

Case 2

A 22-year-old woman presented to clinic with complaints of significant paraxial neck and upper back pain and a progressively stooped over posture. She had a remove history of an intramedullary spinal cord tumor for which she underwent C6 laminectomy and C7-T2 osteoplastic laminotomy. Preoperative imaging (Fig. 9.3) demonstrated significant cervical kyphosis with a positive cervical sagittal vertical axis (cSVA) of 8.8 cm and − 14.2° of C2–7 cervical lordosis. 36″ scoliosis films demonstrated compensatory lumbar hyperlordosis of 64° with a negative C7 SVA (−6.4 cm) and thoracic hypokyphosis (T4–12 kyphosis 14.2°), highlighting her attempt to maintain forward gaze with truncal retroversion. The apex of her deformity was at the level of her prior laminoplasty and CT demonstrated ankylosis of the anterior longitudinal ligament at C6/C7. She was taken to the operating room for circumferential fusion with an anterior first stage for C6/C7 anterior cervical diskectomy and fusion, followed by a C4-T4 posterior instrumented fusion.

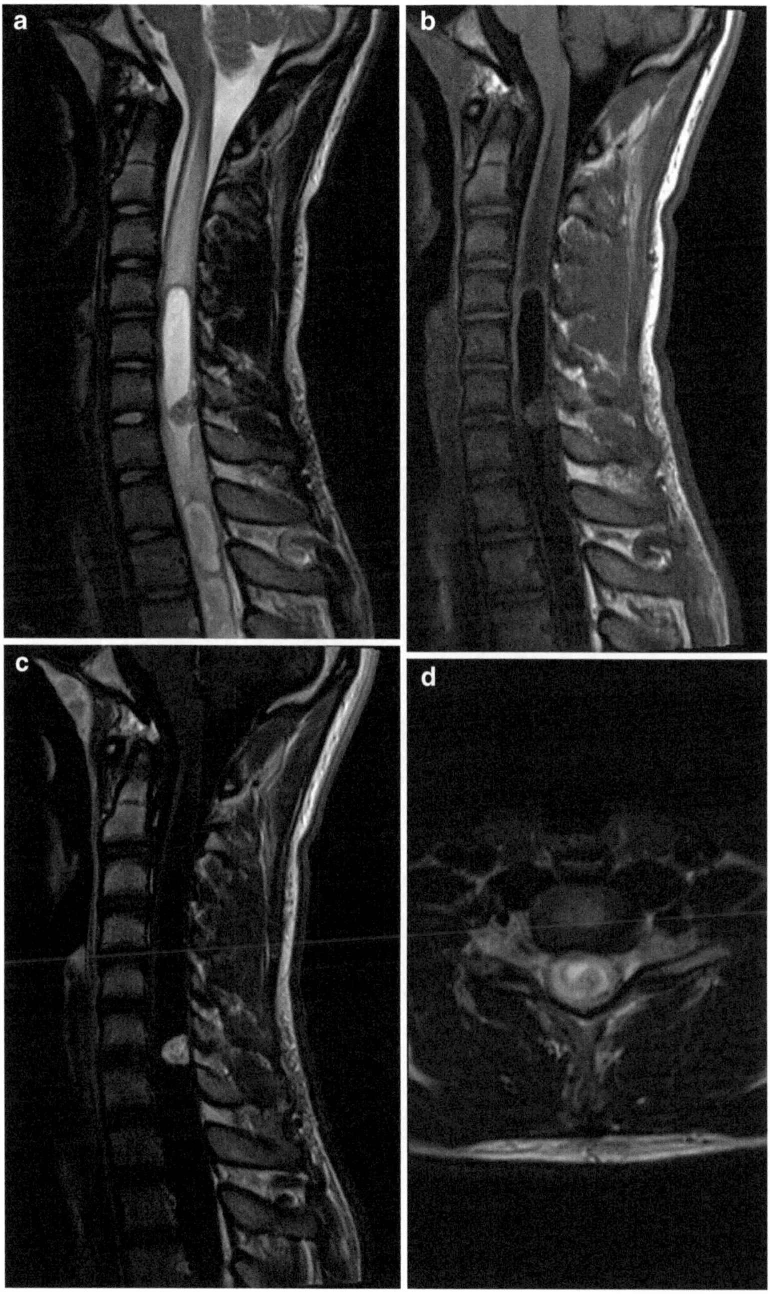

Fig. 9.1 Preoperative magnetic resonance imaging of a 16-year-old patient with von HippelLindau who presented with left upper extremity weakness and was found to have an avidly contrast-enhancing nodule with extensive associated syrinx in the cervical spinal cord. (**a**) sagittal T2-weighted sagittal image; (**b**) sagittal T1-weighted fluid attenuated inversion recovery without contrast; (**c**) sagittal T1-weighted fluid attenuated inversion recovery with contrast; (**d**) axial T2-weighted slice at C6/7

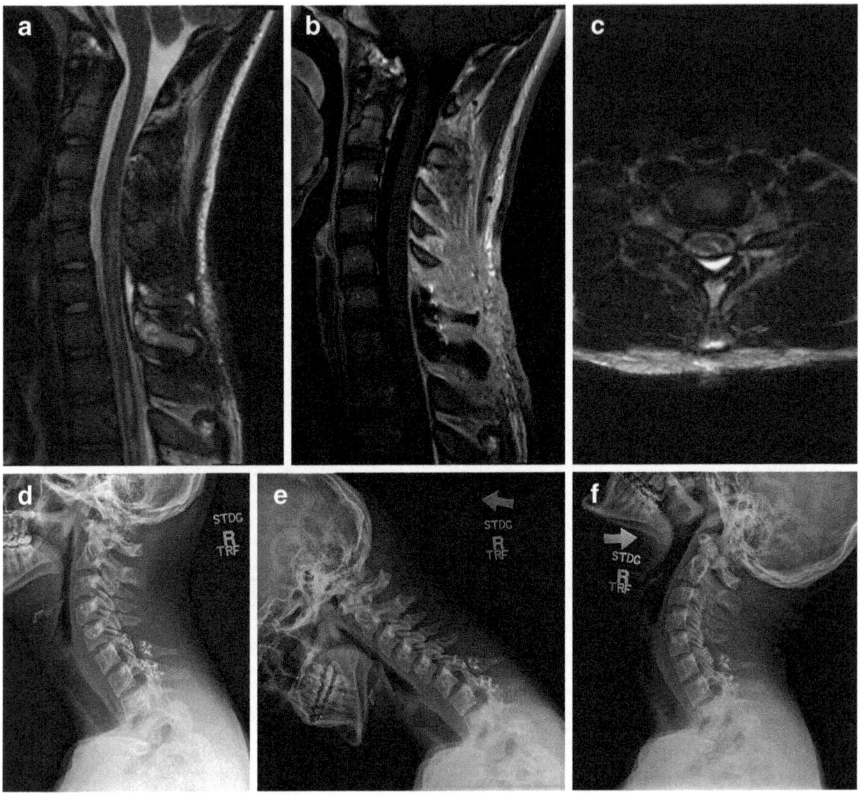

Fig. 9.2 Three-month postoperative magnetic resonance imaging showing complete resection of the lesion and significant improvement in the syrinx. (**a**) sagittal T2-weighted sagittal image; (**b**) sagittal T1-weighted fluid attenuated inversion recovery with contrast and (**c**) axial T2-weighted slice at C6/7. (D–F) Standing neutral, flexion, and extension-view radiographs show a developing focal kyphosis across the laminoplasty site from C6-T1, which is exacerbated in flexion

Postoperative imaging (Fig. 9.4) demonstrated significant improvement in her cervical sagittal alignment (cSVA 5.0 cm) and restoration of normal cervical lordosis (C2–7 lordosis 13.5°). Upright scoliosis films (not shown) also demonstrated reduction in her thoracic hypokyphosis (T4–12 kyphosis 35.2°) and truncal retroversion (C7 SVA 2.06). Clinically, she reported significant improvement in her posture and paraxial neck pain.

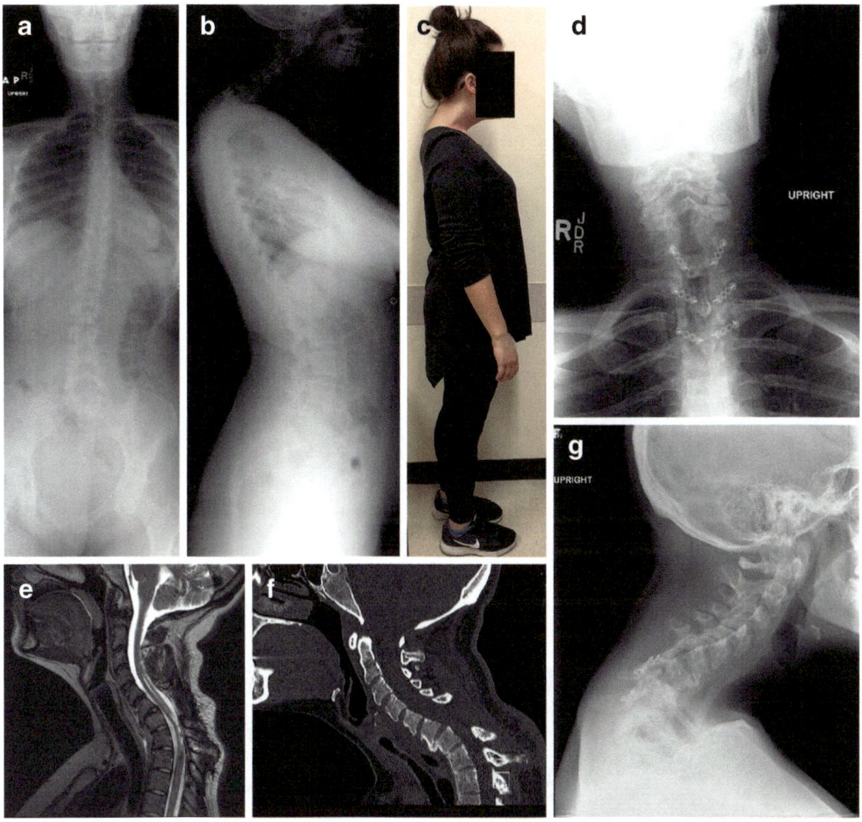

Fig. 9.3 Preoperative upright scoliosis films (**a**, **b**) demonstrated significant positive cervical sagittal balance (cSVA) obvious on clinical exam as a craned forward neck/swan neck deformity (**c**). (**d**, **g**) Upright cervical X-rays show laminoplasty plates from prior osteoplastic laminotomy for her intramedullary lesion. The apex of the deformity was identified at the cervicothoracic junction C6-T1. MR (**e**) showed a persistent small syrinx in the cervical spine immediately proximal to the apex of the deformity but without appreciable cord compression. (**f**) CT demonstrated open disc spaces throughout the cervical and upper thoracic spine, with the exception of ankylosis at the C6/7 segment suggesting a largely flexible deformity

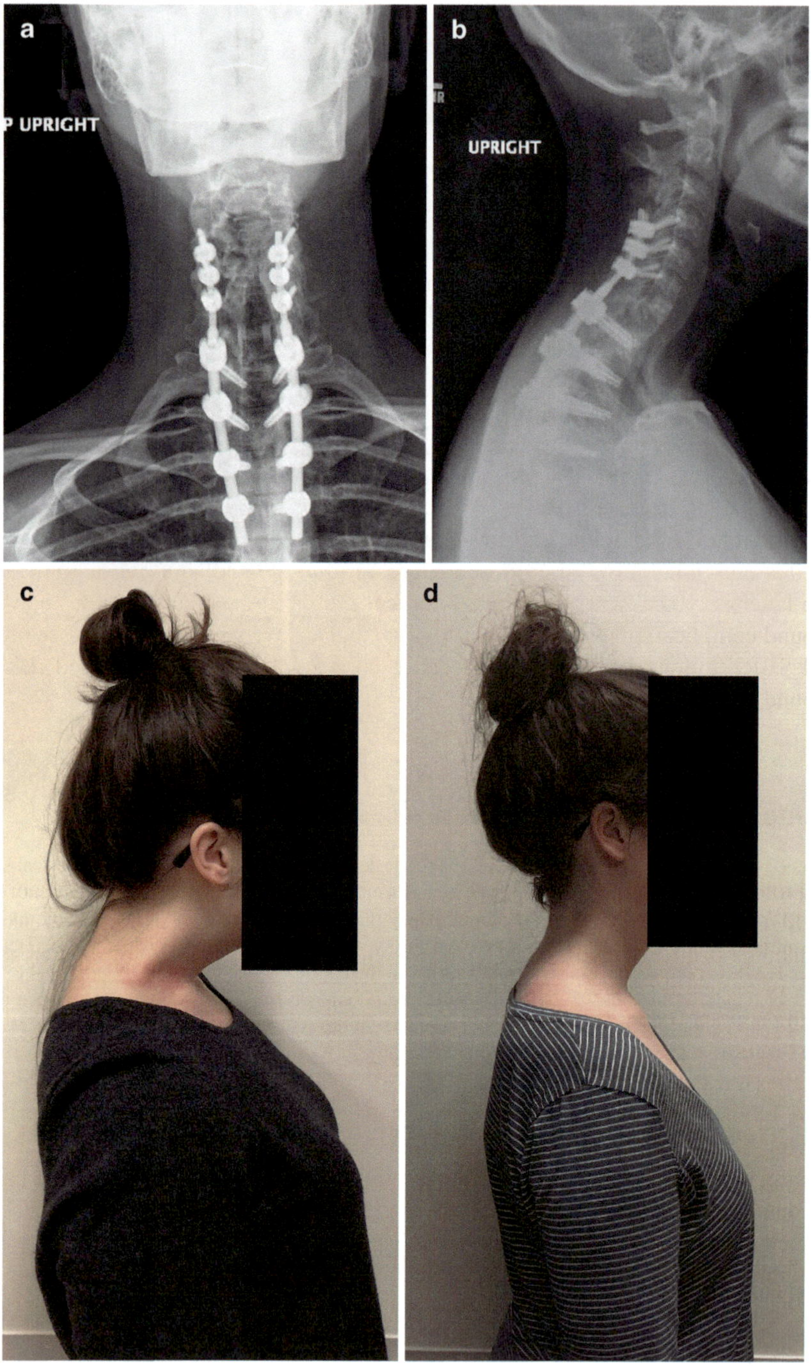

Fig. 9.4 (**a**, **b**) Postoperative upright cervical radiographs after the patient underwent a circumferential fusion with C6/7 anterior cervical diskectomy and fusion followed by a C4-T4 instrumented fusion. (**c**, **d**) Clinical photographs show significant improvement in her upright alignment

Conclusion

Progressive postoperative deformity in the form of postlaminectomy kyphosis is clinically significant sequelae of the management of intradural tumors. Biomechanical testing studies suggest that resection of the posterior ligaments—the supraspinous ligament, interspinous ligament, and ligamentum flavum—and capsular ligaments likely confer much of the risk for this outcome. However, clinical studies have suggested that extensive soft tissue dissection with resultant postoperative paraspinal muscular atrophy, violation or compromise of the facet joints, and elevated T1 slope may additionally contribute. Younger age may also be a contributing factor, though it is unclear if this is due to the flexibility of the juvenile spine or is an artifact of lead time bias, wherein pediatric patients have more time to suffer progressive deformity. One of the most popular strategies to minimize the risk of postoperative progressive deformity is the use of osteoplastic laminotomy (laminoplasty) as opposed to laminectomy. The laminoplasty bone contains biomechanically important ligaments and provides points of attachment to which the dissected muscle can reaffix itself, which may help to restore posterior tension band integrity. Nevertheless, it is likely that in some patients, especially those who undergo multilevel laminectomies/laminoplasties, fusion may be required to prevent later kyphosis.

Devices None.

Previous Presentations None.

Disclosures Zach Pennington None.
Daniel Sciubba Consulting for Baxter, DePuy Synthes, Medtronic, Stryker.
Benjamin D Elder None.

Funding None.

References

1. Ostrom QT, Price M, Neff C et al (2022) CBTRUS statistical report: primary brain and other central nervous system tumors diagnosed in the United States in 2015–2019. Neuro-Oncology 24(Supplement_5):v1–v95. https://doi.org/10.1093/neuonc/noac202
2. Momin AA, Oyem P, Patil N et al (2022) Epidemiology of primary malignant non-osseous spinal tumors in the United States. Spine J 22(8):1325–1333. https://doi.org/10.1016/j.spinee.2022.02.015
3. Hersh AM, Patel J, Pennington Z et al (2022) Perioperative outcomes and survival after surgery for intramedullary spinal cord tumors: a single-institution series of 302 patients. J Neurosurg Spine 37(2):252–262. https://doi.org/10.3171/2022.1.SPINE211235
4. Hersh AM, Antar A, Pennington Z et al (2022) Predictors of survival and time to progression following operative management of intramedullary spinal cord astrocytomas. J Neuro-Oncol 158(1):117–127. https://doi.org/10.1007/s11060-022-04017-4

5. Hersh AM, Patel J, Pennington Z et al (2022) A novel online calculator to predict nonroutine discharge, length of stay, readmission, and reoperation in patients undergoing surgery for intramedullary spinal cord tumors. Spine J 22(8):1345–1355. https://doi.org/10.1016/j.spinee.2022.03.005
6. Lubelski D, Pennington Z, Ochuba A et al (2022) Natural history of brachial plexus, peripheral nerve, and spinal Schwannomas. Neurosurgery 91(6):883–891. https://doi.org/10.1227/neu.0000000000002118
7. Pennington Z, Mikula AL, Lakomkin N et al (2022) Impact of tumor-associated syrinx on outcomes following resection of primary ependymomas of the spinal cord. J Neuro-Oncol 160(3):725–733. https://doi.org/10.1007/s11060-022-04194-2
8. Barrena S, Miguel M, de la Torre CA et al (2011) Late surgery for spinal deformities in children previously treated for neural tumors. Eur J Pediatr Surg 21(01):54–57. https://doi.org/10.1055/s-0030-1267968
9. McGirt MJ, Garcés-Ambrossi GL, Parker SL et al (2010) Short-term progressive spinal deformity following Laminoplasty versus laminectomy for resection of Intradural spinal tumors. Analysis of 238 patients. Neurosurgery 66(5):1005–1012. https://doi.org/10.1227/01.NEU.0000367721.73220.C9
10. Pennington Z, Ahmed AK, Sciubba DM (2020) Deformity secondary to vertebral body metastases. In: Ramakrishna R, Magge RS, Baaj AA, Knisely JPS (eds) Central nervous system metastases, 1st edn. Springer, pp 583–601. https://doi.org/10.1007/978-3-030-42958-4_44
11. Takeshita K, Peterson ETK, Bylski-Austrow D, Crawford AH, Nakamura K (2004) The nuchal ligament restrains cervical spine flexion. Spine (Phila Pa 1976) 29(18):E388–E393. https://doi.org/10.1097/01.brs.0000138309.11926.72
12. Posner I, White AA, Edwards WT, Hayes WC (1982) A biomechanical analysis of the clinical stability of the lumbar and lumbosacral spine. Spine (Phila Pa 1976) 7(4):374–389. https://doi.org/10.1097/00007632-198207000-00008
13. Panjabi MM, Hausfeld JN, White AA (1981) A biomechanical study of the ligamentous stability of the thoracic spine in man. Acta Orthop Scand 52(3):315–326. https://doi.org/10.3109/17453678109050109
14. White AA, Johnson RM, Panjabi MM, Southwick WO (1975) Biomechanical analysis of clinical stability in the cervical spine. Clin Orthop Relat Res 109(109):85–96. https://doi.org/10.1097/00003086-197506000-00011
15. Panjabi MM, White AA III, Johnson RM (1975) Cervical spine mechanics as a function of transection of components. J Biomech 8(5):327–336. https://doi.org/10.1016/0021-9290(75)90085-8
16. Panjabi MM, White AA, Keller D, Southwick WO, Friedlaender G (1978) Stability of the cervical spine under tension. J Biomech 11(4):189–197. https://doi.org/10.1016/0021-9290(78)90012-X
17. Hartman RA, Tisherman RE, Wang C et al (2016) Mechanical role of the posterior column components in the cervical spine. Eur Spine J 25(7):2129–2138. https://doi.org/10.1007/s00586-016-4541-1
18. Adams MA, Hutton WC, Stott JRR (1980) The resistance to flexion of the lumbar intervertebral joint. Spine (Phila Pa 1976) 5(3):245–253. https://doi.org/10.1097/00007632-198005000-00007
19. Barros EMK, Rodrigues CJ, Rodrigues NR, Oliveira RP, Barros TE, Rodrigues AJ (2002) Aging of the elastic and collagen fibers in the human cervical interspinous ligaments. Spine J 2(1):57–62. https://doi.org/10.1016/S1529-9430(01)00167-X
20. Erbulut DU, Zafarparandeh I, Lazoglu I, Ozer AF (2014) Application of an asymmetric finite element model of the C2-T1 cervical spine for evaluating the role of soft tissues in stability. Med Eng Phys 36(7):915–921. https://doi.org/10.1016/j.medengphy.2014.02.020
21. Li Y, Shen Z, Huang M, Wang X (2017) Stepwise resection of the posterior ligamentous complex for stability of a thoracolumbar compression fracture: an in vitro biomechanical investigation. Medicine (Baltimore) 96(35):e7873. https://doi.org/10.1097/MD.0000000000007873
22. Heuer F, Schmidt H, Klezl Z, Claes L, Wilke HJ (2007) Stepwise reduction of functional spinal structures increase range of motion and change lordosis angle. J Biomech 40(2):271–280. https://doi.org/10.1016/j.jbiomech.2006.01.007

23. White AA III, Panjabi MM (1978) The basic kinematics of the human spine: a review of past and current knowledge. Spine (Phila Pa 1976) 3(1):12–20. https://doi.org/10.1097/00007632-197803000-00003
24. Gillespie KA, Dickey JP (2004) Biomechanical role of lumbar spine ligaments in flexion and extension: determination using a parallel linkage robot and a porcine model. Spine (Phila Pa 1976) 29(11):1208–1216. https://doi.org/10.1097/00007632-200406010-00010
25. McGirt MJ, Chaichana KL, Atiba A et al (2008) Incidence of spinal deformity after resection of intramedullary spinal cord tumors in children who underwent laminectomy compared with laminoplasty. J Neurosurg Pediatr 1(1):57–62. https://doi.org/10.3171/PED-08/01/057
26. Yeh JS, Sgouros S, Walsh AR, Hockley AD (2001) Spinal sagittal malalignment following surgery for primary intramedullary Tumours in children. Pediatr Neurosurg 35(6):318–324. https://doi.org/10.1159/000050444
27. Sciubba DM, Chaichana KL, Woodworth GF, McGirt MJ, Gokaslan ZL, Jallo GI (2008) Factors associated with cervical instability requiring fusion after cervical laminectomy for intradural tumor resection. J Neurosurg Spine 8(5):413–419. https://doi.org/10.3171/SPI/2008/8/5/413
28. McGirt MJ, Constantini S, Jallo GI (2008) Correlation of a preoperative grading scale with progressive spinal deformity following surgery for intramedullary spinal cord tumors in children. J Neurosurg Pediatr 2(4):277–281. https://doi.org/10.3171/PED.2008.2.10.277
29. Yao KC, McGirt MJ, Chaichana KL, Constantini S, Jallo GI (2007) Risk factors for progressive spinal deformity following resection of intramedullary spinal cord tumors in children: an analysis of 161 consecutive cases. J Neurosurg Pediatr 107(6):463–468. https://doi.org/10.3171/PED-07/12/463
30. Hersh DS, Iyer RR, Garzon-Muvdi T, Liu A, Jallo GI, Groves ML (2017) Instrumented fusion for spinal deformity after laminectomy or laminoplasty for resection of intramedullary spinal cord tumors in pediatric patients. Neurosurg Focus 43(4):E12. https://doi.org/10.3171/2017.7.FOCUS17329
31. Kim BJ, Cho SM, Hur JW, Cha J, Kim SH (2021) Kinematics after cervical laminoplasty: risk factors for cervical kyphotic deformity after laminoplasty. Spine J 21(11):1822–1829. https://doi.org/10.1016/j.spinee.2021.06.010
32. Muellner M, Haffer H, Moser M et al (2022) Paraspinal musculature impairment is associated with spinopelvic and spinal malalignment in patients undergoing lumbar fusion surgery. Spine J 22(12):2006–2016. https://doi.org/10.1016/j.spinee.2022.07.103
33. Muellner M, Haffer H, Chiapparelli E et al (2022) Differences in lumbar paraspinal muscle morphology in patients with sagittal malalignment undergoing posterior lumbar fusion surgery. Eur Spine J 31(11):3109–3118. https://doi.org/10.1007/s00586-022-07351-3
34. Elysee JC, Lovecchio F, Lafage R et al (2021) The relationship of global sagittal malalignment to fatty infiltration in the aging spine. Eur Spine J 30(9):2480–2485. https://doi.org/10.1007/s00586-021-06759-7
35. Kawaguchi Y, Matsui H, Gejo R, Tsuji H. Preventive measures of Back muscle injury after posterior lumbar spine surgery in rats. Spine *(Phila Pa* 1976*).* 1998;23(21):2282–2287. doi:https://doi.org/10.1097/00007632-199811010-00006
36. Kawaguchi Y, Yabuki S, Styf J et al (1996) Back muscle injury after posterior lumbar spine surgery. Spine (Phila Pa 1976) 21(22):2683–2688. https://doi.org/10.1097/00007632-199611150-00019
37. Ashana AO, Ajiboye RM, Sheppard WL, Sharma A, Kay AB, Holly LT (2017) Cervical Paraspinal muscle atrophy rates following Laminoplasty and laminectomy with fusion for cervical Spondylotic myelopathy. World Neurosurg 107:445–450. https://doi.org/10.1016/j.wneu.2017.07.173
38. Sangala JR, Nichols T, Freeman TB (2011) Technique to minimize paraspinal muscle atrophy after posterior cervical fusion. Clin Neurol Neurosurg 113(1):48–51. https://doi.org/10.1016/j.clineuro.2010.09.001
39. Styf JR, Willén J. The effects of external compression by three different retractors on pressure in the erector spine muscles during and after posterior lumbar spine surgery in humans. Spine (Phila Pa 1976). 1998;23(3):354–358. doi:https://doi.org/10.1097/00007632-199802010-00014
40. Taylor H, H. McGregor A, Medhi-Zadeh S, et al. The impact of self-retaining retractors on the paraspinal muscles during posterior spinal surgery. Spine (Phila Pa 1976). 2002;27(24):2758–2762. doi:https://doi.org/10.1097/00007632-200212150-00004

41. Mukai Y, Takenaka S, Hosono N, Miwa T, Fuji T (2013) Intramuscular pressure of the multifidus muscle and low-back pain after posterior lumbar interbody fusion: comparison of mini-open and conventional approaches. J Neurosurg Spine 19(6):651–657. https://doi.org/10.3171/2013.8.SPINE13183
42. Healy AT, Lubelski D, West JL, Mageswaran P, Colbrunn R, Mroz TE (2016) Biomechanics of open-door laminoplasty with and without preservation of posterior structures. J Neurosurg Spine 24(5):746–751. https://doi.org/10.3171/2015.7.SPINE15229
43. Zdeblick TA, Zou D, Warden KE, McCabe R, Kunz D, Vanderby R (1992) Cervical stability after foraminotomy. A biomechanical in vitro analysis. J Bone Joint Surg Am 74(1):22–27. http://www.ncbi.nlm.nih.gov/pubmed/1734010
44. Subramaniam V, Chamberlain RH, Theodore N et al (2009) Biomechanical effects of Laminoplasty versus laminectomy: stenosis and stability. Spine (Phila Pa 1976) 34(16):E573–E578. https://doi.org/10.1097/BRS.0b013e3181aa0214
45. Kode S, Gandhi AA, Fredericks DC, Grosland NM, Smucker JD (2012) Effect of multilevel open-door Laminoplasty and laminectomy on flexibility of the cervical spine. Spine (Phila Pa 1976) 37(19):E1165–E1170. https://doi.org/10.1097/BRS.0b013e31825e6251
46. Kode S, Kallemeyn NA, Smucker JD, Fredericks DC, Grosland NM (2014) The effect of multi-level laminoplasty and laminectomy on the biomechanics of the cervical spine: a finite element study. Iowa Orthop J 34:150–157. http://www.ncbi.nlm.nih.gov/pubmed/25328475
47. Xu H, Wu J, Xie H et al (2022) Biomechanical behaviour of tension-band-reconstruction titanium plate in open-door laminoplasty: a study based on finite element analysis. BMC Musculoskelet Disord 23(1):851. https://doi.org/10.1186/s12891-022-05804-w
48. Shiraishi T (2002) A new technique for exposure of the cervical spine laminae. J Neurosurg Spine 96(1):122–126. https://doi.org/10.3171/spi.2002.96.1.0122
49. Hosono N, Sakaura H, Mukai Y, Ishii T, Yoshikawa H (2005) En bloc laminoplasty without dissection of paraspinal muscles. J Neurosurg Spine 3(1):29–33. https://doi.org/10.3171/spi.2005.3.1.0029
50. Murphy RF, Mooney JF (2017) The crankshaft phenomenon. J Am Acad Orthop Surg 25(9):e185–e193. https://doi.org/10.5435/JAAOS-D-16-00584
51. Lee CS, Nachemson AL (1997) The crankshaft phenomenon after posterior Harrington fusion in skeletally immature patients with thoracic or thoracolumbar idiopathic scoliosis followed to maturity. Spine (Phila Pa 1976) 22(1):58–67. https://doi.org/10.1097/00007632-199701010-00010

Chapter 10
Chin-On-Chest Deformity from High-Dose Head and Neck Radiation

Michael Shost, Salim Yakdan, Jacob Greenberg, Zachary Wilt, Jetan Badhiwala, Zach Pennington, Darryl Lau, and Jason W. Savage

Background

Cervicothoracic spine deformities can negatively impact patient function and quality of life [1]. Cervical kyphosis is common, being observed in nearly 40% of community dwelling adults [2] and 30% of patients with known thoracolumbar deformity [3]. Most patients are asymptomatic, but with progression cervical kyphosis can result in a "dropped head syndrome" (DHS) or chin-on-chest deformity [4]. DHS appears to be relatively uncommon on the whole, though prior studies of its prevalence are few in number. Of those published series, the literature review by Umapathi noted a 3:2 female-to-male ratio and mean age of 74.5 years, [5] while a more recent review by Drain et al. identified a mean age of 63.3 years, though with a similar 3:2 female-to-male ratio [6].

Patients with chin-on-chest deformity usually present with significant dysfunction, pain, dysphagia, and potentially neurological deficits resulting from ventral compression of the spinal cord as it drapes over the kyphotic spine [7–9]. The sagittal imbalance caused by this condition affects the patient's ability to maintain a

M. Shost (✉) · J. Greenberg · Z. Wilt · J. Badhiwala · J. W. Savage
Cleveland Clinic Center for Spine Health, Cleveland, OH, USA
e-mail: mds244@case.edu; jacobgreenberg@wustl.edu; jetan.badhiwala@sunnybrook.ca; savagej2@ccf.org

S. Yakdan
Department of Neurosurgery, Washington University, St. Louis, MO, USA

Z. Pennington
Department of Neurologic Surgery, Mayo Clinic, Rochester, MN, USA
e-mail: pennington.zachary@mayo.edu

D. Lau
Department of Neurosurgery, New York University, New York, NY, USA
e-mail: darryl.lau@nyulangone.org

D. M. Sciubba (ed.), *Spinal Tumor Associated Deformity*,
https://doi.org/10.1007/978-3-031-87939-5_10

forward gaze or a steady gait, resulting in increased fall risk [10, 11]. In severe cases, the chin-on-chest deformity may even hinder feeding due to the inability of the patient to fully opening the jaw or maintaining a proper posture for swallowing [12, 13]. This can result in continued deconditioning and even global skeletal muscle loss, further exacerbating the condition. Last, the deformity can also have intolerable negative cosmetic and social consequences.

Pathogenesis

Chin-on-chest deformity can occur secondary to multilevel disc degeneration, bony failure (i.e., wedging of the cervical vertebral bodies), [14] multilevel anterolisthesis, cervical paraspinal muscle weakness, [15] or a combination of these factors [16]. Failure of the anterior and middle column (discs and vertebral bodies) leads to a loss of anterior column height relative to the posterior column (lateral masses, facet joints) with resultant kyphosis. In the degenerative population, this is usually due to multilevel disc degeneration, which may also be accompanied by vertebral wedging [17]. However, in the context of neoplastic disease of the spine, anterior and middle column shortening is likely due to pathologic fracture of tumor-infiltrated vertebra(e). However, concurrent disc degeneration may also be seen given that many patients are in the sixth decade of life and beyond. Deformity secondary to disc collapse may show flexibility on preoperative evaluation, but deformity secondary to vertebral body collapse is often fixed, at least to a degree, which influences surgical planning.

Weakness of the posterior cervical musculature—the semispinalis capitis, semispinalis cervicis, splenius capitis, multifidus, and splenius cervicis [18, 19] —has been associated with cervical spine deformity in multiple congenital [20] and neurological conditions, [15, 21–25] along with a handful of endocrinological and metabolic conditions [26–30]. The semispinalis cervicis and capitis play particularly important roles in neck extension with the semispinalis cervicis running from the transverse processes of the upper thoracic vertebra (T3-T5) to the spinous processes of the C2-C5 vertebra [31]. Deformity due to paraspinal musculature weakness is generally flexible at presentation, though with time there can be ossification of the anterior longitudinal ligament, resulting in a fixed deformity [15].

Radiation-induced dropped head syndrome falls into this latter category and is increasingly recognized as an important cause of DHS in the oncology population [32]. Approximately 60% of cancer patients undergo radiotherapy (RT) at some point during their treatment course [33] and high-dose radiotherapy remains an integral part of standard management in head and neck cancer [34]. Patients with metastatic cancer to the spine—the most common site of bony metastasis—also commonly receive radiotherapy to help with pain palliation and local disease control, as do patients undergoing treatment for supradiaphragmatic lymphomas. [35, 36] Given this, the cohort of patients at risk for postradiotherapy DHS is relatively large. Additionally, post-RT DHS can present in a very delayed fashion—5–30 years postradiotherapy [37]. Johansson et al. were the first to report an association between DHS and mantle field RT in patients undergoing treatment for lymphoma [38]. Since then, DHS has been increasingly recognized as a long-term complication of head and neck radiation, and more cases of radiation-induced DHS and also camptocormia were reported [38–41]. The exact etiology of postradiotherapy DHS appears to be multifactorial and may represent a combination of both radiation-induced movement disorders [32] and the fibrosis and atrophy of irradiated muscle [42]. The most recent literature suggests that movement disorders caused by radiotherapy are a combined effect of neuropathy/plexopathy and muscular injury [37, 43]. Both myopathic and neurogenic EMG changes have been reported [37]. In a narrative review done by Stubblefield et al., neuromuscular complications were attributed to the direct and indirect effects of progressive fibrotic sclerosis, which can affect all the neural structures (i.e., brain, spinal cord, nerve root, plexus, peripheral nerves) and the muscles [36].

Clinical and Radiographic Evaluation

Clinical Workup

Evaluation of patients presenting with chin-on-chest deformity should include a detailed clinical history along with a thorough radiographic evaluation and neurological examination. Patient history can be helpful for identifying the potential etiology of the cervical deformity (e.g., progressive postradiation deformity, new onset neck pain concerning for compression fracture). It can also identify relevant medical comorbidities essential for evaluating a patient's surgical candidacy. The neurological exam should focus on signs/symptoms concerning for myelopathy, which may favor more urgent surgical intervention. The patient's exam should also include assessment of the flexibility of the deformity by having the patient move their neck through the full range of motion. In most clinical encounters for severe DHS, a readily noticeable exam finding is an elevated chin-brow vertical angle (CBVA) (Fig. 10.1). This measurement is established by the angle between a line that connects the patient's brow and chin and a vertical line; a CBVA between $-10°$ and $10°$ is considered normal, [44] though some studies of community dwelling individuals have suggested an even narrower range ($-1.5°$ to $5.8°$) [45]. Using a population of patients undergoing surgical evaluation, Lafage et al. [46] found that patients with CBVA less than $-5°$ or greater than $18°$ were both associated with significant disability as measured with the Oswestry Disability Index. It is noted that patients with significant subaxial kyphosis or a high T1 slope attempt to compensate with induced lordosis in the upper cervical spine with resultant posterior neck pain. As the deformity continues, extension fails to be sufficient and patients begin to develop an ever-increasing CBVA with a resultant progressively downward gaze that impairs eye contact, gaze concordance, walking, and many other activities of daily life

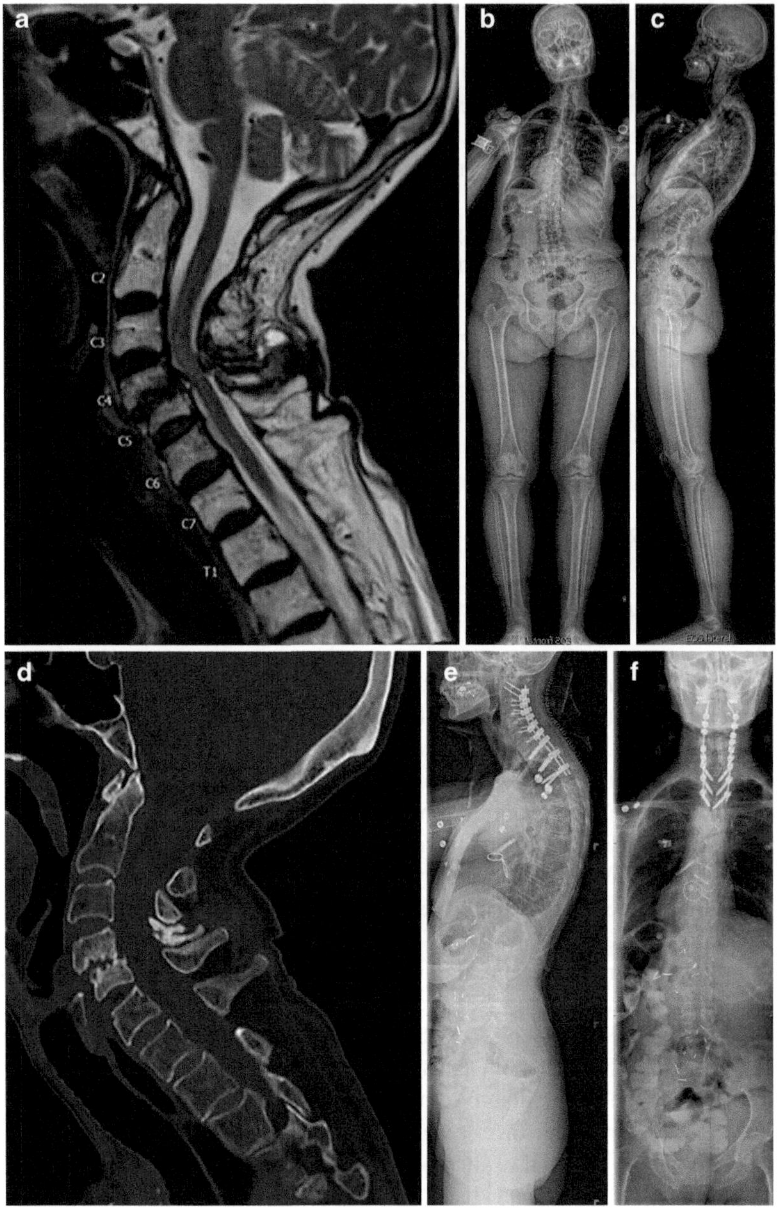

Fig. 10.1 (**a**) T2-weight MR showed stenosis at the C4/5 level with a grade 1–2 spondylolisthesis. (**b**, **c**) Preoperative upright radiographs showed significant lumbar hyperextension with a negative sagittal balance (−11 cm). (**d**) CT showed disc space collapse with erosion of the adjoining endplates and sclerosis of the underlying cancellous bone. (**e, f**) Upright radiographs following C2-T3 instrumented fusion showed good correction with the patient able to maintain a forward gaze without compensatory lumbar hyperlordosis. (**g**) MR, (**h**) CT, and (**i, j**) upright radiographs showed distal junctional failure inside of 12 weeks with a compression fracture of T3. The patient had a resultant high T1 slope (67°) with negative sagittal balance (−12.3 cm) due to lumbar hyperlordosis (84°). (**k, l**) She ultimately underwent extension of her fusion to the pelvis

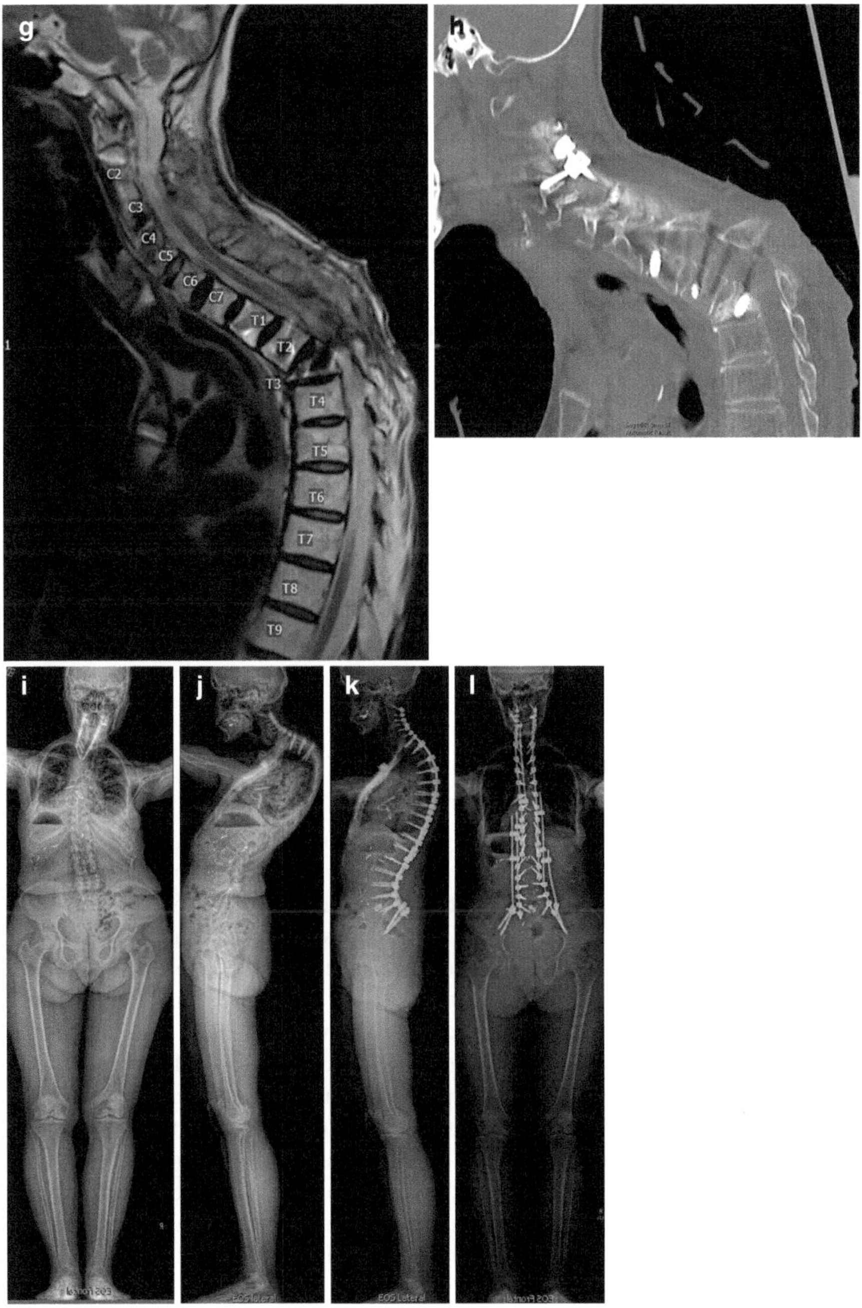

Fig. 10.1 (continued)

solely from the mechanical positioning of the head. Additionally with progression, there can be cord compression. Previous studies have demonstrated a connection between the severity of kyphotic cervical deformities and spinal cord intramedullary pressure. Increased intramedullary pressure can compromise cord vascular supply leading to demyelination and progressive cord injury [9, 47, 48]. Prior studies have shown that increasingly kyphotic deformities of the cervical spine correlate with the severity of myelopathy, so careful monitoring of a patient's clinical exam findings as well as periodic radiographic studies allows for objective measurements of deformity evolution over time [9]. Overly negative CBVA is also maladaptive, as cervical flexion is necessary for many activities, such as using the bathroom and walking [44]. An overly upward gaze prevents patients from seeing their feet and increases their fall risk.

Additionally, cervical deformity is associated with high baseline levels of swallowing dysfunction and patients being considered for surgery should be referred for a preoperative swallow evaluation. At the bedside, this may be performed by having the patient lean against a wall and keep their head in contact with the wall while attempting to drink from a cup of water, though formal evaluation is often recommended. The bedside exam is informative, though in that the patient is prevented from extending/flexing their head; those with difficulty drinking from the cup are at increased likelihood of postoperative swallowing issues if the fusion construct is extended to the occiput.

Radiographic Evaluation

Radiographic assessment is key to surgical planning, not only for identifying the flexibility and severity of the deformity but also for identifying concurrent stenosis that should be addressed during correction of the deformity [49–54]. Not all cervical deformity originates in the cervical spine. Consequently, evaluation of patients with chin-on-chest deformity should include assessment of global alignment to ensure accurate classification of the origins of the deformity. Global alignment is dictated by the combination of craniocervical, cervical, thoracic, and lumbar balance as well as the spinopelvic interaction. To evaluate this, 36-inch standing scoliosis films should be obtained, or if possible, full-length standing radiographs including the knee that allow the surgeon to evaluate the patient's compensatory mechanisms (e.g., pelvic retroversion and knee flexion). Flexion–extension view cervical radiographs should also be considered to help assess the rigidity of the deformity [55]. From these radiographs, the C7-sagittal vertical axis (SVA), lumbar lordosis (LL), pelvic tilt (PT), pelvic incidence (PI), and T4–12 thoracic kyphosis (TK) should all be measured to quantify the thoracolumbar alignment (Fig. 10.2) [47]. SVA is used as a measure of global alignment and for most patients a target SVA <5 cm is sought as this has been associated with improved quality of life outcomes [56]. Some patients may initially present with "normal" SVA but have significantly elevated pelvic tilt (i.e., >25°) or thoracic hypokyphosis, two signs that

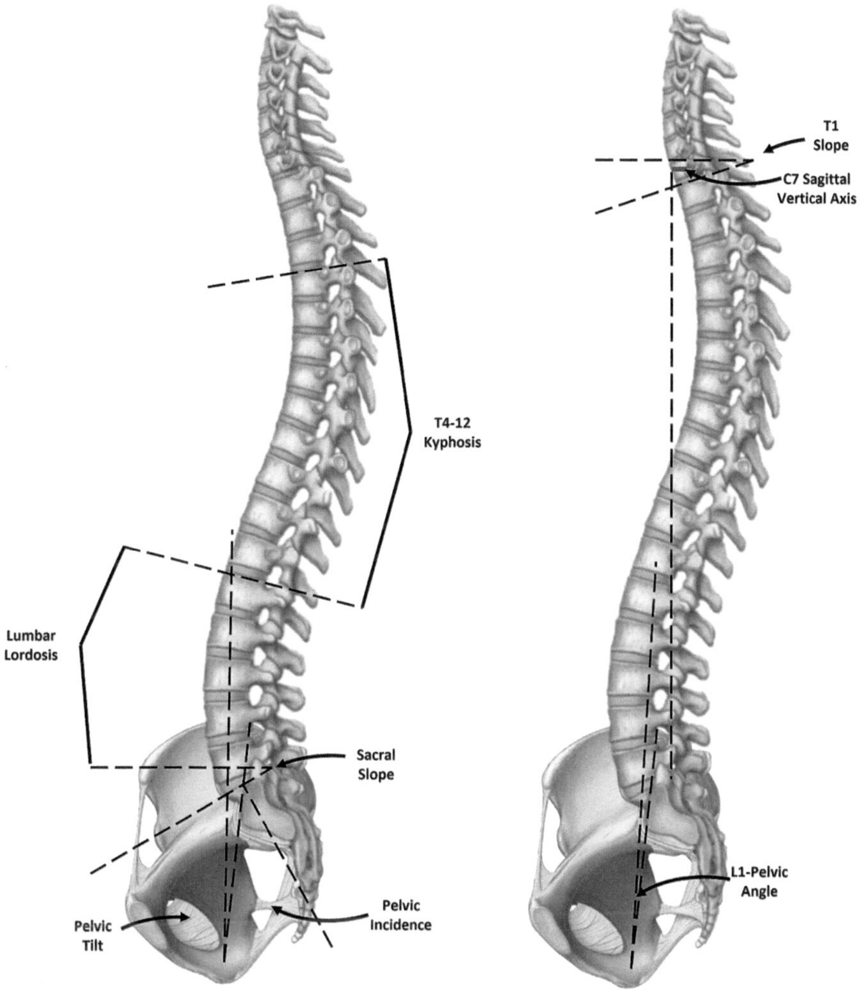

Fig. 10.2 Summary of the sagittal alignment parameters in the cervical, thoracic, and lumbar spine

they may have compensated thoracolumbar sagittal plane deformity. With further deformity progression, these patients develop increasingly positive SVA and suffer concordantly greater disability. Typical thoracolumbar alignment goals therefore include SVA <5 cm, PI-LL mismatch <10°, and PT < 25°.

The cervical spine has some analogous parameters to those employed for the thoracolumbar spine, with T1 slope (T1S) acting as a surrogate for sacral slope (SS), C2–7 lordosis (CL) for lumbar lordosis, C2–7 SVA (cSVA) for SVA, and cervical lordosis T1 slope mismatch (TS-CL) for PI-LL mismatch [44, 54]. The cervical sagittal vertical axis (cSVA) is the horizontal distance between vertical lines drawn through the midpoint of the C2 vertebral body and posterosuperior aspect of the C7 vertebral body. It is a measure of cervical spine sagittal alignment, and more positive cSVA value is associated with increasing strain on the cervical joints and paraspinal muscles. Tang et al. found that cSVA > 4 cm was correlated with increased neck pain and worsened disability postoperatively [51].

Normal cervical lordosis ranges from 20° to 35° with some variation based on measurement technique [9, 55, 57]. While both C1 and C2 have been used as the superior aspect for the measurement, the Ames-ISSG cervical deformity classification [54] employs C2, and it has been reported that measurements using C1 tend to overestimate lordosis [58]. Increased cervical lordosis is a mechanism seen in many aging adults to maintain forward gaze in the setting of progressive thoracolumbar sagittal imbalance and loss of cervical lordosis [59, 60]. Loss of cervical lordosis is a hallmark of DHS and C2–7 lordosis is conventionally measured using the Cobb angle, though other methods (e.g., Jackson physiological stress lines, Harrison posterior tangent method) have been reported and may improve on the accuracy of the Cobb method in addition to providing more discrete information on the lordosis at each cervical level [60, 61].

Assessment of the cervicothoracic junction is key to assessing the etiology of the deformity and its anatomy can be described with the thoracic inlet angle, T1 slope, and neck tilt (Fig. 10.3). The thoracic inlet angle is analogous to PI and is formed by the perpendicular bisector of the superior T1 endplate and a line connecting the midpoint of the superior T1 endplate to the superior aspect of the sternum. T1

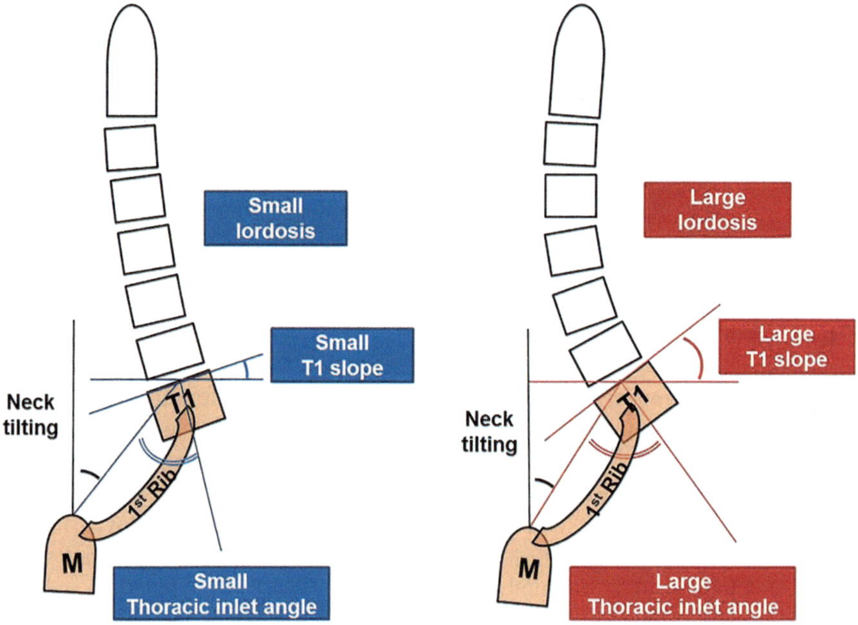

Fig. 10.3 Illustration of how thoracic inlet angle and T1-slope impact the amount of cervical lordosis required to maintain cervical sagittal vertical axis and balance. Reproduced from Sheer et al. Neurosurgery 2021;88:864–883

slope—analogous to sacral slope for the thoracolumbar spine—is subtended by a line through the superior endplate of T1 and a horizontal line. Finally, neck tilt—analogous to pelvic tilt—is the angle between the line that connects the upper sternum and midpoint of the superior end plate of T1 and a vertical line through the upper sternum. A 2012 study by Lee et al. outlined average values for these measurements in asymptomatic adults for thoracic inlet angle, T1 slope, and neck tilt of 69.5°, 25.7°, and 43.7°, respectively [50]. A recent study by Sakamoto et al. showed postoperative T1 slope—cervical lordosis mismatches >20° were associated with poorer quality of life outcomes following surgery [62]. It has also been shown that a high T1 slope requires more cervical lordosis to maintain a "normal" cSVA and overall sagittal plane balance in the cervical spine. Patient with high T1S may have an unrecognized thoracolumbar deformity, though in the content of oncologic disease, chin-on-chest deformity is usually secondary to either pathologic fracture (focal cervical deformity) or weakness of the posterior chain. The latter can occur following previous posterior surgery (see Chaps. 1 and 9) or from radiotherapy, which can cause fibrosis and atrophy of the paraspinal muscles/cervical extensors.

Surgical Treatment

Surgery for cervical kyphosis can be for any of the following indications: (1) neurologic deficits/spinal cord compression related to the deformity, (2) intractable pain secondary to malalignment, or (3) functional disability (e.g., feeding difficulties) caused by the deformity. In many cases, surgery for chin-on-chest deformity is performed for a combination of all three. Although surgical correction of this deformity is frequently morbid, patient satisfaction following the correction is high [63]. When weighing surgical options, there are a number of options to consider such as the positioning of the patient, the approach, the implantable hardware and fixation options, whether an osteotomy is required, and the vertebral levels to include. These considerations are interrelated and are often dictated by the characteristics of the deformity.

Historically, the approaches for correction of cervical kyphosis have been varied and less extensively studied than deformities of the thoracolumbar spine. Multiple cervical deformity classification schema have been developed but all incorporate sagittal alignment parameters, neurological status, cervical spine flexibility, and involvement of the cervicothoracic junction. [52, 54, 64]

Flexible deformities (e.g., postlaminectomy kyphosis and postradiation kyphosis) afford more treatment options as passive positioning of the neck is sufficient to reduce the deformity. The corrected deformity can then be locked in posteriorly with or without an adjunct anterior approach. Bivector traction is often used to help with repositioning of the head/neck once the corrective procedure has been performed. Rigid deformities are more cumbersome, as they cannot be passively corrected and are subdivided based on the presence of ankylosis. In cases of rigidity without ankylosis, anterior discectomies provide flexibility for subsequent reduction of the deformity prior to anterior grafting; a posterior stage is generally then performed to increase the biomechanical stability of the construct (Fig. 10.4). Though anterior grafts alone can be sufficient for flexible or mild deformities, posterior screw-rod instrumentation has been shown to provide long-term maintenance of correction and lordotic alignment in cervical kyphotic deformities [65]. A posterior stage also allows for the performance of osteotomies and posterior column shortening, which can complement the anterior column lengthening performed during the anterior approach. The use of a circumferential approach for complex reductions is common, especially when there are comorbidities that may raise the concern for the development of pseudoarthrosis or the loss of deformity correction [66].

The choice of fixation options has associated benefits and drawbacks. For example, cobalt chrome rods offer the most rigidity, creating a stiffer construct than titanium rods, but may increase the risk of developing junctional kyphosis and/or failure [8, 67–69]. Recent advances in fusion fixation materials also include carbon fiber-reinforced polyetheretherketone (CFR-PEEK) instrumentation [70]. Particularly in the case of oncology patients who may benefit from long-term monitoring with MRI scans, the use of carbon fiber pedicle screws and rods provides similar durability and strength to traditional hardware with significantly smaller imaging artifacts [71, 72]. However, neither of the major vendors currently have FDA-approved cervical systems. Similarly, there are several interbody hardware options including autograft or allograft bone, titanium, PEEK, and CFR-PEEK. These implants can be further augmented with morselized bone, demineralized bone matrix (DBM), or bone morphogenetic protein (BMP) to encourage fusion [73]. However, the use of BMP in the cervical spine remains controversial

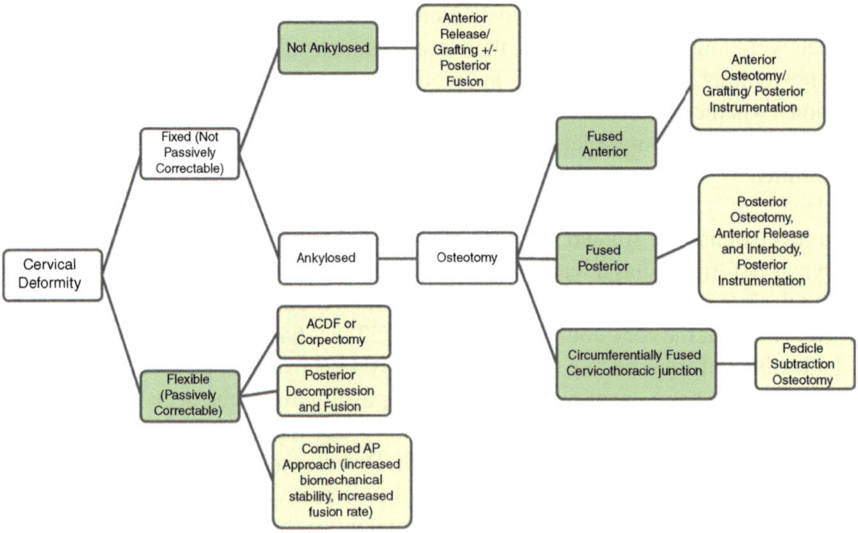

Fig. 10.4 Algorithm for treating cervical deformity. Reproduced from Shannon H, et al. Neurosurg Focus 2014;36:E5

and is not advised in the anterior cervical spine following reports of swelling leading to dysphagia and respiratory distress [74–76]. Additionally, while BMP use in oncology patients has been reported, [77] its use remains contraindicated per FDA labeling owing to the theoretically increased risk of new malignancy, though several studies have failed to demonstrate any association between BMP use and malignancy risk [78, 79]. The addition of BMP to a posterior cervical fusion surgery for patients with chin-on-chest deformity following oncology treatment should involve careful surgical decision-making on a case-by-case basis that weighs the risks and benefits for each individual patient. The addition of vertebral augmentation with cement is another option that may be used to help correct postradiation cervical kyphosis, [80] though its use in the cervical spine has been limited owing to the difficulty with performing transpedicular augmentation of cervical vertebrae. Nevertheless, it has been widely used in the thoracolumbar spine [81] and so may be a valuable technique for reducing loss of fixation at the distal construct end in patients undergoing treatment for cervical deformity. [82] Additionally, a handful of authors [83] have described the use of cement augmentation of anterior cervical plate screws as a method for improving purchase in patients with weak bone, placing the cement into the pilot holes prior to screw placement. Such a strategy may be feasible for patients with postradiation deformity undergoing circumferential fusion.

The main goals of surgery are reduction/correction of the deformity and restoration of horizontal gaze. Consequently, when developing a surgical plan, the surgeon must ask what is driving the deformity (e.g., high T1 slope, multilevel kyphosis, focal subaxial kyphosis as in the case of pathologic fracture), which helps with level determination. The surgeon should also ask whether the deformity appears to be driven by anterior column collapse (e.g., pathologic fracture), which requires anterior column lengthening, subluxation/spondylolisthesis (generally requires a posterior stage to maintain the reduction), or a combination of the two. Additionally, the degree to which the deformity is fixed, i.e., irreducible w positioning, is important as it guides decisions regarding osteotomy use. Ames and colleagues [84] described a nomenclature system with seven grades of increasing invasiveness. Grades 1 (partial facet resection) and 2 (complete facet resection) are posterior-based osteotomies capable of achieving up to 10° of lordosis per level [85] but require an unfused anterior column [84]. These osteotomies can be combined with ACDFs performed anteriorly to further increase correction. When compressing across the posterior column osteotomy, care must be taken to ensure the nerve roots are thoroughly decompressed so as to avoid injury. Grades 3–4 are anterior-only bony resections, with grade 3 being a partial or complete corpectomy and grade 4 being an anterior osteotomy through the lateral vertebral body and uncovertebral joints. Grade 4 osteotomies pose increased risk of injury to the vertebral arteries, which may often need to be skeletonized to complete the osteotomy. Grades 5 and 6 are posterior-only opening wedge and closing wedge three-column osteotomies, respectively. Grade 5 osteotomy resects the posterior elements and then employs an osteoclastic fracture into the anterior column to use the middle column as a fulcrum for segmental correction. It is generally employed in the ankylosed spine and so may not be needed for postradiotherapy cervical kyphosis. Grade 6 osteotomy is the cervical equivalent of a pedicle subtraction osteotomy and allows for significant segmental correction. Last, grade 7 (vertebral column resection) is a combined antero-posterior osteotomy that completely resection the vertebral body and posterior elements. It allows for significant sagittal and coronal correction, and grade 6 is ideally suited for fixed deformities with focal kyphosis. Vertebral column resections in the upper thoracic spine can be done from an all-posterior approach though. These more invasive osteotomies are generally reserved for the most-severe deformities [86].

Osteotomies in the cervical spine carry greater intrinsic risk than thoracic spine osteotomies given the presence of the vertebral artery, which generally enters the vertebral foramina at the level of C6. As a result, many surgeons will perform osteotomies at the level of C7 or below to ensure that the vertebral artery remains anterior and is less likely to be injured [87]. Radiographically, the more caudal osteotomy site has the added advantage of providing maximal cSVA correction [53]. Other advantages of osteotomies at the cervicothoracic junction include that the spinal canal is wider at more caudal levels of the cervical spine [88] and the relative occupancy ratio of the spinal cord is lower, [89] theoretically reducing the risk of spinal cord injury. Additionally, in the case of injury during osteotomy, a more caudal osteotomy level would correspond to greater preservation of function, including potential partial preservation of hand grip and function [90]. This approach was supported by Yuk et al., [87] who reported their experience in a small series of patients treated for cervicothoracic deformity. We likewise prefer performing PSO in the upper thoracic versus lower cervical spine, as it avoids the potential for irritation/injury to the C8 or T1 nerve roots. It also allows for the PSO to be closed with pedicle screws above and below the osteotomy site, which are more powerful fixation tools than either lateral mass or pedicle screws of the subaxial cervical spine.

The selection of instrumentation levels is dependent on the location of the deformity within the cervical spine or potentially cervicothoracic spine. For patients requiring a large cSVA correction or with significant preoperative T1S-CL mismatch, [6] selecting a lower instrumented vertebra (LIV) within the proximal thoracic spine [versus cervicothoracic junction] may improve long-term fusion outcomes and reduce revision risk. Kim and colleagues [91] from the International Spine Study Group (ISSG) recently compared outcomes between cervical deformity patients with an LIV in the cervicothoracic junction or proximal thoracic spine. The authors noted similar radiographic and clinical outcomes at 1 year but acknowledged the cohort was relatively small and those with proximal thoracic LIVs underwent greater deformity correction and more commonly required a three-column osteotomy. C2 is a commonly selected UIV for cervical deformity as it allows for preservation of movement at the atlantooccipital and atlantoaxial joints, which account for greater than 50% of motion in the cervical spine. C2 additionally often has large pedicles relative to other cervical segments, which allows for placement of pedicle screws that afford stronger purchase relative to lateral mass screws and so can facilitate greater correction. Subaxial cervical spine pedicle screws may be preferred in cases of severe deformity as they have lower rates of bone-screw interface loosening and higher fatigue strength. They can therefore better facilitate correction and help to offload mechanical stresses on other levels [92, 93].

Overall, severe kyphotic cervical deformities such as chin-on-chest represent a complex surgical challenge, and there is a lack of consensus in the field on approach, fusion levels, or osteotomies [94]. Therefore, these cases should be approached with a thoughtful evaluation of the patient's clinical status and goals for treatment. This is especially important in the oncology population, where surgeons must also consider the patient's overall disease burden and prognosis, as recovery from significant cervical deformity correction may be 12 months longer.

Case Example

A 69-year-old female with prior history of mantle radiation treatment (treatment field chest to abdomen) for Hodgkin's lymphoma came to clinical attention after undergoing open heart surgery for aortic stenosis. She underwent placement of mechanical mitral and aortic valve replacements along with augmentation of the noncoronary sinus with a Dacron patch (on Warfarin). After surgery, the patient endorsed difficulty maintaining upright head posture; she endorsed her head dropping forward with a loss of posterior cervical muscle control. She sought neurosurgical evaluation and was initially managed with a combination of exercise and physical therapy, which allowed her to maintain normal cervical alignment. However, she developed worsening head posture along with weakness of the arms and hands, clumsiness of bilateral hands, spasms of the left greater than right upper arms, and paresthesias of the bilateral upper extremities that had become constant. She underwent MR (Fig. 10.1a) that showed collapsed of the C4/5-disc space and compression of the cervical cord. Upright scoliosis films (Fig. 10.1b, c) showed lumbar hyperextension as compensatory mechanisms to maintain foreword gaze; she had a − 11 cm SVA. She ultimately presented to the emergency department with 2–3 weeks of significant symptom progression, noted for worsening hand weakness and clumsiness, and an inability to ambulate due to gait unsteadiness. On exam, she had 4/5 weakness of the hand grip and interossei, along with a left-sided Hoffman. She underwent C2-T3 posterior instrumented fusion and C4–5 laminectomy (Fig. 10.1e, f).

Unfortunately, the patient suffered distal junctional failure with MR and CT (Fig. 10.1g, h) showed a wedge compression fracture of the T3 body. Upright scoliosis films (Fig. 10.1i, j) showed significant thoracic hyperkyphosis (113°) with an apex at the fracture, a high T1-slope (67°), negative sagittal alignment (SVA −12.3 cm), and lumbar hyperlordosis (84°). The patient was taken to the OR for extension of her fusion to the pelvis (Fig. 10.1k, l) with a PSO at the fracture site (T3). This resulted in overall improvement in her sagittal alignment (−2.9 cm), reduction of the T1 slope (31°), and thoracic kyphosis (61°).

Summary

Chin-on-chest deformity is a clinically disabling condition, the treatment of which often involves highly morbid, staged surgery. The etiology is often multifactorial and in the context of postradiation kyphosis, the deformity may occur secondary to a combination of anterior column failure (i.e., pathologic fracture) and weakness of the posterior chain due to fibrosis and atrophy of the paraspinal musculature following radiotherapy. The exact strategy for correction is based on the focality of the deformity, location of the deformity apex, and relative rigidity of the deformity. Treatment seeks to restore horizontal gaze and sagittal alignment, and the surgical plan may require a combination of interbody placement to restore anterior column height and osteotomies to correct fixed deformities. Complications occur in a non-trivial proportion of patients—up to 40% of patients suffer intraoperative complications, [95] over 50% experience perioperative complications, [96] and more than a third require surgical revision [95]. Therefore, thorough preoperative evaluation and patient counseling are essential to achieve an optimal outcome in this high-risk population.

References

1. Smith JS, Line B, Bess S et al (2017) The Health Impact of Adult Cervical Deformity in Patients Presenting for Surgical Treatment: Comparison to United States Population Norms and Chronic Disease States Based on the EuroQuol-5 Dimensions Questionnaire. Neurosurgery 80:716–725
2. Ao S, Liu Y, Wang Y, Zhang H, Leng H (2019) Cervical kyphosis in asymptomatic populations: incidence, risk factors, and its relationship with health-related quality of life. J Orthop Surg Res 14:322
3. Smith JS, Lafage V, Schwab FJ et al (2014) Prevalence and Type of Cervical Deformity Among 470 Adults With Thoracolumbar Deformity. Spine (Phila Pa 1976) 39:E1001–E1009
4. Marcon RM, Ono AH de A, Zelada FGB, Cristante AF, Barros Filho TEP (2018) Surgical correction of severe and fixed chin-on-chest deformity. Acta Ortopédica Bras 26:415–417
5. Umapathi T (2002) Head drop and camptocormia. J Neurol Neurosurg Psychiatry 73:1–7
6. Drain JP, Virk SS, Jain N, Yu E (2019) Dropped Head Syndrome: A Systematic Review. Clin Spine Surg 32:423–429
7. Koller H, Hartmann S (2018) Die fixierte zervikale hochgradige Kyphose. Orthopade 47:505–517
8. Miyamoto H, Ikeda T, Aoyama S, Toriumi K, Akagi M (2023) Dropped head syndrome: a treatment strategy and surgical intervention. Eur Spine J 32:1275–1281
9. Ames CP, Blondel B, Scheer JK et al (2013) Cervical Radiographical Alignment: comprehensive assessment techniques and potential importance in cervical myelopathy. Spine (Phila Pa 1976) 38:S149–S160
10. McDaniels-Davidson C, Nichols JF, Vaida F, Marshall LM, Kado DM (2020) Kyphosis and 3-year fall risk in community-dwelling older men. Osteoporos Int 31:1097–1104
11. Kado DM, Huang M-H, Nguyen CB, Barrett-Connor E, Greendale GA (2007) Hyperkyphotic Posture and Risk of Injurious Falls in Older Persons: The Rancho Bernardo Study. J Gerontol Ser A Biol Sci Med Sci 62:652–657

12. Moses MJ, Tishelman JC, Zhou PL, Moon JY, Beaubrun BM, Buckland AJ, Protopsaltis TS (2019) McGregor's slope and slope of line of sight: two surrogate markers for Chin-Brow vertical angle in the setting of cervical spine pathology. Spine J 19:1512–1517
13. Iyer S, Kim HJ, Bao H et al (2019) Cervical Deformity Patients Have Baseline Swallowing Dysfunction but Surgery Does Not Increase Dysphagia at 3 Months: Results From a Prospective Cohort Study. Glob Spine J 9:532–539
14. Remes V, Marttinen E, Poussa M, Kaitila I, Peltonen J (1999) Cervical Kyphosis in Diastrophic Dysplasia. Spine (Phila Pa 1976) 24:1990
15. Sharan AD, Kaye D, Charles Malveaux WMS, Riew DK (2012) Dropped Head Syndrome: Etiology and Management. J Am Acad Orthop Surg 20:766–774
16. McKay SD, Al-Omari A, Tomlinson LA, Dormans JP (2012) Review of Cervical Spine Anomalies in Genetic Syndromes. Spine (Phila Pa 1976) 37:E269–E277
17. Hiratzka J, Ching A, Hart R (2011) Degenerative Cervical Kyphosis: Anatomy, Biomechanics, and Etiology. Semin Spine Surg 23:170–172
18. Zhang J, Tsuzuki N, Hirabayashi S, Saiki K, Fujita K (2003) Surgical Anatomy of the Nerves and Muscles in the Posterior Cervical Spine. Spine (Phila Pa 1976) 28:1379–1384
19. Bogduk N (1982) The Clinical Anatomy of the Cervical Dorsal Rami. Spine (Phila Pa 1976) 7:319–330
20. Rose MR, Levin KH, Griggs RC (1999) The dropped head plus syndrome: quantitation of response to corticosteroids. Muscle Nerve 22:115–118
21. Kuncl RW, Cornblath DR, Griffin JW (1988) Assessment of thoracic paraspinal muscles in the diagnosis of ALS. Muscle Nerve 11:484–492
22. Hoffman D, Gutmann L, Griggs RC, Mendell JR, Miller RG (1994) The dropped head syndrome with chronic inflammatory demyelinating polyneuropathy. Muscle Nerve 17:808–810
23. Jaster JH, Bertorini TE, Swims MP, Dohan FC, Menke PG, Becske T, Mönkemüller KE (1996) Cervical Kyphosis after resolution of myopathic head drop. A Case Report Spine (Phila Pa 1976) 21:2023–2025
24. Oliveira A, Massano J, Rosas MJ (2013) Dropped head syndrome in early-onset Parkinson disease treated with bilateral subthalamic stimulation: clinical, imaging, EMG, and biopsy findings. Neurol Sci 34:593–594
25. Katz JS, Wolfe GI, Burns DK, Bryan WW, Fleckenstein JL, Barohn RJ (1996) Isolated neck extensor myopathy. Neurology 46:917–921
26. Mano T (2017) Reversal of Dropped Head Syndrome After the Cessation of Dopaminergic Agonist Treatment in Parkinson Disease. Clin Neuropharmacol 40:219–220
27. Bleck TP (1993) Dropped head syndrome. Neurology 43:846
28. Yoshida S, Takayama Y (2003) Licorice-induced hypokalemia as a treatable cause of dropped head syndrome. Clin Neurol Neurosurg 105:286–287
29. Askmark H, Olsson Y, Rossitti S (2000) Treatable dropped head syndrome in hypothyroidism. Neurology 55:896–897
30. Beekman R, Tijssen CC, Visser LH, Schellens RLLA (2002) Dropped head as the presenting symptom of primary hyperparathyroidism. J Neurol 249:1738–1739
31. Nolan JP, Sherk HH (1988) Biomechanical Evaluation of the Extensor Musculature of the Cervical Spine. Spine (Phila Pa 1976) 13:9–11
32. Seidel C, Kuhnt T, Kortmann R-D, Hering K (2015) Radiation-induced camptocormia and dropped head syndrome. Strahlentherapie und Onkol 191:765–770
33. Morris ZS, Harari PM (2014) Interaction of Radiation Therapy With Molecular Targeted Agents. J Clin Oncol 32:2886–2893
34. Alterio D, Marvaso G, Ferrari A, Volpe S, Orecchia R, Jereczek-Fossa BA (2019) Modern radiotherapy for head and neck cancer. Semin Oncol 46:233–245
35. Waldstein C (2023) Radiotherapy update: current role of radiotherapy in the treatment of lymphomas. Mag Eur Med Oncol 16:62–66
36. Stubblefield MD (2011) Radiation Fibrosis Syndrome: Neuromuscular and Musculoskeletal Complications in Cancer Survivors. PM&R 3:1041–1054

37. Grimm S, Chamberlain M (2011) Hodgkin's Lymphoma: A Review of Neurologic Complications. Adv Hematol 2011:1–7
38. Johansson AS, Erlanson M, Lenner P, Lindh J, Osterman B (1998) Late side-effects are common after treatment of Hodgkin's disease. Muscular atrophy following radiotherapy is a neglected risk. Lakartidningen 95:44–47
39. Kelly L, Perju-Dumbrava LD, Thyagarajan D, Lee YC (2013) Delayed postirradiation camptocormia. BMJ Case Rep 2013:bcr2013200083
40. Psimaras D, Maisonobe T, Delanian S, Leclercq D, Lenglet T, Feuvret L, Ricard D, Hoang-Xuan K, Pradat P-F (2011) Late onset radiation-induced camptocormia. J Neurol 258:1723–1725
41. Schlienger M, Ferroir J-P, Huguet F, Deluen F, Pène F, Marseguerra R, Touboul E (2013) Syndrome de la tête tombante après traumatisme cervical dans le cadre d'un lymphome de Hodgkin irradié en mantelet. Cancer/Radiothérapie 17:44–49
42. Collao N, D'Souza D, Messeiller L et al (2023) Radiation induces long-term muscle fibrosis and promotes a fibrotic phenotype in fibro-adipogenic progenitors. J Cachexia Sarcopenia Muscle 14:2335–2349
43. Khan MY (1974) Radiation-induced changes in skeletal muscle. An electron microscopic study. J Neuropathol Exp Neurol 33:42–57
44. Sivaganesan A, Smith JS, Kim HJ (2020) Cervical deformity: evaluation, classification, and surgical planning. Neurospine 17:833–842
45. Yan Y-Z, Shao Z-X, Pan X-X, Chen S-Q, Wu A-M, Tian N-F, Wu Y-S, Wang X-Y (2018) Acceptable Chin–Brow vertical angle for neutral position radiography: preliminary analyses based on parameters of the whole sagittal spine of an asymptomatic chinese population. World Neurosurg 120:e488–e496
46. Lafage R, Challier V, Liabaud B et al (2016) Natural head posture in the setting of sagittal spinal deformity. validation of chin-brow vertical angle, slope of line of sight, and McGregor's slope with health-related quality of life. Neurosurgery 79:108–115
47. Savage JW, Schroeder GD, Hsu WK, Patel AA (2014) Cervical deformity: Pre-operative evaluation and surgical treatment options. Semin Spine Surg 26:172–179
48. Shimizu K, Nakamura M, Nishikawa Y, Hijikata S, Chiba K, Toyama Y (2005) Spinal kyphosis causes demyelination and neuronal loss in the spinal cord: a new model of kyphotic deformity using juvenile Japanese small game fowls. Spine (Phila Pa 1976) 30:2388–2392
49. Suk K-S, Kim K-T, Kim J-M, Chung KH (2002) Significance of Chin-brow vertical angle in correction of kyphotic deformity of ankylosing spondylitis patients. J Korean Soc Spine Surg 9:115
50. Lee S-H, Kim K-T, Seo E-M, Suk K-S, Kwack Y-H, Son E-S (2012) The influence of thoracic inlet alignment on the craniocervical sagittal balance in asymptomatic adults. J Spinal Disord Tech 25:E41–E47
51. Tang JA, Scheer JK, Smith JS, Deviren V, Bess S, Hart RA, Lafage V, Shaffrey CI, Schwab F, Ames CP (2012) The impact of standing regional cervical sagittal alignment on outcomes in posterior cervical fusion surgery. Neurosurgery 71:662–669
52. Hann S, Chalouhi N, Madineni R, Vaccaro AR, Albert TJ, Harrop J, Heller JE (2014) An algorithmic strategy for selecting a surgical approach in cervical deformity correction. Neurosurg Focus 36:E5
53. Nemani VM, Derman PB, Kim HJ (2016) Osteotomies in the cervical spine. Asian Spine J 10:184
54. Ames CP, Smith JS, Eastlack R et al (2015) Reliability assessment of a novel cervical spine deformity classification system. J Neurosurg Spine 23:673–683
55. Scheer JK, Lau D, Smith JS, Lee S-H, Safaee MM, Fury M, Ames CP (2021) Alignment, classification, clinical evaluation, and surgical treatment for adult cervical deformity: a complete guide. Neurosurgery 88:864–883
56. Schwab F, Patel A, Ungar B, Farcy J-P, Lafage V (2010) Adult spinal deformity-postoperative standing imbalance: how much can you tolerate? An overview of key parameters in assessing alignment and planning corrective surgery. Spine (Phila Pa 1976) 35:2224–2231

57. El Fegoun AB, Schwab F, Gamez L, Champain N, Skalli W, Farcy J-P (2005) Center of gravity and radiographic posture analysis: a preliminary review of adult volunteers and adult patients affected by scoliosis. Spine (Phila Pa 1976) 30:1535–1540
58. Martini ML, Neifert SN, Chapman EK, Mroz TE, Rasouli JJ (2021) Cervical spine alignment in the sagittal axis: a review of the best validated measures in clinical practice. Glob Spine J 11:1307–1312
59. Hardacker JW, Shuford RF, Capicotto PN, Pryor PW (1997) Radiographic standing cervical segmental alignment in adult volunteers without neck symptoms. Spine (Phila Pa 1976) 22:1472–1479
60. Gore DR, Sepic SB, Gardner GM (1986) Roentgenographic findings of the cervical spine in asymptomatic people. Spine (Phila Pa 1976) 11:521–524
61. Harrison DE, Harrison DD, Cailliet R, Troyanovich SJ, Janik TJ, Holland B (2000) Cobb method or Harrison posterior tangent method. Spine (Phila Pa 1976) 25:2072–2078
62. Sakamoto R, Nakamoto H, Yoshida Y et al (2022) Does T1 slope minus cervical lordosis mismatch affect surgical outcomes of cervical laminoplasty in the absence of preoperative severe kyphosis? BMC Musculoskelet Disord 23:810
63. Etame AB, Wang AC, Than KD, La Marca F, Park P (2010) Outcomes after surgery for cervical spine deformity: review of the literature. Neurosurg Focus 28:E14
64. Kim HJ, Virk S, Elysee J et al (2020) The morphology of cervical deformities: a two-step cluster analysis to identify cervical deformity patterns. J Neurosurg Spine 32:353–359
65. Heary RF, Choudhry OJ, Jalan D, Agarwal N (2013) Analysis of cervical sagittal alignment after screw-rod fixation. Neurosurgery 72:983–992
66. Mummaneni PV, Dhall SS, Rodts GE, Haid RW (2008) Circumferential fusion for cervical kyphotic deformity. J Neurosurg Spine 9:515–521
67. Dubousset J, Diebo BG (2023) Proximal junctional Kyphosis in modern spine surgery: why is it so common? Spine Surg Relat Res 7:2022–0100
68. Shega FD, Zhang H, Manini DR, Tang M, Liu S (2020) Comparison of effectiveness between Cobalt Chromium rods versus titanium rods for treatment of patients with spinal deformity: a systematic review and meta-analysis. Adv Orthop 2020:1–10
69. Scheer JK, Tang JA, Deviren V, Acosta F, Buckley JM, Pekmezci M, McClellan RT, Ames CP (2011) Biomechanical analysis of cervicothoracic junction osteotomy in cadaveric model of ankylosing spondylitis: effect of rod material and diameter. J Neurosurg Spine 14:330–335
70. Boriani S, Pipola V, Cecchinato R, Ghermandi R, Tedesco G, Fiore MR, Dionisi F, Gasbarrini A (2020) Composite PEEK/carbon fiber rods in the treatment for bone tumors of the cervical spine: a case series. Eur Spine J 29:3229–3236
71. Murthy NK, Wolinsky J-P (2021) Utility of carbon fiber instrumentation in spinal oncology. Heliyon 7:e07766
72. Porras JL, Pennington Z, Hung B, Hersh A, Schilling A, Goodwin CR, Sciubba DM (2021) Radiotherapy and surgical advances in the treatment of metastatic spine tumors: a narrative review. World Neurosurg 151:147–154
73. Chong E, Pelletier MH, Mobbs RJ, Walsh WR (2015) The design evolution of interbody cages in anterior cervical discectomy and fusion: a systematic review. BMC Musculoskelet Disord 16:99
74. Perri B, Cooper M, Lauryssen C, Anand N (2007) Adverse swelling associated with use of rh-BMP-2 in anterior cervical discectomy and fusion: a case study. Spine J 7:235–239
75. Mendenhall SK, Priddy BH, Mobasser J-P, Potts EA (2021) Safety and efficacy of low-dose rhBMP-2 use for anterior cervical fusion. Neurosurg Focus 50:E2
76. Cole T, Veeravagu A, Jiang B, Ratliff JK (2014) Usage of recombinant human bone morphogenetic protein in cervical spine procedures: analysis of the MarketScan longitudinal database. J Bone Jt Surg 96:1409–1416
77. De la Garza RR, Nakhla J, Echt M et al (2018) Use of bone morphogenetic protein-2 in vertebral column tumor surgery: a national investigation. World Neurosurg 117:e17–e21

78. Mazur-Hart DJ, Yamamoto EA, Yoo J, Orina JN (2023) Bone morphogenetic protein and cancer in spinal fusion: a propensity score–matched analysis. J Neurosurg Spine 39:1–7
79. Wijaya JH, Tjahyanto T, Alexi R, Purnomo AE, Rianto L, Arjuna YYE, Tobing JFL, Yunus Y, Faried A (2023) Application of rhBMP in spinal fusion surgery: any correlation of cancer incidence? A systematic review and meta-analysis. Eur Spine J 32:2020–2028
80. Mitchell SL, Donaldson CJ, El Dafrawy MH, Kebaish KM (2019) Difficulties in treating post-irradiation Kyphosis in adults: a series of five cases. Spine Deform 7:937–944
81. Ehresman J, Pennington Z, Elsamadicy AA et al (2021) Fenestrated pedicle screws for thoracolumbar instrumentation in patients with poor bone quality: case series and systematic review of the literature. Clin Neurol Neurosurg 206:106675
82. Hoffmann J, Preston G, Whaley J, Khalil JG (2023) Vertebral Augmentation in Spine Surgery. J Am Acad Orthop Surg 31:477–489
83. Oppenlander ME, Bina R, Snyder LA, Dickman CA (2014) Intravertebral polymethylmethacrylate augmentation of anterior cervical discectomy fusion and plating in the setting of osteoporosis. J Spinal Disord Tech 27:185–188
84. Ames CP, Smith JS, Scheer JK et al (2013) A standardized nomenclature for cervical spine soft-tissue release and osteotomy for deformity correction. J Neurosurg Spine 19:269–278
85. Bin ZG, Hong Z, Wang Z, Zheng B (2022) A novel technique of transpedicular opening-wedge osteotomy for treatment of rigid kyphosis in patients with ankylosing spondylitis. BMC Surg 22:155
86. Garg S, Kipper E, LaGreca J, Carry P, Erickson M (2015) Are routine postoperative radiographs necessary during the first year after posterior spinal fusion for idiopathic scoliosis? a retrospective cohort analysis of implant failure and surgery revision rates. J Pediatr Orthop 35:33–38
87. Yuk FJ, Rasouli JJ, Arginteanu MS, Steinberger AA, Moore FM, Yao KC, Caridi JM, Gologorsky Y (2020) The case for T2 pedicle subtraction osteotomy in the surgical treatment of rigid cervicothoracic deformity. J Neurosurg Spine 32:248–257
88. Tatarek NE (2005) Variation in the human cervical neural canal. Spine J 5:623–631
89. Okada Y, Ikata T, Katoh S, Yamada H (1994) Morphologic analysis of the cervical spinal cord, durai tube, and spinal canal by magnetic resonance imaging in normal adults and patients with cervical spondylotic myelopathy. Spine (Phila Pa 1976) 19:2331–2335
90. Dru AB, Lockney DT, Vaziri S, Decker M, Polifka AJ, Fox WC, Hoh DJ (2019) Cervical spine deformity correction techniques. Neurospine 16:470–482
91. Kim HJ, Piyaskulkaew C, Riew KD (2014) Anterior cervical osteotomy for fixed cervical deformities. Spine (Phila Pa 1976) 39:1751–1757
92. Jones EL, Heller JG, Silcox DH, Hutton WC (1997) Cervical pedicle screws versus lateral mass screws: anatomic feasibility and biomechanical comparison. Spine (Phila Pa 1976) 22:977–982
93. Johnston TL, Karaikovic EE, Lautenschlager EP, Marcu D (2006) Cervical pedicle screws vs. lateral mass screws: uniplanar fatigue analysis and residual pullout strengths. Spine J 6:667–672
94. Smith JS, Klineberg E, Shaffrey CI et al (2016) Assessment of surgical treatment strategies for moderate to severe cervical spinal deformity reveals marked variation in approaches, osteotomies, and fusion levels. World Neurosurg 91:228–237
95. Passias PG, Horn SR, Jalai CM et al (2017) Comparative analysis of perioperative complications between a multicenter prospective cervical deformity database and the Nationwide Inpatient Sample database. Spine J 17:1633–1640
96. Smith JS, Buell TJ, Shaffrey CI et al (2020) Prospective multicenter assessment of complication rates associated with adult cervical deformity surgery in 133 patients with minimum 1-year follow-up. J Neurosurg Spine 33:588–600

Chapter 11
Postoperative Scoliosis After Chest Wall Tumor Resection

Christian Schroeder, Ki-Eun Chang, Tianyi Niu, Margot Martinez Moreno, Zach Pennington, Patricia Sullivan, and Ziya L. Gokaslan

Introduction

Surgical approaches to chest wall tumors must balance the need for aggressive surgical resection with the anatomical limitations of the thoracic spine and ribs. Without surgical fixation, postoperative deformity can result after excision of chest wall tumors via disruption of the innervation to intercostal musculature or destruction of bony anatomy. This effect is most extreme on the developing pediatric spine, and the occurrence of postoperative scoliosis following lateral thoracotomy, also known as thoracogenic scoliosis, has been well-documented in the literature [1]. The surgical approach is dictated by the tumor type, including intramedullary, extramedullary, intradural, and extradural tumors. This chapter will review relevant surgical anatomy when approaching a chest wall tumor, surgical decision-making, and the recommended extent of fusion.

C. Schroeder · K.-E. Chang · T. Niu · M. M. Moreno · P. Sullivan · Z. L. Gokaslan (✉)
Department of Neurosurgery, Brown University, Warren Alpert Medical School/Rhode Island Hospital, Lifespan Health, Providence, RI, USA
e-mail: christian_schroeder@brown.edu; tniu@lifespan.org; margot_martinez_moreno@brown.edu; patricia_sullivan@brown.edu; ziya_gokaslan@brown.edu

Z. Pennington
Department of Neurologic Surgery, Mayo Clinic, Rochester, MN, USA
e-mail: pennington.zachary@mayo.edu

D. M. Sciubba (ed.), *Spinal Tumor Associated Deformity*,
https://doi.org/10.1007/978-3-031-87939-5_11

Anatomic Considerations

The thoracic cavity is composed of 12 sets of ribs, each articulating with a thoracic vertebra posteriorly and the sternum anteriorly. In some cases, elongated transverse processes of the lumbar spine may be characterized as riblets, and lumbar ribs have been reported in approximately 0.2–5.8% of patients, [2–4] most commonly in those with lumbarized S1 vertebrae [2, 3]. As rib counting is a common technique for intraoperative localization, careful review of patient anatomy is necessary to avoid wrong-level surgery.

Each vertebra is composed of the anterior body, two pedicles, and the posterior elements: spinous process, lamina, pars, superior and inferior articulating facets, demi facets, and costal facet (Fig. 11.1). The ribs serve multiple functions in addition to their protective function for the thoracic and mediastinal viscera (i.e., heart, lungs). Biomechanical models have demonstrated that the rib cage provides significant support to the thoracic spine, though the degree of stabilization has varied from study to study and is dependent upon the extent of resection [5, 6]. In one cadaveric study, Feiertag et al. [7] demonstrated that single-level unilateral rib head resection alone was insufficient to increase range of motion for lateral bending, flexion, or extension. By contrast, Oda et al. showed significant increases in flexion/extension, lateral bending, and axial rotation following rib head and costovertebral joint resection in their cadaveric study. In a similar study using functional spine units instead of whole thoracic spine preparations, Oda and colleagues again showed the importance of the costovertebral joints [8]. Addition of unilateral rib head and

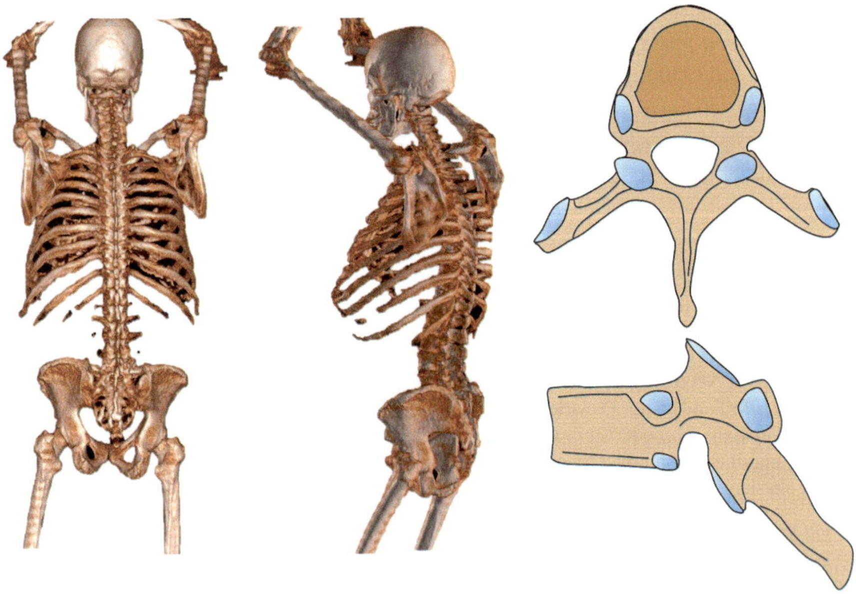

Fig. 11.1 Spinal anatomy, dorsal view. Sagittal and axial view of the thoracic vertebral body

costovertebral joint resection to total facetectomy increased a 43% increase in flexion/extension, a 32% increase in lateral bending, and a 58% increase in axial rotation relative to laminectomy and mesial facetectomy alone. Another cadaveric study by Liebsch and colleagues [6] found that sixth to eighth rib head removal resulted in significant increases in lateral bending and axial rotation but not flexion/extension. As lateral bending and axial rotation are the two primary shifts associated with scoliosis, this provides a possible etiology for thoracogenic scoliosis.

The ribs are also important for their capacity to assist in respiration as the anchor point for the intercostal muscles. The external, internal, and innermost intercostal muscles assist in inspiration and forced expiration. Some studies have also found them to provide significant stabilization, with their resection resulting in significant increases in motion for lateral bending and axial rotation [5, 6]. When removing ribs during an *en bloc* or gross total resection, the intercostal nerve is traditionally ligated within the neurovascular bundle, leading to denervation of the intercostal muscles. The combination of loss of the physical support of the rib as well as the weakening of the intercostal muscles contributes to asymmetrical ventilation, which can lead to postoperative complications, such as pneumonia and respiratory dysfunction. With tumor resection and subsequent asymmetrical intercostal function, patients may hypoinflate the ipsilateral lung. This hypoinflation may synergize with the increased range of motion following rib resection and so allow for the occurrence of progressive thoracic coronal scoliosis, especially in the pediatric population [9, 10].

The number of ribs removed plays a role in the likelihood of developing scoliosis [5, 6, 11–13]. Studies have shown that the removal of the posterior aspect of three or more ribs is most associated with the development of scoliosis in children [12–14]. In contrast, removal of the anterior aspect of the ribs was not associated with developing scoliosis; however, an increase in the number of ribs removed was correlated with the degree of spine curvature [11, 15]. If posterior rib resection is needed for tumor resection, postoperative scoliosis can be prevented through prophylactic measures such as a spinal fusion [16]. Spinal instrumentation with pedicle screw fixation can reconstitute the strength of the posterior tension band, and anterior reconstruction with a metallic cage or cement can reduce the risk of postoperative kyphotic deformity.

In addition to the rib cage, the thoracic spine is also unique in that its nerve roots can be sacrificed with relatively little resultant disability. The thoracic nerve roots play a crucial role in the innervation of the paraspinal musculature and muscles for inspiration; however, they do not directly innervate the limbs (except for T1) and thus can be sacrificed when necessary for gross total resection. In contrast, the roots C5-T1 and L1-S1 are considered functional motor roots and thus sacrifice risks, a functional motor deficit that can impair upper and lower extremity function with a concordant significant limitation in patient function. For this reason, a thoracic vertebral corpectomy is possible via a posterior approach, as nerve roots can be sacrificed without upper or lower extremity impairment, facilitating placement of a cage construct through a corridor obliquely oriented to the pedicle.

The ability to employ posterior-only approaches for thoracic corpectomy is fortunate, as the viscera of the thoracic cavity (i.e., lungs, heart, great vessels) pose a significant obstacle for anterior approaches [17]. When an anterior approach to the spine is needed, or where the tumor incorporates portions of the chest wall, a multidisciplinary surgical team incorporating a cardiothoracic surgeon allows for the design of the optimal approach. Intraoperatively, dual-lumen endotracheal tubes may be utilized to create a surgical corridor within the chest cavity by allowing selective deflation of a single lung; this can significantly improve visualization and access to the tumor. Figure 11.2 demonstrates the anatomical challenges posed when a tumor closely approximates critical structures at the superior sulcus.

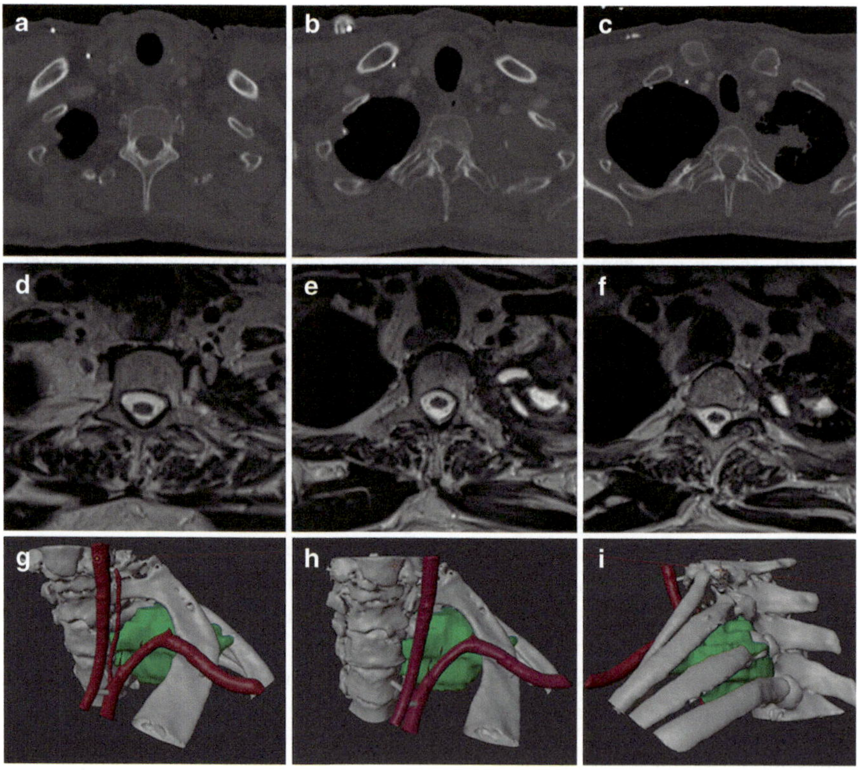

Fig. 11.2 Preoperative axial computed tomography (**a–c**) and T2-weighted magnetic resonance imaging (**d–f**) displaying multiple two-dimensional axial views of the left superior sulcus lesion with vertebral and chest wall involvement. An integrated three-dimensional model was prepared based on preoperative CT and MRI and virtually rendered for 360° visualization of the Pancoast tumor (green) and surrounding vertebral, costal, and vascular anatomy (**g–i**)

Pediatric Considerations

Pediatric patients require additional considerations when considering tumor access and resection. Scoliosis is a progressive disease, and it has been known for the better part of a century that the younger the age of the patient at the time of tumor resection, the more severe the postoperative scoliosis and the more likely corrective surgery will be needed [1, 12, 15, 18, 19]. Additionally, the craniocaudal location of the chest wall resection appears to influence the risk of thoracogenic scoliosis. Glotzbecker and colleagues [20] examined 21 juvenile patients who underwent chest wall resection and noted that resections extending cephalad to the sixth rib demonstrated a more than tenfold higher risk of thoracogenic scoliosis as compared to those in which the chest wall resection is confined to the region below the sixth rib. This was more important than gender, age at resection, or the presence of baseline scoliosis at the time of the deformity. They conjectured that scoliosis develops with the concavity ipsilateral to the resection for two main reasons. First, the ribs present on the side contralateral to the resection exert greater force on the thoracic spinal column than the discontinuous ribs ipsilateral to the resection, creating a net force vector toward the side of resection. Second, they report that there is likely scarring at the resection site with resultant contraction that is not present on the contralateral side, again favoring curvature of the spine toward the resection side. This latter mechanism was also favored by Kergin and Dewar in their 1950 description of thoracogenic scoliosis among pediatric patients who underwent pleural decortication for lung empyema [19]. It was similarly cited by DeRosa, Kawakami et al., and other groups as the mechanism by which curve convexity is consistently ipsilateral to the rib resection [1, 11, 15, 21]. However, Scalabre et al. [12] reported the scoliotic curve consistently developing with the convexity ipsilateral to the defect in their series of 40 pediatric patients who underwent chest wall tumor resection. Ahmed et al. [13] similarly noted the curve to be convex toward the resection side in 21 of their 64 patients who underwent chest wall tumor resection. It is therefore unclear if the relative influence of the aforementioned traction mechanism is dependent upon features of the initial chest wall surgery. A third potential contributory mechanism to thoracogenic scoliosis that is supported by the biomechanical data [5, 6, 8] is the increased range of motion for lateral flexion and axial rotation following resection of the costovertebral joints. Such increased mobility is likely a necessary permissive state for the onset of progressive postoperative thoracogenic scoliosis. A fourth mechanism put forth based upon studies of pediatric patients undergoing thoracotomy for congenital heart disease is neuromuscular paralysis of the operated side of the trunk, [21] which was supported in a rabbit model of progressive scoliosis by Langenskiold and Michelsson [22]. Authors argue that damage to the intercostal nerve and muscles results in an imbalance of strength between the operated and nonoperated sides, which favors the nonoperated side. This net imbalance leads to progressive lateral truncal shift and scoliotic curve development.

Like adults, posterior rib resection is highly associated with developing scoliosis; however, instrumented fusion can be challenging in children, and the child's growth trajectory must be taken into consideration when designing a construct. Unlike the more well-known adolescent idiopathic scoliosis, conservative management with bracing is generally not an option because of the rib cage defect [15]. The defect precludes pad placement at this site, which is necessary to help resist the forces applied on the spine by the ribs contralateral to the resection. Early intervention or prevention of spinal deformity is essential for treating pediatric patients, as thoracogenic scoliosis is known to be progressive, with the rate of progression being most rapid within the first 10 years postresection [1, 15]. In one recent series by Sacco et al. [23], the authors described 307 patients treated with lateral thoracotomy, of whom 32 suffered thoracogenic scoliosis. Thirteen developed curves with the convexity ipsilateral to the surgery, and 19 developed curves with the convexity contralateral to the surgery, with a median time to diagnosis of 4.3 and 5.6 years following thoracotomy. In the most severe cases (curve >45°), curve progression was more rapid, with a median time to diagnosis of only 13 months. The authors noted a lower risk of thoracogenic scoliosis with patient age > 5 years and use of a left-sided versus right-sided lateral thoracotomy. Such interventions can be identified through methods like pulmonary function tests and the Lansky play-performance scale to assess and improve patient quality of life [24].

Surgical Approaches

Management of Lesions in Patients Without Pre-existing Deformity

Chest wall tumors may be approached via *en bloc* or gross total resection if the goal is oncologic cure. Primary spinal tumors such as chordomas require *en bloc* surgical resection to provide the greatest opportunity for long-term recurrence-free survival [25–27]. Previous studies by the senior author have reported on the precise surgical technique for multilevel *en bloc* spondylectomy in primary tumors [28]. Briefly, *en bloc* surgical approaches may require two separate stages, with a posterior decompression and fusion to stabilize the spinal column and perform posterior release followed by an anterolateral/lateral approach to complete resection and delivery of the tumor followed by anterior column reconstruction (Figs. 11.3 and 11.4). During the first [posterior] stage, nerve roots are also sectioned to facilitate tumor delivery during the second stage. While thoracic root sectioning does not lead to significant weakness (i.e., no weakness of the extremities), multilevel root sectioning increases the risk of spinal cord ischemia, as demonstrated by Fujimaki et al. [29] and Kato et al. [30] in canine models. Additionally, preoperative angiography should be considered to look for the location of the artery of Adamkiewicz, ligation of which can cause a spinal cord infarct [31].

The use of preoperative 3D-printed models can help to conceptualize the tumor margins and surgical corridor for preoperative planning [32, 33]. The authors

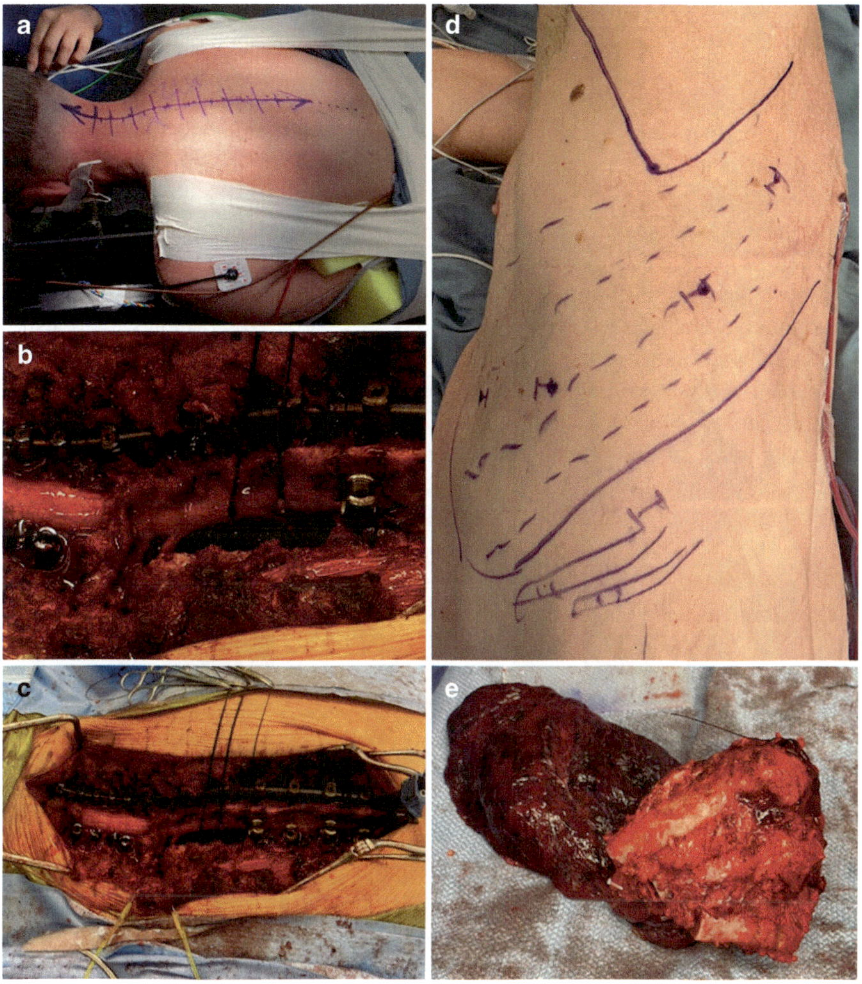

Fig. 11.3 The patient was positioned prone for posterior approach to instrumented fusion, partial corpectomies, and mobilization of the tumor (**a**). Implanted posterior segmental instrumentation (**b**, **c**) is shown. For stage 2, the patient was placed in lateral decubitus position and extensive planning for five thoracoscopic ports and plans for a subcostal incision extending through the diaphragm for delivery of the intact specimen (**d**). The Pancoast tumor was resected successfully with partial T2–4 vertebrae, adjacent chest wall, and left upper lobe of the lung (**e**)

recommend anterior reconstruction with a metallic cage or cement when the vertebral body is excised, with posterior instrumented fixation 2–3 levels above and below the level of the tumor. Some groups recommend vascularized fibular strut autograft due to a theoretically increased rate of bony fusion, [34, 35] though the small cross-sectional area of the fibular strut graft may increase the risk of implant subsidence [36]. When selecting levels for the posterior instrumentation, it is generally recommended to avoid stopping the construct at either the cervicothoracic or

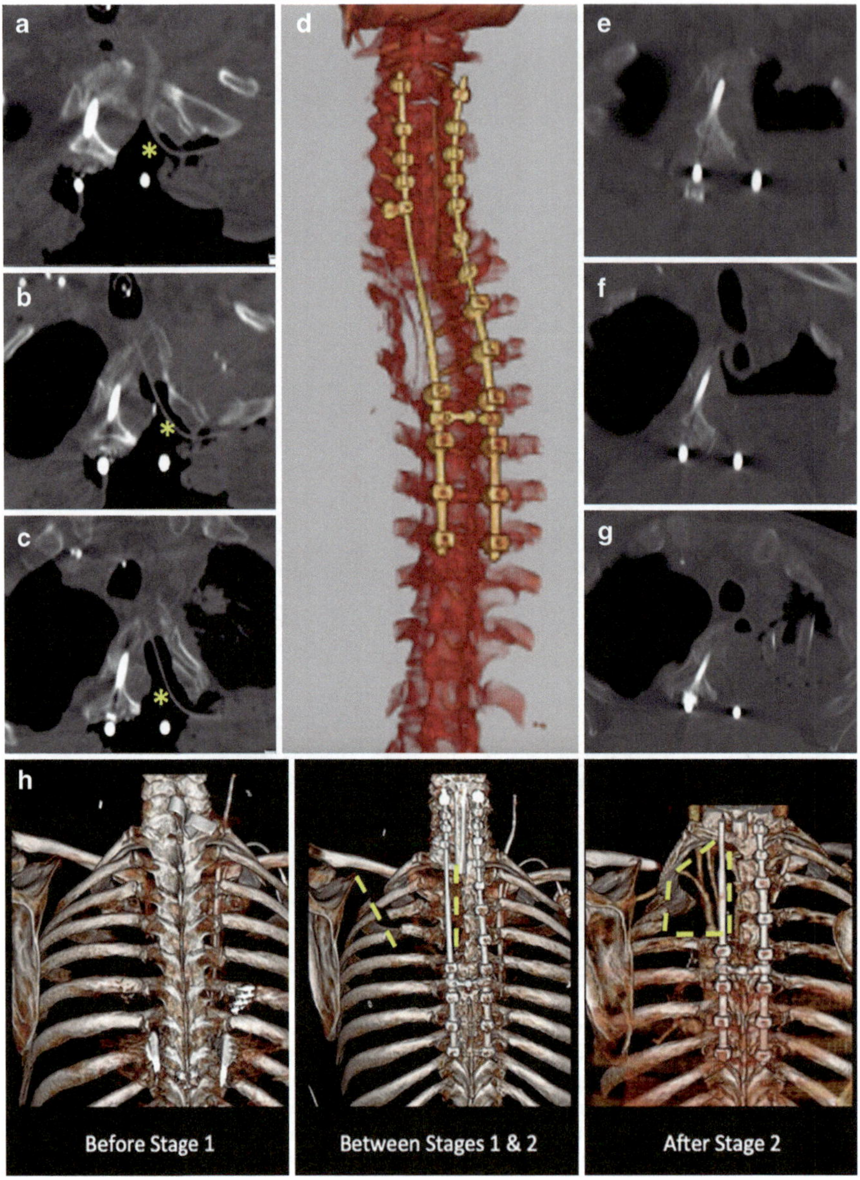

Fig. 11.4 Computed tomography (CT) between stages 1 and 2, showing posterior separation of the tumor from the spinal column with placement of a Silastic sheet (*) to be retrieved anteriorly during stage 2 (**a**–**c**). The thoracic defect (T2-T4) where the left-sided tumor was separated from the spinal column is visualized in 3D (**d**). Following stage 2, a second CT demonstrated the resection cavity, bovine pericardial patch, and intact instrumentation (**e**–**g**). 3D reconstruction of the ribs before stage 1, between stages, and after stage

thoracolumbar junction. Crossing these junctions (i.e., not ending the posterior fusion construct at C7-T1 or T12-L1 when possible) is generally recommended at the author's institution owing to the potential increased risk of adjacent segment disease associated with constructs ending at these junctional points. However, the ideal length of a fusion construct is debated. Regardless of the levels selected, hardware failure is a major concern after a large tumor resection. Chest wall tumors and construct length more than six vertebral levels are just two factors associated with increased construct failure [37]. Patients who have comorbidities such as osteoporosis and Parkinson's are also at a higher risk for construct failure and reoperation [38, 39]. Pedicle screw augmentation with cement may be used to further reinforce the construct in patients at risk of failure [40]. Advances in minimally invasive surgery (MIS) techniques, e.g., video-assisted thoracic surgery (VATS), may allow for resection of chest wall lesions without rib resection or substantial destabilization of the thoracic spine [23, 41–44]. However, oncologic principles must still be observed, and an open approach accompanied by instrumented fusion is our preference over an attempted MIS technique if *en bloc* resection is required.

Vertebral column metastases seldom require *en bloc* resection and are commonly amenable to a posterior-only approach. Increasingly, many patients with radiosensitive tumors are being managed with separation surgery, which describes posterior decompression and epidural disease debulking as a neoadjuvant for definitive radiotherapy [45–48]. These patients may also have underlying instability, which is addressed with percutaneous instrumentation. Where anterior column support is needed in patients with metastatic disease, a posterior-only approach can generally be used, as *en bloc* resection is not required. Consequently, the surgeon is able to work through the window created between adjacent nerve roots. Again, a titanium mesh cage is our preferred approach, especially in light of the increased availability of expandable titanium cages with wide footprints [49]. In cases requiring anterior column reconstruction, a mini-open [50] or open approach can be employed depending upon surgeon comfort. The construct generally involves instrumentation two levels above and below the targeted segment. In patients who do not present with instability, care must be taken to evaluate the extension of tumor invasion into the posterolateral elements and the degree of posterolateral element resection that will be performed intraoperatively. Instability of the posterolateral elements at multiple levels, whether iatrogenic or oncologic in origin, can theoretically increase the risk of postoperative scoliosis, though clinical data to support this is wanting.

Nerve sheath tumors—neurofibromas and schwannomas—can also cause spinal instability with progressive enlargement and erosion of the pedicle and facet joint. Surgical resection may also instigate instability if the posterolateral elements are removed to access the tumor and lateral root sleeve [51]. As with chest wall tumor, usually multiple posterior ribs need to be removed to place the patient at appreciable risk of postoperative scoliosis [12]. Reports of scoliosis following nerve sheath tumor resection have been uncommon, but several groups have reported it. One series by Nakamura et al. described new scoliosis in three patients who underwent facet joint resection and partial vertebral body resection as part of surgery for their dumbbell schwannoma [52]. Fixation should be considered to provide stabilization and support. Minimally invasive surgery (MIS) is also a viable approach for some tumors [53–55].

Correction of Thoracogenic Scoliosis

In patients who present with thoracogenic scoliosis following prior chest wall tumor resection, thorough clinical and radiographic evaluations are necessary, as in the case of any deformity. Clinically, patients should undergo a thorough neurological examination, including a full sensorimotor exam, as well as pulmonary function testing, as poor pulmonary function, specifically reduced vital capacity, is a known risk factor for complications during the surgical correction of thoracogenic scoliosis [15]. Patients with thoracogenic scoliosis often demonstrate a restrictive pattern on pulmonary function testing due to contractions (postsurgical and postradiation-induced changes), which may make ventilation more complex during surgery. Radiographic evaluation should include upright scoliosis films; bending scoliosis films or supine films utilizing a bolster are also helpful to help demonstrate the flexibility of the lesion. In addition to evaluating the flexibility of the deformity, radiographs should be reviewed to characterize the severity (Cobb angle) and directionality of the deformity and to identify the apical, neutral, and stable vertebrae to help with level selection. Other authors have shown that the apex of the deformity tends to be at the level of the thoracotomy [21]. In some cases of early-onset scoliosis and adolescent idiopathic scoliosis, growth-preserving interventions are preferred, including growing rods and the vertical expandable prosthetic titanium rib (VEPTR). The use of the VEPTR device has been reported in the work by the Children's Spine Study Group [56]. In their series of 41 patients with thoracogenic scoliosis, 17 underwent surgery, with 15 being treated with the VEPTR device. Of these 15, only 2 patients had worsening of their deformity. Of the remaining 12 with follow-up, 11 had improvement in their deformity, and the remaining patient demonstrated relative stability of their deformity (56° → 58°). Complications were relatively common though, with 13 complications in 7 patients, of which 5 were pneumonia and 1 patient suffered device failure 3 times.

The chief advantage of growth-preserving techniques, such as VEPTR, in pediatric patients is that they can allow for relatively normal growth until skeletal maturity. At such time, a definitive fusion operation can be performed. VEPTR instrumentation can be performed between ribs, between the rib and spine, or between the rib and pelvis [57]. Descriptions of VEPTR placement can be found elsewhere [57], but, in short, patients are placed prone or in the lateral decubitus position on the operating table, and a J-shaped incision is made starting over the second to fifth ribs 2–3 cm lateral to the midline and extending inferiorly to the planned distal instrumented segment. After incising the trapezius, the chest wall is palpated, and the point just lateral to the erector spinae is felt. The erector spinae are then elevated medially until the portion of the rib just lateral to the transverse process can be palpated. This is the strongest portion of the rib and the segment best able to transfer distraction forces from the VEPTR device to the spine. The parietal pleura is then stripped from the underside of the upper and lower ribs, taking care to try and preserve the periosteum. The cranial locking hook is then placed on the superior edge of the upper rib, and the caudal hook is placed on the inferior edge of the lower rib. The hooks are brought together, secured with the compression device, capturing the proximal ribs. The same procedure is then performed for the cranial and caudal ribs of the lower instrumented level. If the spine is chosen as the distal attachment point, a laminar hook is placed on the superior surface of the lamina, taking care to place the hook between the bone and ligamentum flavum. Alternatively, if a pelvic distal segment is chosen (unlikely for thoracogenic scoliosis), a 4 cm incision is made over the ipsilateral posterior superior iliac spine, and an S-hook is placed over top of the iliac crest. After placing the proximal and distal fixation points, the chest wall is distracted on the concave site with a rib retractor. A rib sleeve matching the distance between the proximal and distal fixators is then selected and secured to the superior and then inferior implant. With distal fixation points in the spine or pelvis, two separate incisions are commonly used, and the rib sleeve is tunneled through the paraspinal muscles to the distal attachment.

For adult patients, instrumented fusion is the treatment of choice for symptomatic patients. As spine reconstruction is generally performed at the time of tumor resection where there is concern for spine destabilization, adult patients presenting with thoracogenic scoliosis are uncommon. Additionally, the risk for progressive scoliosis outside of the growing period is low. For adult patients who do present with thoracogenic scoliosis, management can largely rely on the same principles as adult degenerative scoliosis. Specifically, the upper instrumented vertebra (UIV) should be the stable vertebra—the vertebra that is bisected by the central sacral vertical line [58]. If the UIV is at the apex of the patient's kyphosis though, a more proximal UIV level may be beneficial to reduce the risk of adjacent segment disease or proximal junctional kyphosis. The lower instrumented vertebra should be a stable and neutral vertebra—one in which there is no appreciable rotation in the axial plane [59, 60].

Conclusions

Chest wall tumor resection can result in postoperative scoliosis, also known as thoracogenic scoliosis. Most common in pediatric patients, the curve can occur with the convexity ipsilateral to the site of resection or, more commonly, contralateral. Thoracogenic scoliosis is progressive in nature, and risk factors include younger age, surgery during periods of peak growth, and resection of three or more ribs. In pediatric patients, upfront instrumentation is generally avoided due to growth concerns. Where deformity develops and continues to progress, growth-permissive instrumentation techniques such as the vertical expandable prosthetic titanium rib (VEPTR) are preferred. Definitive fusion can then be performed at skeletal maturity. In adults, thoracogenic scoliosis is far less common. Patients with concern for postoperative spinal instability can be instrumented upfront with pedicle screw instrumentation so as to reduce the risk of progressive postoperative scoliosis. In both populations though, there is an interplay between preservation of motion segments and achieving optimal deformity correction, and the decision to perform instrumented fusion requires thoughtful conversation between the surgeon and patient.

References

1. Sacco R, Bonnevalle M, Nectoux E, Fron D, Ould-Slimane M, Sharma D, Lucchesi G, Canavese F (2022) Thoracogenic scoliosis: a retrospective review of 129 pediatric patients with a mean follow-up of 10 years. Eur Spine J 31:2287–2294
2. Nakajima A, Usui A, Hosokai Y, Kawasumi Y, Abiko K, Funayama M, Saito H (2014) The prevalence of morphological changes in the thoracolumbar spine on whole-spine computed tomographic images. Insights Imaging 5:77–83
3. Doo AR, Lee J, Yeo GE, Lee KH, Kim YS, Mun JH, Han YJ, Son J-S (2020) The prevalence and clinical significance of transitional vertebrae: a radiologic investigation using whole spine spiral three-dimensional computed tomographic images. Anesth Pain Med 15:103–110
4. Chiu CK, Chin TF, Chung WH, Chan CYW, Kwan MK (2023) Variations in the number of vertebrae, prevalence of lumbosacral transitional vertebra and prevalence of cervical rib among surgical patients with adolescent idiopathic scoliosis. Spine (Phila Pa 1976) 49:64–70
5. Liebsch C, Wilke H-J (2022) How does the rib cage affect the biomechanical properties of the thoracic spine? A systematic literature review. Front Bioeng Biotechnol 10:904539
6. Liebsch C, Graf N, Appelt K, Wilke H-J (2017) The rib cage stabilizes the human thoracic spine: an in vitro study using stepwise reduction of rib cage structures. PLoS One 12:e0178733
7. Feiertag MA, Horton WC, Norman JT, Proctor FC, Hutton WC (1995) The effect of different surgical releases on thoracic spinal motion. A cadaveric study. Spine (Phila Pa 1976) 20:1604–1611
8. Oda I, Abumi K, Cunningham BW, Kaneda K, McAfee PC (2002) An in vitro human cadaveric study investigating the biomechanical properties of the thoracic spine. Spine (Phila Pa 1976) 27:E64–E70
9. Cooper DM, Rojas JV, Mellins RB, Keim HA, Mansell AL (1984) Respiratory mechanics in adolescents with idiopathic scoliosis. Am Rev Respir Dis 130:16–22
10. Tsiligiannis T, Grivas T (2012) Pulmonary function in children with idiopathic scoliosis. Scoliosis 7:7
11. DeRosa GP (1985) Progressive scoliosis following chest wall resection in children. Spine (Phila Pa 1976) 10:618–622
12. Scalabre A, Parot R, Hameury F, Cunin V, Jouve J-L, Chotel F (2014) Prognostic risk factors for the development of scoliosis after chest wall resection for malignant tumors in children. J Bone Joint Surg Am 96:e10
13. Ahmed G, Emran IM, Rashad I, Zaghloul MS, Mahrous MR, Tabl YA, Elshafiey M (2024) Scoliosis after resection of primary pediatric chest wall tumors. J Pediatr Surg 59:1754–1758
14. Harris CJ, Helenowski I, Murphy AJ et al (2022) Implications of tumor characteristics and treatment modality on local recurrence and functional outcomes in children with chest wall sarcoma. Ann Surg 276:e969–e975
15. Kawakami N, Winter RB, Lonstein JE, Denis F (1994) Scoliosis secondary to rib resection. J Spinal Disord 7:522–527

16. Haghshenas V, Moghimi M, Haghshenas MP, Shin C, Holderread BM, Hirase T, Hanson DS, Rhines L, Marco R (2022) Scoliosis following chest wall resection for tumor with and without prophylactic fixation: case series. Cureus 14:e21115
17. Pennington Z, Westbroek EM, Lo S-FL, Sciubba DM (2021) Surgical approaches to tumors of the occipito-cervical, subaxial cervical, and cervicothoracic spine: an algorithm for standard versus extended anterior cervical access. World Neurosurg 156:e41–e56
18. Saltsman JA, Danzer E, Hammond WJ, Rhee D, Berhe S, Monteagudo J, Price AP, Heaton TE, Jones DR, LaQuaglia MP (2021) Survival and scoliosis following resection of chest wall tumors in children and adolescents. Ann Surg 274:e167–e173
19. Kergin FG, Dewar FP (1950) Pleural decortication in the prevention and treatment of thoracogenic scoliosis. Arch Surg 61:705–712
20. Glotzbecker MP, Gold M, Puder M, Hresko MT (2013) Scoliosis after chest wall resection. J Child Orthop 7:301–307
21. Roclawski M, Sabiniewicz R, Potaz P, Smoczynski A, Pankowski R, Mazurek T, Daibo B (2009) Scoliosis in patients with aortic coarctation and patent ductus arteriosus: does standard posterolateral thoracotomy play a role in the development of the lateral curve of the spine? Pediatr Cardiol 30:941–945
22. Langenskiöld A, Michelsson J-E (1961) Experimental progressive scoliosis in the rabbit. J Bone Joint Surg Br 43-B:116–120
23. Sacco R, Ould-Slimane M, Bonnevalle M, Nectoux E, Zago A, Dujardin F, Canavese F (2023) Thoracogenic scoliosis: coronal deformity progression in paediatric patients. Eur Spine J 32:639–650
24. Patil N, Kadamba P, Somashekhar M, Shetty J, Rama S (2023) Thoracic tumors in children and their long-term outcomes: a single-center experience. J Indian Assoc Pediatr Surg 28:18
25. Gokaslan ZL, Zadnik PL, Sciubba DM et al (2016) Mobile spine chordoma: results of 166 patients from the AOSpine knowledge forum tumor database. J Neurosurg Spine 24:644–651
26. Barber SM, Sadrameli SS, Lee JJ, Fridley JS, Teh BS, Oyelese AA, Telfeian AE, Gokaslan ZL (2021) Chordoma – current understanding and modern treatment paradigms. J Clin Med 10:1054
27. Boriani S, Bandiera S, Biagini R, Bacchini P, Boriani L, Cappuccio M, Chevalley F, Gasbarrini A, Picci P, Weinstein JN (2006) Chordoma of the mobile spine: fifty years of experience. Spine (Phila Pa 1976) 31:493–503
28. Sciubba DM, Gokaslan ZL, Black JH, Simmons O, Suk I, Witham TF, Bydon A, Wolinsky J-P (2011) 5-level spondylectomy for en bloc resection of thoracic chordoma: case report. Oper Neurosurg 69:onsE248–onsE256
29. Fujimaki Y, Kawahara N, Tomita K, Murakami H, Ueda Y (2006) How many ligations of bilateral segmental arteries cause ischemic spinal cord dysfunction? An experimental study using a dog model. Spine (Phila Pa 1976) 31:E781–E789
30. Kato S, Kawahara N, Tomita K, Murakami H, Demura S, Fujimaki Y (2008) Effects on spinal cord blood flow and neurologic function secondary to interruption of bilateral segmental arteries which supply the artery of Adamkiewicz: an experimental study using a dog model. Spine (Phila Pa 1976) 33:1533–1541
31. Westbroek EM, Ahmed AK, Pennington Z, Goodwin ML, Xia Y, Boone C, Gailloud P, Sciubba DM (2019) Hypervascular metastatic spine tumor angiographic relationships with the artery of Adamkiewicz and other radiculomedullary arteries. World Neurosurg 126:e480–e485
32. Mikula AL, Rhines LD, Patel SS et al (2024) Utility of 3D-printed models in the surgical planning for primary spine tumors: a survey of international spinal oncology experts. Glob Spine J. 21925682241278324
33. Ahmed AK, Pennington Z, Molina CA, Xia Y, Goodwin CR, Sciubba DM (2019) Multidisciplinary surgical planning for en bloc resection of malignant primary cervical spine tumors involving 3D-printed models and neoadjuvant therapies: report of 2 cases. J Neurosurg Spine 30:424–431

34. Ackerman DB, Rose PS, Moran SL, Dekutoski MB, Bishop AT, Shin AY (2011) The results of vascularized-free fibular grafts in complex spinal reconstruction. J Spinal Disord Tech 24:170–176
35. Moran SL, Bakri K, Mardini S, Shin AY, Bishop AT (2009) The use of vascularized fibular grafts for the reconstruction of spinal and sacral defects. Microsurgery 29:393–400
36. Bongers MER, Ogink PT, Chu KF, Patel A, Rosenthal B, Shin JH, Lee S-G, Hornicek FJ, Schwab JH (2021) The use of autologous free vascularized fibula grafts in reconstruction of the mobile spine following tumor resection: surgical technique and outcomes. J Neurosurg Spine 34:283–292
37. Amankulor NM, Xu R, Iorgulescu JB, Chapman T, Reiner AS, Riedel E, Lis E, Yamada Y, Bilsky MH, Laufer I (2014) The incidence and patterns of hardware failure after separation surgery in patients with spinal metastatic tumors. Spine J 14:1850–1859
38. Lehman RA, Kang DG, Wagner SC (2015) Management of osteoporosis in spine surgery. J Am Acad Orthop Surg 23:253–263
39. Babat LB, McLain RF, Bingaman W, Kalfas I, Young P, Rufo-Smith C (2004) Spinal surgery in patients with parkinson's disease: construct failure and progressive deformity. Spine (Phila Pa 1976) 29:2006–2012
40. Ehresman J, Pennington Z, Elsamadicy AA et al (2021) Fenestrated pedicle screws for thoracolumbar instrumentation in patients with poor bone quality: case series and systematic review of the literature. Clin Neurol Neurosurg 206:106675
41. Court C, Boulate D, Missenard G, Mercier O, Fadel E, Bouthors C (2021) Video-assisted thoracoscopic en bloc vertebrectomy for spine tumors. J Bone Joint Surg 103:1104–1114
42. Hireche K, Moqaddam M, Lonjon N, Marty-Ané C, Solovei L, Ozdemir BA, Canaud L, Alric P (2022) Combined video-assisted thoracoscopy surgery and posterior midline incision for en bloc resection of non-small-cell lung cancer invading the spine. Interact Cardiovasc Thorac Surg 34:74–80
43. Yamamoto S, Hirose M, Oyaizu T, Muramatsu A, Suzuki M, Ohta S (2022) Leiomyosarcoma of the chest wall mimicking schwannoma resected by a video-assisted thoracoscopic approach: a case report. J Surg Case Rep 2022:rjab563
44. Yamamoto S, Sogabe M, Endo S (2021) Video-assisted thoracoscopic surgery lobectomy and en bloc resection of the chest wall with incision of the costovertebral joints for non-small cell lung cancer. J Surg Case Rep 2021:rjab190
45. Laufer I, Iorgulescu JB, Chapman T, Lis E, Shi W, Zhang Z, Cox BW, Yamada Y, Bilsky MH (2013) Local disease control for spinal metastases following "separation surgery" and adjuvant hypofractionated or high-dose single-fraction stereotactic radiosurgery: outcome analysis in 186 patients. J Neurosurg Spine 18:207–214
46. Barzilai O, Laufer I, Robin A, Xu R, Yamada Y, Bilsky MH (2019) Hybrid therapy for metastatic epidural spinal cord compression: technique for separation surgery and spine radiosurgery. Oper Neurosurg 16:310–318
47. Pennington Z, Ehresman J, Szerlip NJ, Sciubba DM (2021) Hybrid therapy for metastatic disease. Clin Spine Surg 34:369–376
48. Sciubba DM, Pennington Z, Colman MW et al (2021) Spinal metastases 2021: a review of the current state of the art and future directions. Spine J 21:1414–1429
49. Stinchfield T, Vadapalli S, Pennington Z, Sivagnanam R, Prevost J, Schroeder G, Sciubba DM (2019) Improvement in vertebral endplate engagement following anterior column reconstruction using a novel expandable cage with self-adjusting, multiaxial end cap. J Clin Neurosci 67:249–254
50. Lau D, Chou D (2015) Posterior thoracic corpectomy with cage reconstruction for metastatic spinal tumors: comparing the mini-open approach to the open approach. J Neurosurg Spine 23:217–227
51. Jeon JH, Hwang HS, Jeong JH, Park SH, Moon JG, Kim CH (2008) Spinal schwannoma; analysis of 40 cases. J Korean Neurosurg Soc 43:135

52. Nakamura M, Iwanami A, Tsuji O, Hosogane N, Tsuji T, Ishii K, Toyama Y, Chiba K, Matsumoto M, Watanabe K (2013) Long-term surgical outcomes of cervical dumbbell neurinomas. J Orthop Sci 18:8–13
53. Salame K, Lidar Z, Khashan M, Ofir D, Regev GJ (2022) Minimally invasive resection of benign osseous tumors of the spinal column: 10 years' experience and long-term outcomes of a specialized center. Medicina (Kaunas) 58:1840
54. Saifuddin A, White J, Sherazi Z, Shaikh MI, Natali C, Ransford AO (1998) Osteoid osteoma and osteoblastoma of the spine. Factors associated with the presence of scoliosis. Spine (Phila Pa 1976) 23:47–53
55. Pennington Z, Ahmed AK, Molina CA, Ehresman J, Laufer I, Sciubba DM (2018) Minimally invasive versus conventional spine surgery for vertebral metastases: a systematic review of the evidence. Ann Transl Med 6:103
56. Eby SF, Hilaire TS, Glotzbecker M, Smith J, White KK, Larson AN (2018) Thoracogenic spinal deformity: a rare cause of early-onset scoliosis. J Neurosurg Spine 29:674–679
57. Akçalı Ö (2024) Vertical expandable prosthetic titanium Rib (VEPTR) procedure for early-onset scoliosis. In: Zileli M, Yaman O, Aebi M (eds) Correction techniques for spinal deformity, 1st edn. Thieme Medical and Scientific, Noida, pp 73–77
58. Dalton J, Fourman MS, Lyons K, Sarmiento JM, Lovecchio F, Akosman I, Shaw J, Dowdell J (2022) Level selection for optimal adult spinal deformity correction: a narrative review. Semin Spine Surg 34:100987
59. King HA, Moe JH, Bradford DS, Winter RB (1983) The selection of fusion levels in thoracic idiopathic scoliosis. J Bone Joint Surg Am 65:1302–1313
60. Mistovich RJ, Blumenschein LA, Glotzbecker MP (2023) Surgical level selection in adolescent idiopathic scoliosis: an evidence-based approach. J Am Acad Orthop Surg 31:373–381

Chapter 12
Flatback Deformity from Lumbosacral Tumor Surgery

Thomas A. Pieters, Gabrielle Santangelo, Zach Pennington, Sheng-Fu Larry Lo, and Daniel M. Sciubba

Introduction and Early Descriptions of Flatback Deformity

Flatback syndrome or flatback deformity describes the loss of normal lumbar lordosis, which can result in increased sagittal imbalance with associated back pain, as well as thigh pain from compensatory measures. Loss of lumbar lordosis following lumbar fusion was first described in 1973 by Doherty, when he reported increased truncal inclination and loss of lumbar lordosis in patients who had undergone Harrington rod instrumentation for thoracolumbar scoliosis [1]. Subsequently, Moe and Denis described a similar phenomenon, which they called "flatback syndrome," in their series of 16 patients who had undergone thoracolumbar fusion [2]. The syndrome they described was clinically characterized by muscular pain in the upper back and lower cervical area, knee pain, and inability to stand upright. The authors reported treating these patients with extension osteotomies with good short-term results [2]. Another early study by LaGrone et al. employed a similar strategy in their series of 55 patients with loss of lumbar lordosis following lumbar fusion [3]. Fifty-two of the patients had experienced

T. A. Pieters
Department of Neurosurgery, University of Massachusetts, Worcester, MA, USA

G. Santangelo
Department of Neurosurgery, University of Rochester, Rochester, NY, USA
e-mail: gabrielle_santangelo@urmc.rochester.edu

Z. Pennington
Department of Neurologic Surgery, Mayo Clinic, Rochester, MN, USA
e-mail: pennington.zachary@mayo.edu

S.-F. L. Lo · D. M. Sciubba (✉)
Department of Neurosurgery, Donald and Barbara Zucker School of Medicine at Hofstra/Northwell, Great Neck, NY, USA
e-mail: larrylo@northwell.edu; dsciubba1@northwell.edu

D. M. Sciubba (ed.), *Spinal Tumor Associated Deformity*,
https://doi.org/10.1007/978-3-031-87939-5_12

flatback deformity following Harrington rod instrumentation and presented with an inability to stand erect. All were treated with extension osteotomies (19 multilevel) and Harrington compression rods (41) or a combination of compression and distraction rods, with an average increase in lumbar lordosis from 5° to 27° postoperatively and 21° at minimum 2-year follow-up. Importantly, they noted that failure to restore sagittal plane balance led to a higher rate of pseudoarthrosis and recurrent deformity (Fig. 12.1).

There has subsequently been increased acceptance of the negative impact of positive sagittal balance on patient clinical outcomes. And over the past 20 years, there has been increased research linking sagittal imbalance and patient quality of life, with many citing the seminal study by Glassman et al. associating greater SVA with poorer SF-12 physical health scores and greater disability on the Oswestry Disability Index. [4] While there has been widespread acceptance of the key role of adequate spinopelvic balance restoration in the deformity literature, such investigations have been limited in spine oncology [5]. Oftentimes the oncologic aspects of the operation may be prioritized, especially in the case of metastatic tumor treatment, where patients have historically had limited survival [6]. However, given the significant improvements in survival seen in patients with spinal metastases, [7] such concerns should be less prominent, and greater attention should be paid to ensuring proper spinopelvic alignment when instrumenting patients for vertebral column neoplasms.

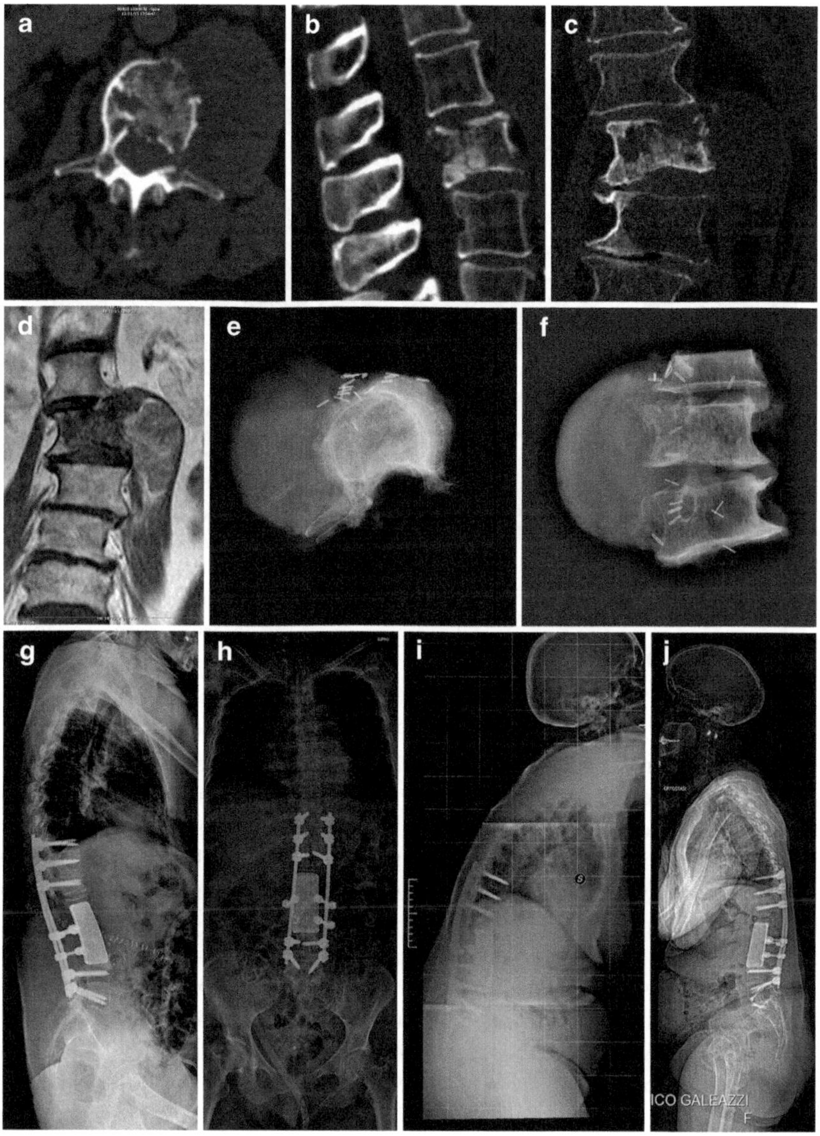

Fig. 12.1 Woman, age 55, L2 chordoma. Loss of balance after *en bloc* vertebrectomy and T10–L5 fusion. Reproduced in this form with the express written permission of original publishing authors. (**a**) CT-scan, transverse section. Lytic, infiltrating lesion producing a huge soft tissue mass. (**b**) CT-scan, sagittal midline section showing the discontinuity of the cortex and the cancellous bone infiltration. (**c**) CT-scan coronal view: the tumor occurred on a degenerative deformity. (**d**) MRI best shows the tumor growing inside the psoas muscle fascia. (**e**) *En bloc* resection, tumor-free margin. (**f**) *En bloc* resection included three vertebral bodies. (**g**) Postop standing radiograph, lateral view. Anterior column reconstruction was performed by 3D-printed titanium cage and posterior T10–L5 fixation. (**h**) Postop standing radiograph, coronal view. (**i**) 20 months follow-up standing radiograph showing progressive kyphotic deformity (associated with increasing pain). (**j**) The patient underwent revision thoracolumbar fusion with a circumferential approach to restore the lumbar lordosis using an L5–S1 ALIF, (**k**, **l**) followed by a posterior thoracolumbar fusion with extension of the posterior instrumentation to the pelvis using a dual rod construct [19]

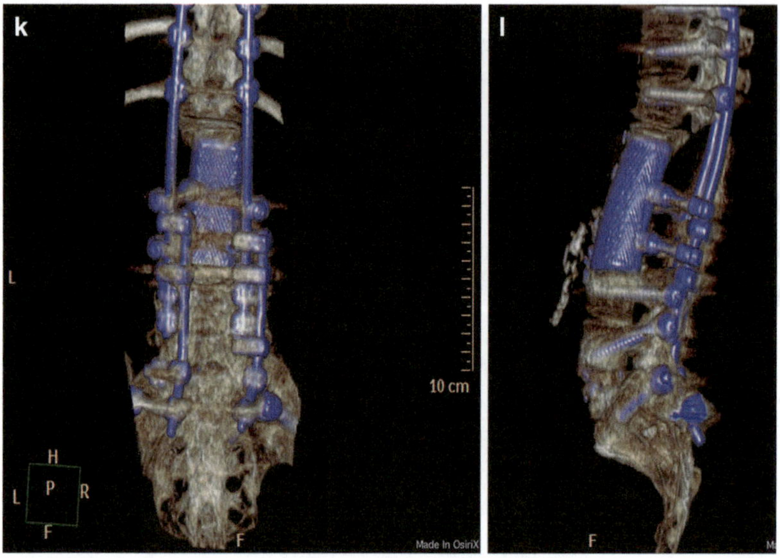

Fig. 12.1 (continued)

Etiology of Flatback Deformity

Flatback deformity can result from multiple causes, though iatrogenic flatback deformity—which occurs secondary to prior lumbar fusion—was the first described. Early series often documented iatrogenic flatback following the placement of Harrington rod distraction instrumentation for scoliosis [3, 8–10]. Placement of this instrumentation with a lower instrumented vertebra (LIV) in the lower lumbar or lumbosacral spine was a powerful strategy for reducing coronal deformity; however, it was often associated with loss of lumbar lordosis and thoracic kyphosis [3, 11, 12]. Farcy and Schwab [10] described a similar iatrogenic syndrome, which they termed "kyphotic decompensation syndrome," and described it as a syndrome of pain and imbalance that was due to an iatrogenic cause other than distraction instrumentation for scoliosis. However, in modern parlance, most group both classes as iatrogenic flatback syndrome.

Modern pedicle screw-based systems eliminate distraction instrumentation as a potential cause of iatrogenic flatback syndrome; nevertheless, many patients require treatment for this condition annually. Wiggins et al. [8] argued that the primary risk factor for iatrogenic flatback deformity with modern pedicle screw-based systems is inadequate patient positioning. Specifically, the use of patient positions with flexed hips results in loss of lumbar lordosis that is then fixed *in situ* when the instrumentation is place. Avoidance of flatback deformity therefore demands patients be placed in a prone position with the hips fully extended [8]. Segmental distraction, e.g., that caused by interlaminar and interspinous devices [13] or that employed for posterior or transforaminal lumbar interbody placement (PLIF/TLIF) can also contribute to loss of lordosis. Avoidance of these interlaminar/interspinous process devices and ensuring anterior interbody placement can help to avoid these potential causes of iatrogenic flatback. Two additional iatrogenic contributions to flatback deformity appear to be pseudoarthrosis at adjacent segments after fusion [8, 14] and selective thoracic fusion for scoliosis [15].

Noniatrogenic contributions to flatback deformity have also been described. Among the general population, multilevel degenerative changes with resultant disc height loss have been described as a cause of flatback deformity [16]. Within the oncologic population, vertebral body collapse due to neoplastic involvement is also observed. In contrast to degenerative flatback deformity, such oncologic cases have a focal malalignment, which will impact the surgical plan selected. Last, new carbon fiber-reinforced PEEK (CFR-PEEK) instrumentation cannot be curved like conventional titanium or cobalt chrome instrumentation. So while such CFR-PEEK instrumentation offers superior radiographic follow-up and facilitates planning for radiotherapy [17, 18] the use of CFR-PEEK longitudinal elements may create constructs with insufficient lumbar lordosis, creating a flatback deformity.

Loss of Sagittal Balance During Spine Tumor Surgery

Prioritization of the oncologic goals in spine tumor surgery may lead surgeons to neglect focus on prevention or correction of deformity [19]. Sagittal imbalance after spine tumor surgery can result from multiple factors both in the primary setting and in a delayed fashion [19]. In the former context, deformity results from insufficient correction or restoration of alignment at the time of surgery. Lumbopelvic parameters have been historically neglected in oncologic spine surgery, [5] so prevention of primary deformity depends upon proper positioning on the table with hips in extension and achievement of lumbopelvic harmony. Sagittal alignment goals for corrective surgery should be the same as for degenerative surgery, generally held as pelvic tilt (PT) $< 25°$, a sagittal vertical axis (SVA) less than 5 cm, and a pelvic incidence (PI) lumbar lordosis mismatch (LL) $<10°$. Deformity in the delayed setting can result from nonunion of anterior column reconstruction, adjacent segment disease (proximal or distal junctional kyphosis), or subsidence of the anterior column reconstruction (e.g., fibular strut graft) [5]. Fibular strut grafts appear to have increased subsidence risk relative to titanium corpectomy cages due to the smaller cross-sectional area [5, 20]. Nonunion appears to be a more common reason following large or multilevel spondylectomies given the greater stresses placed on the corpectomy graft [21, 22]. Longer spondylectomy defects may also increase the risk of adjacent segment disease by shifting greater amounts of stress to the adjacent segments [19].

En bloc resection of primary spinal tumors with negative margins has been shown to offer patients long-term tumor control with reduced recurrence and tumor-related morbidity [23–25]. Such resections, when combined with improvements in radiotherapy, are promising longer survival in this patient population. With this comes an increased risk of progressive postoperative deformity, along with a greater resultant deficit where the patient's native alignment is not restored at the time of tumor resection [19]. A similar dilemma is also manifest in the metastatic spine population, which has similarly seen an improvement in overall survival [26]. For these patients, surgical intervention has increasingly shifted toward minimally invasive separation surgery, which is limited in its ability to provide significant sagittal plane realignment [27, 28]. However, some centers have shown improved local control with more extensive resection including removal of anterior column disease [29]. The open approaches employed for these cases offer substantial ability to correct sagittal and coronal alignment and may merit consideration in patients being treated for spinal metastases who have concurrent deformity.

Presentation of Flatback Deformity

As originally described by Moe and Denis, flatback syndrome was clinically characterized by pain in the upper back and lower cervical spine, pain in the knees, and an inability to stand erect. Radiographically, it was characterized by a positive sagittal balance, which they defined as a horizontal distance greater than 2 cm between the C7 plumbline and sacral promontory [2]. Subsequent descriptions [8, 12, 16] have characterized the flatback syndrome by forward truncal inclination, an inability to stand fully upright with the knees fully extended, and axial pain, often with a subjective sense of imbalance and difficulty with horizontal gaze. The loss of lumbar lordosis leads patients to subconsciously extend their thoracic and cervical spine [30, 31] in order to maintain horizontal gaze [12]. However, continued paraspinal muscle activation leads to progressive pain and fatigue throughout the day. Patients also flex their knees [11] and hips, retroverting the pelvis [32] so as to bring the spine into an upright posture. Again, consistent activation of the knee and hip flexors creates strain in the upper thighs, leading to fatigue and anterior thigh pain [33]. Patients may also extend their ankles to shift their upper body center of mass over their feet in an attempt to stay within the "cone of economy." [32]With continued progression of the deformity, patients adopt a more stooped posture and may be at risk for falls.

However, the drive for patients with flatback deformity to seek clinical attention, namely nonspecific low back pain (NSLBP), may result from a combination of poor spinal alignment and degeneration of the paraspinal musculature. Paraspinal muscular degeneration has consistently been shown to have an association with NSLBP [34] and in one study, Han et al. [35] showed paraspinal muscle integrity is key to maintaining correction, noting that patients suffering recurrent deformity had significantly smaller multifidus cross-sectional area and greater fatty infiltration.

Patient Evaluation

In patients with complaints consistent with flatback syndrome, careful radiographic evaluation is necessary to both identify the nature of the deformity and the patient's compensatory mechanisms. Barrey et al. proposed three steps to analyze such patients including (1) understanding the pelvic incidence, (2) understanding if the patient is globally balanced in terms of their sagittal alignment, and (3) understanding the compensatory mechanisms in the spine, the pelvis, or the lower limbs [31]. Radiographic evaluation should include standing 36″ scoliosis films; full body radiographs (e.g., EOS films) are preferred, if available, as they allow for simultaneous visualization of the patient's compensatory measures (i.e., hip flexion, knee flexion). Global balance can be assessed with the C7 sagittal vertical axis (SVA), and detailed analysis of the spinopelvic balance should be assessed, taking stock of the pelvic incidence (PI), pelvic tilt (PT), sacral slope (SS), and total lumbar and lower lumbar lordosis (LL). For patients presenting with tumor and de novo flatback deformity (e.g., due to pathologic fracture or concomitant multilevel degenerative disease), MR and CT of the lumbar spine should be acquired. MR helps to visualize the presence of concurrent neural element compression, and CT can be used to assess underlying bone quality, [36–38] as well as to look for the presence of fixed deformity (i.e., ankylosis of one or more segments). Fixed deformities may require bone work in addition to that necessary for oncologic treatment. In patients who present with flat back deformity in the setting of a prior fusion, CT lumbar spine should be acquired to look for underlying bone quality and the presence of fusion within the prior construct. Patients who have been fused into a flatback deformity will require a three-column osteotomy to change their global alignment, whereas those with multilevel pseudoarthrosis may be able to have their deformity corrected adequately with multilevel interbody fusion. Flexion/extension upright lumbar radiographs can also be useful for assessing the flexibility of the deformity and to interrogate the presence of successful fusion.

Clinical evaluation should include a full sensorimotor exam, and patients with any evidence of focal deficits require an MR to look for points of potential compression. For those presenting with a flatback deformity and newly diagnosed tumor, biopsy is required prior to surgical planning unless the patient has a known history of metastatic disease. Management of primary and metastatic vertebral column tumors varies significantly regarding resection planning, and patients with primary lesions can have significantly longer prognoses if treated with Enneking-appropriate resection. It is therefore of paramount importance to avoid creation of new deformity in these patients. In patients with a known history of cancer who present with a new vertebral column tumor, patients should undergo repeat staging imaging, as the new spinal metastasis may represent a failure of their current chemotherapy regimen or recurrence of disease. Such staging imaging can be performed with PET/CT. The results of the staging imaging may significantly impact patient counseling, as those with widespread/disseminated disease and a concordantly poor prognosis may be too frail to tolerate an operation to correct their flatback deformity. They may instead be best served by vertebral body augmentation or a shorter-segment construct designed solely to stabilize the affected segment [5, 39]. Last, in patients who present with flatback deformity following a prior operation, repeat staging imaging should also be performed to rule out the presence of widespread metastatic disease and to look for the presence of other affected vertebrae. Such tumor-infiltrated vertebrae will have poorer bony purchase, which could affect the choice of upper and lower instrumented vertebrae (UIV and LIV).

Prevention of Malalignment

It is important to understand that spine tumor surgery has special considerations that may result in type 1 and/or type 2 deformity [40]. Type 1 (segmental) deformity refers to regional relative kyphosis usually with a distal hyperkyphosis, and type 2 (global) deformity refers to patients with positive overall sagittal imbalance [41]. Type 1 deformity is relatively common in the context of spine tumors as tumor infiltration of the vertebral body bone weakens its load-bearing capacity, which can result in pathologic fracture and focal kyphosis. It may also result from instrumented fusion with insufficient lumbar lordosis, creating a flatback deformity. By contrast, type 2 deformity is less common and is often the result of a combination of pathologic fracture and adult degenerative deformity. Treatment of global deformity often require a far more involved surgical correction with instrumentation to the pelvis. Preoperative surgical planning is accordingly more involved and necessitates a thorough understanding of spinopelvic parameters, such as T1-pelvic angle and C7 sagittal vertical axis [42]. In a recent study, Massier et al. used the global alignment and proportion (GAP) score to evaluate the presence of global sagittal plane imbalance in 35 patients who had undergone *en bloc* resection. [43, 44] They found that all 35 patients had moderate to severe sagittal disproportion, and this was associated with poor patient reported health status [43]. Given that sagittal spinal alignment has an influence on postoperative health-related quality of life, full assessment of patient alignment is an important step in presurgical planning and is paramount in patients with favorable prognoses, who will live with the resultant alignment for years [19, 43]. For patients with metastatic disease, in whom overall prognosis is highly dependent upon resumption of their chemoradiation regimen, the desire to correct global alignment must be weighed against the accordant morbidity of such an intervention and its associated delay in the resumption of chemoradiation [29, 45–47]. For those with poor or intermediate prognoses, the cost/benefit discuss with the patient may favor correction of only any associated segmental deformity. In these patients, correction of global deformity may need to be deferred until a time when the patient's disease is better controlled, and they can tolerate the interruption of chemoradiation required to undergo a large deformity operation. Additionally, patients undergoing global deformity correction generally require instrumentation with titanium or cobalt chrome rods, as CFR-PEEK instrumentation cannot undergo the *in situ* bending used in much of deformity surgery. Such instrumentation generates far greater radiographic artifact though. Consequently, the decision to pursue global deformity correction at the time of tumor resection must balance the need for improved surveillance and more accurate radiotherapy planning against the desire to obtain deformity correction.

Regardless of whether a segmental or global deformity is being corrected, surgeons must understand the relative mobility of the segments abutting the tumor-affected level. UIV and LIV should be selected so as to avoid ending a construct at a junctional level, which can increase the risk of proximal and distal kyphosis [19]. Consideration of the UIV orientation and slope as well as the Hounsfield units have been shown to be helpful in choosing an UIV in an attempt to avoid proximal junctional kyphosis and failure [37, 48–50]. If the surgical planning for lumbar tumor resection does not have sacropelvic involvement, careful selection of the LIV may similarly help to prevent distal junctional kyphosis. However, in patients with high PI and those undergoing significant deformity correction, pelvic fixation should be considered due to the high stresses placed on the pedicle screw construct [51].

Correction of Flatback Deformity After Tumor Surgery

When considering a patient with pain from flatback deformity, regardless of the etiology, initial treatment in nonoperative focuses on physical therapy and medical pain management. [8] If conservative management fails, or there is progressive deformity, surgical intervention can be considered assuming the patient's disease status and overall health make them an appropriate surgical candidate. Increasing emphasis has been placed on creating a harmonious spinopelvic balance—the proper balance and interaction between all spinopelvic parameters [52, 53]. Keeping this in mind, surgical planning is based upon the level, severity, and focality of the deformity [8]. Patient radiotherapy history should also be considered given the negative impact of radiotherapy on bone health (see discussion in Chap. 8) and the likely commensurate decrease in screw pullout strength. For cases of flatback deformity without thoracolumbar kyphosis, osteotomies can be made below the level of the conus to minimize the risk of spinal cord injury [8]. For patients with flatback deformity and multilevel pseudoarthrosis, restoration of lumbar lordosis can be achieved through multilevel posterior column osteotomies and the placement of interbodies, which also create an additional fusion surface. In cases of rigid or fixed flatback deformity, a three-column osteotomy is likely required. Global deformity correction prioritizes more caudal placement of this three-column osteotomy as it allows for greater overall sagittal plane correction. If the prior fusion has left the patient with a fused kyphotic deformity, consideration should be made for placing the osteotomy at the apex of the kyphosis, which allows for the maximum correction of the focal deformity [8, 19].

If there is concurrent proximal junctional kyphosis or adjacent segment disease, the construct should be extended into the thoracic spine. Similarly, distal junctional kyphosis in the context of flatback deformity merits extension of the construct caudally, often with sacropelvic fixation [19, 54]. The use of a sacral dome osteotomy has also been described in cases of flatback deformity where extensive correction is needed [55]. Said maneuver can be effective for patients with high PI, but significant stress is placed on the sacral implants, which can result in sacral fracture. Consideration should also be made for anterior column release as it has been shown to successfully restore lumbar lordosis in patients with sagittal imbalance [56]. It may be preferred to three-column osteotomy in spinal oncology patients with reduced physiological reserve; [19, 54] however, it is only an effective option for patients with mobile disc spaces.

Case Example

The following case example is taken from a recent paper by Dr. Berjano and colleagues [19] and is reproduced in this form with the express written permission from this group. A 55-year-old woman was diagnosed with an L2 neoplasm, histologically defined as chordoma after a CT-guided biopsy. Associated with the tumor, the patient presented with a degenerative deformity of the spine. She was submitted to type 3b *en bloc* resection with an anterior–posterior staged approach performed under a single episode of anesthesia. The resected specimen included the portions of tumor involving the caudal L1 body to the cranial L3 body. The margin was histologically confirmed disease-free. Reconstruction was performed with T10-L5 pedicle screw instrumented fusion and anterior column reconstruction with a 3D-printed titanium cage. Two symptomatic and malpositioned pedicle screws (left T10 and T11) were immediately replaced as soon as visualized on postop CT scan. The postoperative upright radiograph was satisfactory, though there was a mild postoperative lumbopelvic mismatch (PI 68°, LL −46°). The patient started a successful rehabilitation program and went back to daily activities with moderate lumbar pain. Twenty-one months later, the patient presented with increasing pain and a progressive kyphotic deformity. Upright radiographs showed positive sagittal balance with a loss of lumbar lordosis and increased pelvic tilt. CT demonstrated subsidence of the caudal part of the prosthesis with loosening of the screws. The patient was submitted to revision surgery with a restoration of the lumbar lordosis using an L5–S1 ALIF, followed by the extension of the posterior fixation to the pelvis using a delta rod system. Postoperative radiographs showed a significant improvement in lumbar lordosis and overall sagittal balance.

Conclusions

Flatback deformity, originally described in the deformity population, describes a loss of lumbar lordosis that leads patients to present with fatigue, a stooped forward posture, inability to stand upright without flexing the knees, and progressive axial pain and fatigue that worsens throughout the day. In the spine tumor population, flatback deformity can result from anterior column collapse due to vertebral body tumor involvement, failure to adequately restore native alignment during tumor resection, or loss of correction during the postoperative period. The occurrence of flatback deformity within the spine tumor population can be minimized by thoroughly evaluating patient alignment preoperatively and obeying alignment principles established by the spinal deformity literature. Some patients may be too frail to tolerate a large deformity operation, in which case surgical planning must still focus on maintaining alignment (i.e., not worsening any associated deformity) even if global deformity correction cannot be achieved with a tolerable level of morbidity. Last, within this population consideration must be made to the decreased bone quality of previously irradiated vertebrae and the need to balance the superior radiographic characteristics of CFR-PEEK instrumentation against the superior ability of conventional screw-rod constructs to achieve deformity correction.

References

1. Doherty JH (1973) Complications of fusion in lumbar scoliosis. J Bone Jt Surg 55:438
2. Moe JH, Denis F (1977) The iatrogenic loss of lumbar lordosis. Orthop Trans 1:131
3. Lagrone MO, Bradford DS, Moe JH, Lonstein JE, Winter RB, Ogilvie JW (1988) Treatment of symptomatic flatback after spinal fusion. J Bone Joint Surg Am 70:569–580
4. Glassman SD, Bridwell K, Dimar JR, Horton W, Berven S, Schwab F (2005) The impact of positive sagittal balance in adult spinal deformity. Spine 30:2024–2029
5. Sankey EW, Park C, Howell EP, Pennington Z, Abd-El-Barr M, Karikari IO, Shaffrey CI, Gokaslan ZL, Sciubba D, Goodwin CRR (2019) Importance of spinal alignment in primary and metastatic spine tumors. World Neurosurg 132:118–128
6. Pennington Z, Ehresman J, Cottrill E, Lubelski D, Lehner K, Feghali J, Ahmed AK, Schilling A, Sciubba DM (2021) To operate, or not to operate? Narrative review of the role of survival predictors in patient selection for operative management of patients with metastatic spine disease. J Neurosurg Spine 34:135–149
7. Rothrock RJ, Barzilai O, Reiner AS, Lis E, Schmitt AM, Higginson DS, Yamada Y, Bilsky MH, Laufer I (2020) Survival trends after surgery for spinal metastatic tumors: 20-year cancer center experience. Neurosurgery 88:402–412
8. Wiggins GC, Ondra SL, Shaffrey CI (2003) Management of iatrogenic flat-back syndrome. Neurosurg Focus 15:1–9
9. Potter BK, Lenke LG, Kuklo TR (2004) Prevention and management of iatrogenic flatback deformity. J Bone Joint Surg Am 86:1793–1808
10. Farcy J-PC, Schwab FJ (1997) Management of flatback and related kyphotic decompensation syndromes. Spine 22:2452–2457
11. Boody BS, Rosenthal BD, Jenkins TJ, Patel AA, Savage JW, Hsu WK (2017) Iatrogenic flatback and flatback syndrome: evaluation, management, and prevention. Clin Spine Surg 30:142–149
12. Lu DC, Chou D (2007) Flatback syndrome. Neurosurg Clin N Am 18:289–294
13. Pennington Z, Lakomkin N, Mikula AL, Elsamadicy AA, Astudillo Potes M, Fogelson JL, Grossbach AJ, Elder BD (2024) Decompression alone versus interspinous/interlaminar device placement for degenerative lumbar pathologies: systematic review and meta-analysis. World Neurosurg 185:417–434
14. Bridwell KH, Lenke LG, Lewis SJ (2001) Treatment of spinal stenosis and fixed sagittal imbalance. Clin Orthop Relat Res 384:35–44
15. Matsumoto H, Colacchio ND, Schwab FJ, Lafage V, Roye DP, Vitale MG (2015) Flatback revisited: reciprocal loss of lumbar lordosis following selective thoracic fusion in the setting of adolescent idiopathic scoliosis. Spine Deform 3:345–351
16. Jang J-S, Lee S-H, Min J-H, Maeng DH (2007) Changes in sagittal alignment after restoration of lower lumbar lordosis in patients with degenerative flat back syndrome. J Neurosurg Spine 7:387–392
17. Porras JL, Pennington Z, Hung B, Hersh A, Schilling A, Goodwin CR, Sciubba DM (2021) Radiotherapy and surgical advances in the treatment of metastatic spine tumors: a narrative review. World Neurosurg 151:147–154
18. Pennington Z, Ehresman J, Elsamadicy AA, Shin JH, Goodwin CR, Schwab JH, Sciubba DM (2021) Systematic review of charged-particle therapy for chordomas and sarcomas of the mobile spine and sacrum. Neurosurg Focus 50:E17

19. Berjano P, Cecchinato R, Pun A, Boriani S (2020) Revision surgery for tumors of the thoracic and lumbar spine: causes, prevention, and treatment strategy. Eur Spine J 29:66–77
20. Bongers MER, Ogink PT, Chu KF, Patel A, Rosenthal B, Shin JH, Lee S-G, Hornicek FJ, Schwab JH (2021) The use of autologous free vascularized fibula grafts in reconstruction of the mobile spine following tumor resection: surgical technique and outcomes. J Neurosurg Spine 34:283–292
21. Luzzati A, Conti S, Sperduti I, Scotto Di Uccio A, Mazzoli S, Cannavò L, Scotto G, Zoccali C (2024) En-bloc spondylectomy in the lumbar spine: indications, results and complications in a series of 47 patients affected by primary malignant bone tumors. Arch Orthop Trauma Surg 144:2027–2038
22. Akamaru T, Kawahara N, Sakamoto J, Yoshida A, Murakami H, Hato T, Awamori S, Oda J, Tomita K (2005) The transmission of stress to grafted bone inside a titanium mesh cage used in anterior column reconstruction after total spondylectomy: a finite-element analysis. Spine 30:2783–2787
23. Amendola L, Cappuccio M, De Iure F, Bandiera S, Gasbarrini A, Boriani S (2014) En bloc resections for primary spinal tumors in 20 years of experience: effectiveness and safety. Spine J 14:2608–2617
24. Gokaslan ZL, Zadnik PL, Sciubba DM et al (2016) Mobile spine chordoma: results of 166 patients from the AOSpine knowledge forum tumor database. J Neurosurg Spine 24:644–651
25. Tomita K, Kawahara N, Baba H, Tsuchiya H, Fujita T, Toribatake Y (1997) Total en bloc spondylectomy. A new surgical technique for primary malignant vertebral tumors. Spine 22:324–333
26. Park S-J, Park J-S, Lee C-S, Kang B-J, Jung C-W (2023) Trends in survival and surgical methods in patients surgically treated for metastatic spinal tumors: 25-year experience in a single institution. Clin Orthop Surg 15:109
27. Laufer I, Iorgulescu JB, Chapman T, Lis E, Shi W, Zhang Z, Cox BW, Yamada Y, Bilsky MH (2013) Local disease control for spinal metastases following "separation surgery" and adjuvant hypofractionated or high-dose single-fraction stereotactic radiosurgery: outcome analysis in 186 patients. J Neurosurg Spine 18:207–214
28. Sciubba DM, Pennington Z, Colman MW et al (2021) Spinal metastases 2021: a review of the current state of the art and future directions. Spine J 21:1414–1429
29. Pennington Z, Pairojboriboon S, Chen X et al (2022) Utility of expanded anterior column resection versus decompression-alone for local control in the management of carcinomatous vertebral column metastases undergoing adjuvant stereotactic radiotherapy. Spine J 22:835–846
30. Barrey C, Jund J, Noseda O, Roussouly P (2007) Sagittal balance of the pelvis-spine complex and lumbar degenerative diseases. A comparative study about 85 cases. Eur Spine J 16:1459–1467
31. Barrey C, Roussouly P, Perrin G, Le Huec J-C (2011) Sagittal balance disorders in severe degenerative spine. Can we identify the compensatory mechanisms? Eur Spine J 20:626–633
32. Lafage V, Schwab F, Skalli W, Hawkinson N, Gagey P-M, Ondra S, Farcy J-P (2008) Standing balance and sagittal plane spinal deformity. Spine 33:1572–1578
33. Klimo P, Astur N, Gabrick K, Warner WC, Muhlbauer MS (2013) Occipitocervical fusion using a contoured rod and wire construct in children: a reappraisal of a vintage technique. J Neurosurg Pediatr 11:160–169
34. Kalichman L, Carmeli E, Been E (2017) The association between imaging parameters of the Paraspinal muscles, spinal degeneration, and low Back pain. Biomed Res Int 2017:1–14
35. Han G, Wang W, Zhou S, Li W, Zhang B, Sun Z, Li W (2023) Paraspinal muscle degeneration as an independent risk for loss of local alignment in degenerative lumbar scoliosis patients after corrective surgery. Glob Spine J 13:1186–1193
36. Mikula AL, Pennington Z, Lakomkin N et al (2022) Independent predictors of vertebral compression fracture following radiation for metastatic spine disease. J Neurosurg Spine 37:617–623
37. Pennington Z, Mikula AL, Lakomkin N et al (2023) Comparison of Hounsfield units and vertebral bone quality score for the prediction of time to pathologic fracture in mobile spine metastases treated with radiotherapy. J Neurosurg Spine 40:19–27

38. Pennington Z, Ehresman J, Lubelski D, Cottrill E, Schilling A, Ahmed AK, Feghali J, Witham TF, Sciubba DM (2021) Assessing underlying bone quality in spine surgery patients: a narrative review of dual-energy X-ray absorptiometry (DXA) and alternatives. Spine J 21:321–331
39. Dea N, Versteeg AL, Sahgal A et al (2020) Metastatic spine disease: should patients with short life expectancy be denied surgical care? An international retrospective cohort study. Neurosurgery 87:303–311
40. Booth KC, Bridwell KH, Lenke LG, Baldus CR, Blanke KM (1999) Complications and predictive factors for the successful treatment of Flatback deformity (fixed sagittal imbalance). Spine 24:1712
41. Angevine PD, Bridwell KH (2006) Sagittal Imbalance. Neurosurg Clin N Am 17:353–363
42. Protopsaltis T, Schwab F, Bronsard N et al (2014) The T1 pelvic angle, a novel radiographic measure of global sagittal deformity, accounts for both spinal inclination and pelvic tilt and correlates with health-related quality of life. J Bone Jt Surg 96:1631–1640
43. Massier JRA, Ogink PT, Schlösser TPC, Ferrone ML, Hershman SH, Cha TD, Shin JH, Schwab JH (2019) Sagittal spinal parameters after en bloc resection of mobile spine tumors. Spine J 19:1606–1612
44. Yilgor C, Sogunmez N, Boissiere L et al (2017) Global alignment and proportion (GAP) score: development and validation of a new method of analyzing spinopelvic alignment to predict mechanical complications after adult spinal deformity surgery. J Bone Jt Surgery-American 99A:1661–1672
45. Fanous AA, Fabiano AJ (2017) Surgical management of spinal metastatic disease. J Neurosurg Sci 61:316–324
46. Hell AK, Kühnle I, Lorenz HM, Braunschweig L, Lüders KA, Bock HC, Kramm CM, Ludwig HC, Tsaknakis K (2020) Spinal deformities after childhood tumors. Cancers (Basel) 12:3555
47. Verla T, Vedantam A, North RY, Xu DS, Raber MR, Fuentes A, Liou NE, Ropper AE (2021) Surgical management of Postradiation, dropped head spinal deformity in patients with head and neck cancer. World Neurosurg 156:e1–e8
48. Mikula AL, Fogelson JL, Lakomkin N et al (2021) Lower Hounsfield units at the upper instrumented vertebrae are significantly associated with proximal junctional kyphosis and failure near the thoracolumbar junction. Oper Neurosurg 21:270–275
49. Im S-K, Lee KY, Lee J-H (2022) The impact of upper instrumented vertebra orientation on proximal junctional kyphosis: a novel and fixed parameter, fused spinopelvic angle. Spine 47:1651–1658
50. Mikula AL, Lakomkin N, Pennington Z et al (2022) Association between lower Hounsfield units and proximal junctional kyphosis and failure at the upper thoracic spine. J Neurosurg Spine 37:694–702
51. Marciano GF, Simhon ME, Lehman RA, Lenke LG (2023) Strategies to avoid distal junctional pathology. Neurosurg Clin N Am 34:585–597
52. Jean L (2014) Influence of age and sagittal balance of the spine on the value of the pelvic incidence. Eur Spine J 23:1394–1399
53. Vaz G, Roussouly P, Berthonnaud E, Dimnet J (2002) Sagittal morphology and equilibrium of pelvis and spine. Eur Spine J 11:80–87
54. Cecchinato R, Redaelli A, Martini C, Morselli C, Villafañe JH, Lamartina C, Berjano P (2017) Long fusions to S1 with or without pelvic fixation can induce relevant acute variations in pelvic incidence: a retrospective cohort study of adult spine deformity surgery. Eur Spine J 26:436–441
55. Pennington Z, Ahmed AKK, Goodwin CRR, Westbroek EM, Sciubba DM (2019) The use of sacral osteotomy in the correction of spinal deformity: technical report and systematic review of the literature. World Neurosurg 130:285–292
56. Turner JD, Akbarnia BA, Eastlack RK, Bagheri R, Nguyen S, Pimenta L, Marco R, Deviren V, Uribe J, Mundis GM (2015) Radiographic outcomes of anterior column realignment for adult sagittal plane deformity: a multicenter analysis. Eur Spine J 24:427–432

Chapter 13
Occipitocervical Misalignment Following Fusion

Danielle Golub, Daniel G. Lynch, Daniel Schneider, Sheng-Fu Larry Lo, Thomas A. Pieters, and Daniel M. Sciubba

Introduction

Occipitocervical fusion (OCF) is the standard surgical management of craniovertebral junction (CVJ) instability that results from neoplastic osseous destruction or aggressive cytoreductive surgery. Neoplasms of the CVJ are rare, accounting for only 0.5% of all spinal tumors [1]. The most commonly observed tumors at the CVJ include chordomas, meningiomas, schwannomas, metastatic lesions, chondrosarcomas, and plasmacytomas [2, 3]. Locally infiltrative and destructive lesions are much more likely to necessitate OCF than benign pathologies [3]. The intricate anatomic and kinematic relationships at the CVJ facilitate the majority of complex head and neck movements and make achieving rigid surgical fixation a challenge, especially in the setting of abnormal bony anatomy due to tumor infiltration or after tumor resection [4]. The development and refinement of occipital plates along with screw and rod-based rigid instrumentation in the 1990s and early 2000s have facilitated robust stabilization at the CVJ, allowing for more aggressive tumor resection with associated improvements in survival [5].

Outside of acute traumatic dislocation of the atlantooccipital joint, occipitocervical dislocation typically presents as a slowly progressive and refractory occipital and neck pain syndrome. This can often be accompanied by worsening myelopathy (from lower medullary or upper cervical cord compression) or even lower cranial nerve dysfunction. Large case series have demonstrated good functional outcomes after OCF, with a relatively consistent 85–90% improvement in myelopathy

D. Golub · D. G. Lynch · D. Schneider · S.-F. L. Lo · D. M. Sciubba (✉)
Department of Neurosurgery, Northwell Health, Great Neck, NY, USA
e-mail: dgolub1@northwell.edu; DLynch8@northwell.edu; dschneider5@northwell.edu; larrylo@northwell.edu; dsciubba1@northwell.edu

T. A. Pieters
Department of Neurological Surgery, UMass Memorial Health, Worcester, MA, USA

D. M. Sciubba (ed.), *Spinal Tumor Associated Deformity*,
https://doi.org/10.1007/978-3-031-87939-5_13

symptoms [6, 7]. Long-term fusion rates with modern occipital plate and rod-based fixation are estimated around 77%, with lower rates of revision surgery for pseudoarthrosis [8]. Anterior bony fusion across the clivus, anterior arch of C1, and the atlantoaxial joints tend to occur more readily and serve as the primary site of bony arthrodesis after OCF [8]. Recent refinements in OCF techniques, from patient selection to instrumentation, have expanded our ability to effectively treat CVJ neoplasms, offering these historically challenging patients both extended survival and improved function—key developments that this chapter will examine in detail.

Anatomy and Predictors of Instability

The CVJ is comprised of the occiput (O), atlas (C1), and axis (C2). The atlantooccipital (O-C1) junction is formed by the cup-shaped bilateral occipital condyles and the superior articulating facets of the C1 lateral masses and allows for nearly 25 degrees of head flexion and extension [9]. This convex–concave joint and its capsule resist anterior–posterior translation as well as compressive forces. The atlantoaxial (C1-C2) joint involves the articulation of the dens and the anterior ring of C1 (and foramen magnum superiorly), which also limits posterior translation, as well as the bilateral facet joints, which have a bi-convex shape that allows for significant axial rotation [10]. The alar ligaments and transverse ligaments are both critical to maintaining occipitocervical stability in the anterior–posterior plane, and the alar ligaments are central to preventing hyperrotation [11]. The tectorial membrane and apical ligament also contribute modestly, but their disruption alone has not been shown to be sufficient to generate clinical or radiographic CVJ instability [9].

A handful of cadaveric studies have systematically examined the degree of condylar resection required to generate CVJ instability necessitating OCF. From a lateral transcranial approach, progressive unilateral condylectomy reliably produced instability after an approximately 2/3 resection, typically involving the insertion point of the alar ligament just inferior to the hypoglossal canal [12]. Another cadaveric study examining anterior endoscopic transclival approaches demonstrated that only a modest increase in mobility was routinely generated by this approach (as long as the anterior atlantoaxial joint elements—C1 anterior arch and dens—remained intact) [13]. The occipital condyle joint capsule is thickest and provides the most support at its most posterolateral aspect [14]. A recent systematic review of surgical series describing the anatomic predictors of OCF after skull base chordoma resection accordingly found that a smaller degree of condylar resection from a lateral approach, as compared to the amount resected from an anterior or medial approach, necessitated OCF. Additionally, a total unilateral condylectomy, bilateral 50% condylectomy, or resection of the C1–2 anterior joint elements and associated transverse or alar ligaments reliably predicted OCF [15].

Illustrative Cases

Case 1

A 27-year-old female presented with increasing frequency of headaches and progressive neck pain over several months. MRI of the brain and cervical spine revealed a large T2-hyperintense, minimally enhancing, lower clival mass extending to C2 with ventral cervicomedullary cord compression concerning for chordoma (Fig. 13.1a, b). CT of the cervical spine demonstrated corresponding lucencies in the lower clivus, occipital condyles, and C1 lateral masses (Fig. 13.1c). Given the extensive involvement of the C1 anterior arch and dens, aggressive tumor resection was expected to generate occipitocervical instability, and a two-stage procedure was planned with anterior endoscopic transclival resection followed by posterior OCF.

The first stage endoscopic endonasal transclival approach for resection of the tumor was performed in conjunction with an otolaryngologist to maximize exposure and assist with a multilayer closure involving a vascularized nasopharyngeal flap. The lower clivus, C1 anterior arch, superior odontoid, the associated ligaments, and surrounding soft tissue, as well as the involved anterior dura, were resected (Fig. 13.1d). The intradural portion was carefully resected off the vertebral arteries

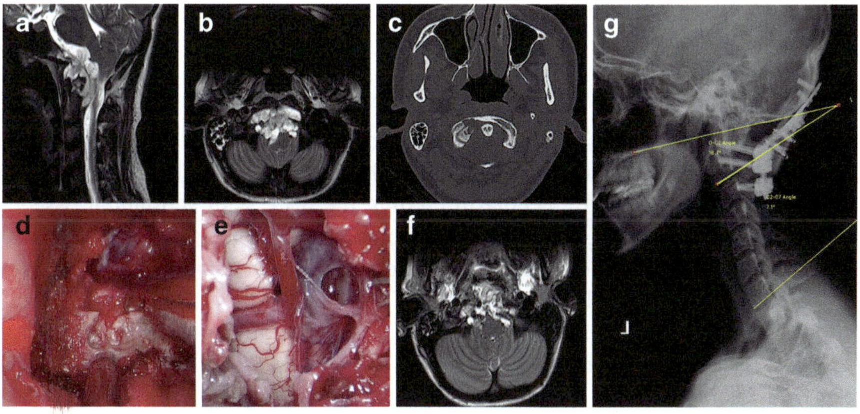

Fig. 13.1 (**a**) Preoperative mid-sagittal and (**b**) axial T2-weighted MRI of the cervical spine demonstrating a T2-hyperintense multilobulated lesion at the inferior clivus extending to the odontoid with mass effect on the ventral medulla and upper cervical spinal cord. (**c**) Preoperative axial CT of the cervical spine at the level of C1 and the tip of the odontoid process showing a lytic lesion involving the right C1 anterior arch and occipital condyle. (**d**) Intraoperative endoscopic view of the anterior approach to the lesion demonstrating resection of the C1 anterior arch, which was involved by tumor. (**e**) Completion of the intradural tumor resection revealed the vertebrobasilar junction and the takeoff of the anterior spinal artery at the cervicomedullary junction. (**f**) Postoperative T2-weighted axial MRI showing gross total resection of tumor with postoperative changes with fat and soft tissue grafts in the area of the inferior clivus previously occupied by tumor. (**g**) Standing cervical X-ray at 3-month follow-up demonstrating evidence of some early bony fusion along the construct with maintained cervical lordosis as well as an O-C2 angle of approximately 18 degrees

and the vertebrobasilar junction using an angled endoscope (Fig. 13.1e). A lumbar drain was also placed for cerebrospinal fluid (CSF) diversion and was kept in place postoperatively to facilitate healing of the skull base repair.

Postoperatively, the patient showed a mild bilateral nystagmus that eventually resolved, and she was maintained in a hard cervical collar. Imaging demonstrated gross total resection of the lesion and atlantooccipital junction bony structures as expected, and pathology confirmed chordoma (Fig. 13.1f). After 6 days of lumbar drainage with no evidence of CSF leak, the lumbar drain was removed, and the patient underwent second-stage OCF from occiput to C3 on postoperative day 7. In order to place C1 lateral mass screws, the bilateral C2 nerve roots were sectioned to optimize visualization of the C1-C2 joints. An occipital plate was secured at the external occipital protuberance, followed by placement of C2 pedicle screws and C3 lateral mass screws. After fixation of the plate and rod system from O-C3, fibular strut allografts were placed along the construct bilaterally and held in place with cables to promote bony fusion and absorb some axial stress from the rods. The patient was discharged home neurologically intact on hospital day 15 with plans for adjuvant proton beam radiotherapy. At 3-month follow-up, she still reported some neck stiffness, but her headaches had resolved, and her cervical X-rays showed early evidence of bony fusion with an ideal O-C2 angle of approximately 18 degrees with maintained physiological cervical lordosis (Fig. 13.1g).

Case 2

A 47-year-old female presented with a history of progressive malignant transformation of an inverted papilloma at the skull base, extending to the CVJ. Imaging revealed an aggressive lytic neoplasm eroding the CVJ, with substantial osseous destruction compromising the atlantoaxial complex (Fig. 13.2a). After resection of the tumor, she acutely developed a severe atlantoaxial dislocation (Fig. 13.2b), characterized by lateral displacement of the C1 arch into the spinal canal. Three-dimensional reconstruction of her CT imaging demonstrated extensive cranial–cervical displacement with profound instability (Fig. 13.2c). Despite urgent posterior internal fixation (Fig. 13.2d), the patient experienced devastating neurological compromise, underscoring the challenges of managing CVJ instability in the setting of advanced oncologic disease. This case highlights the propensity for malignant processes at the CVJ to cause rapid structural deterioration and catastrophic outcomes, necessitating vigilant monitoring and timely intervention in spinal oncology patients.

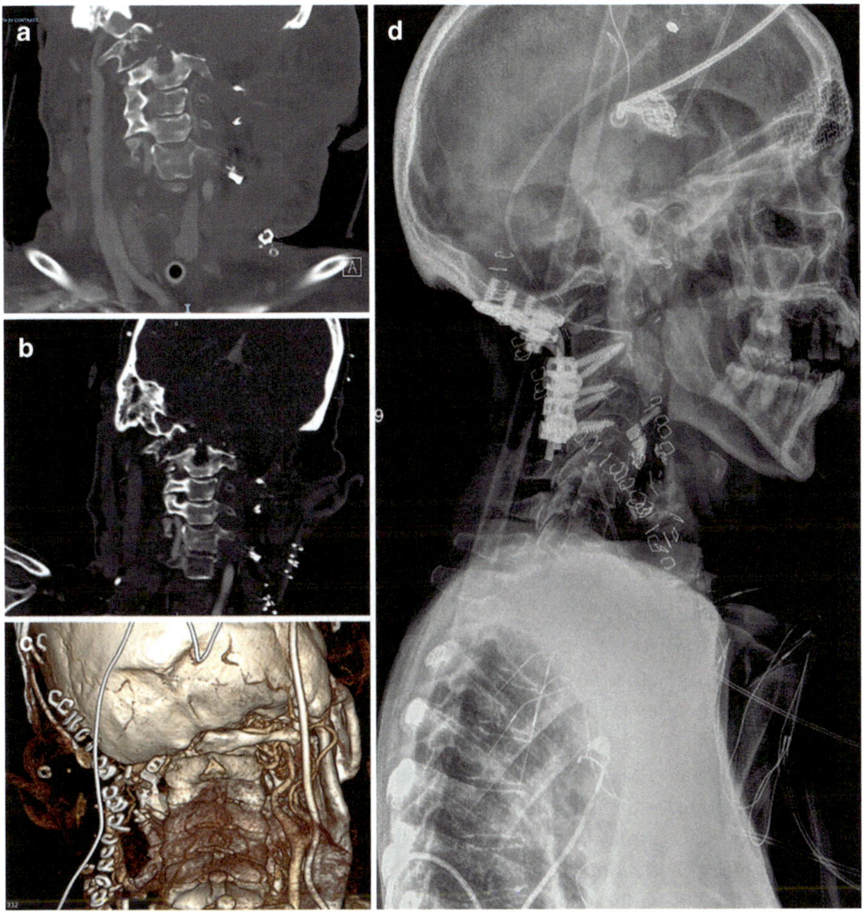

Fig. 13.2 Illustrative case of a 47-year-old female with a malignant skull base neoplasm causing progressive craniocervical junction (CVJ) instability and neurological decline. (**a**) Coronal CT scan demonstrating extensive lytic destruction of the CVJ by the malignantly transformed inverted papilloma. (**b**) Coronal CT scan showing acute severe CVJ dislocation with lateral displacement of the C1 arch into the spinal canal. (**c**) Three-dimensional CT reconstruction illustrating the cranial–cervical instability and structural compromise. (**d**) Lateral postoperative radiograph depicting posterior internal fixation. Despite intervention, the patient sustained severe neurological deficits, emphasizing the complexity of managing oncologic CVJ instability

Occipitocervical Instrumentation

The instrumentation options available for OCF have expanded greatly since the procedure was first reported by Foerster in 1927 [16]. Early techniques involved simple onlay bone grafting of tibial, fibular, and/or iliac crest grafts, which, while effective in promoting fusion, require extended periods of external immobilization [17]. This technique was later modified to include stabilization of the bone grafts with wiring, providing increased stability [18, 19]. Rod-and-wire constructs were subsequently developed in which a U-shaped rod is affixed to the occiput via wires threaded through burr holes and to the cervical spine via sublaminar wiring [20, 21]. Further advances in instrumentation in the 1990s allowed for the development of plate-and-screw systems that resulted in immediate postoperative rigidity at the CVJ and reduced need for postoperative external immobilization [22]. However, these plate-and-screw systems could not be easily adapted to patient anatomy, and rigid fixation with rod-and-screw systems became more prevalent in the late 1990s and early 2000s [23] but were complicated by occipital screw pullout [24]. Combining these two techniques, plate-and-rod systems were developed consisting of an occipital plate and titanium rods for fixation via lateral mass screws [25]. Occipital condyle screws have also been described as an alternative to occipital plating systems for CVJ fixation when the occipital bone is inadequate, such as in expansile tumors [26].

Several important differences between these instrumentation methods are notable. Rigid fixation methods such as rod-and-screw systems were shown to have superior biomechanical stability and clinical outcomes compared to nonrigid systems, such as wiring [27, 28]. In a systematic review, instrumentation failure and neurologic outcomes were also superior with rigid systems compared to nonrigid [29]. Notably, the same review found that patients undergoing OCF in the setting of tumor had the lowest rates of fusion following OCF regardless of method used.

As an area of active study, there are several notable recent advances in OCF instrumentation relevant to spinal oncologic surgeons. Modem adjunctive techniques including robotic guided screw placement and intraoperative O-arm-based navigation have also been demonstrated to be safe and effective in improving instrumentation accuracy during OCF [30, 31]. To prevent implant failure associated with rod bending to accommodate the occipital–cervical angle, a hinged rod system has been developed with similar long-term stability to contoured rods [32]. Carbon fiber-reinforced polyether ether ketone implants offer several advantages over traditional titanium instrumentation, most notably improved radiation therapy planning and delivery, as well as improved assessment of surveillance imaging, with comparable safety and functionality to titanium [33, 34]. It is not yet clear, however, whether these benefits improve long-term oncologic outcomes [35].

Variability exists in the extent of CVJ instrumentation and fusion recommended, with some groups [24] advocating for routine inclusion of the subaxial spine to C3 or C4 in the construct, while others [25] suggest that C2 is a reasonable lower instrumented vertebrae in the OCF construct. While a case series suggested equivalent fusion rates between OCF constructs with and without subaxial extension, biomechanical studies suggest increased construct stability with subaxial extension, particularly in flexion [36, 37]. In the spinal oncology population, the effect of bony erosion, cytoreductive surgery, and chemoradiation may all impact OCF construct stability, and construct extension to the subaxial spine may therefore be of greater importance in these patients as compared to those with congenital or inflammatory pathologies.

Timing of Instrumentation Around Tumor Resection

With respect to skull base tumor resection, OCF (when required) is most commonly performed as a second-stage procedure during the same index admission [15]. The increased risk of complications due to prolonged surgical time when performing single-stage resection and instrumentation is well-established, especially when patient repositioning is required. The delay between the initial tumor resection case and the second stage for instrumentation is usually determined by patient hemodynamic stability and the resolution of any cerebrospinal fluid leak encountered and repaired during the initial surgery (as described in the illustrative case example). Some authors even recommend OCF as the first stage in patients who would definitively require stabilization after tumor resection; this strategy has been suggested to shorten rehabilitation time and decrease the risk of postoperative infection [38, 39]. Additionally, staging the OCF prior to resection provides the benefit of working with intact anatomical landmarks for instrumentation and potentially improved fusion rates but may limit visibility and access during second-stage tumor resection [38]. Further investigation into the optimal timing strategy with larger cohort studies is still warranted.

Considerations for Radiation Therapy

There is likewise limited data on the optimal time interval between OCF and radiation treatment, although most small series suggest around a 3-month delay to allow for some degree of radiographic fusion to occur [1, 2]. Another option, recently described in a single series of five skull base chordoma patients, is to delay second-stage OCF until after the completion of radiation treatment [40]. In this study, patients were placed in hard collars through radiation treatment and until OCF, which was performed an average of 185 days after tumor resection. The goal of delaying OCF was to maximize radiation precision with optimized MRI-based plans not distorted by metallic artifacts and minimize the dose scattering effect associated with treating adjacent to metallic implants [41, 42]. Additionally, small residuals or early recurrence could be identified more easily on follow-up imaging.

While the advent of titanium implants has significantly reduced the issue of metallic artifact on postoperative imaging when compared to older stainless-steel implants, they still produce a radiation "shielding" effect that results in dose attenuation during treatment [43]. The even more novel and radiolucent carbon fiber/polyether ether ketone (PEEK)-based rod and screw systems seem to have particular imaging and treatment benefits for patients requiring radiation therapy. Dosimetric studies have demonstrated increased radiation plan accuracy and enhanced dose delivery, especially for proton beam radiation, with carbon fiber/PEEK-based instrumentation as compared to traditional metal implants [44]. This treatment precision can potentially be further enhanced by contouring the rods in a lateral convex fashion to establish a wider central treatment corridor centered on the tumor resection cavity or residual [45]. Furthermore, Cofano et al. recently published a series comparing functional outcomes and hardware-related complications in patients with spinal metastases after using either carbon fiber-reinforced PEEK implants or traditional titanium implants and observed no differences [46]. Future comparative studies are necessary to determine if there is a clinically significant local tumor control benefit to using these novel implants, but the existing data seems promising.

Occipitocervical Alignment Parameters

While the clinical consequences of thoracolumbar malalignment are well-described, the impact of postinstrumentation cervical alignment parameters on functional outcomes and quality of life remain relatively understudied. Cervical sagittal balance and the maintenance of horizontal gaze are posited to depend on the relationship between angle and alignment of the cranium and cervical spine on the thoracic inlet (TI) [47]. Cervical sagittal vertical axis (cSVA) is determined by the sagittal offset from the plumb line drawn from the center of the C2 inferior endplate margin and the most superior aspect of C7. The O-C2 angle, most reproducibly measured at the intersection of McGregor's line (a line drawn from the posterosuperior aspect of the hard palate to the most caudal point on the midline occipital curve on a midsagittal cervical spine CT or lateral cervical X-ray) and a line drawn along the inferior margin of the C2 endplate, contributes to over 70% of cervical lordosis [48, 49]. The remainder is mostly dependent on the subaxial C2-C7 angle, measured as the angle between the inferior margin of the C2 endplate to the inferior margin of the C7 endplate [50]. The T1 slope, the angle between the superior endplate of T1 and a horizontal line drawn from midpoint of the T1 superior endplate, is directly related to the TI angle or TIA, a fixed morphological parameter that directly influences cervical lordosis. Similar to pelvic incidence (PI), the TIA—the angle between a vertical line drawn at the center of the T1 superior endplate and a line connecting the center of the T1 superior endplate to the upper sternum—can also be geometrically calculated by the sum of the T1 slope and neck tilt (NT), the angle between the same line connecting the upper sternum and the middle of the T1 superior endplate and a vertical line from the upper sternum/manubrium [47] T1 slope can also be calculated by the sum of cranial tilt, the angle between a vertical T1 plumb line and a line drawn from the tip of the dens to the midpoint of the T1 superior endplate, and cervical tilt, the angle formed between the line drawn from the tip of the dens to the midpoint of the T1 superior endplate and a line perpendicular to the slope of the T1 superior endplate (Fig. 13.3). The optimal ratio of cervical tilt to cranial tilt to maintain horizontal gaze with minimal energy expenditure has been estimated at 7:3 [47].

The C2-C7 angle is more variable in asymptomatic individuals while the O-C2 angle tends to be more constant between 15 and 30 degrees [51, 52]. In other words, the C2-C7 angle is the first to regionally compensate for thoracolumbar malalignment in order to maintain horizontal gaze. However, when there is severe cSVA

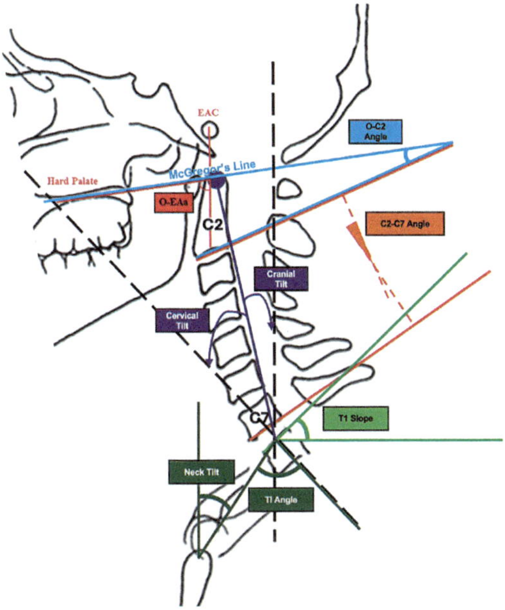

Fig. 13.3 Illustrative schematic of the critical craniocervical alignment parameters relevant to OCF as described in the literature

malalignment and true cervical deformity, the O-C2 angle may demonstrate a secondarily compensatory increase [53]. After OCF, a handful of studies have noted that fixation tends to increase the O-C2 angle, which provokes a corresponding decrease in the subaxial cervical lordosis, or the C2-C7 angle, to maintain horizontal gaze against the T1 slope [49, 54]. In some cases, iatrogenic O-C2 hyperlordosis can induce progressive cervical kyphosis, an increased incidence of cervicothoracic degenerative disease, and negatively affect patient-reported quality of life and functional outcomes [54]. Prior to instrumentation, each patient's baseline cervical lordosis should be considered in relation to their T1 slope, and an O-C2 angle of around 15 degrees should be pursued [49].

Postoperative Dysphagia

Postoperative dysphagia, reported in 17–35% of cases, is perhaps the most commonly reported complication of malalignment after OCF [55]. The association between prolonged hospitalizations, diminished quality of life, and generally increased morbidity and mortality and new postoperative dysphagia is well-described. A significantly decreased postoperative O-C2 angle, particularly when decreased by more than 10 degrees as compared to preoperative parameters, is highly associated with the development of postoperative dysphagia due to the iatrogenic mechanical stenosis created in the oropharyngeal space [56–59]. A reduction in the O-C2 angle makes the mandible shift posteriorly and the bony ring surrounding the oropharyngeal space becomes compromised. Some surgeons utilize the occipital and external acoustic meatus axis angle (O-EAa, measured between McGregor's line and a line connecting the external auditory canal to the midpoint of the C2 endplate) as another validated metric for occipitocervical alignment, with the added advantage of maintaining reliability in cases where significant atlantoaxial translational deformity might compromise traditional O-C2 measurements. Its correlation with oropharyngeal space dimensions offers surgeons an additional tool for preoperative planning. A recent systematic review of the literature on postoperative dysphagia after OCF in 329 patients suggested there while there may be some correlation between a small postoperative O-C2 angle and dysphagia, the strongest predictor of postoperative dysphagia was a postsurgical decrease in the O-C2 angle [55]. Additionally, preoperative dysphagia was also unsurprisingly associated with worsened postoperative dysphagia, and the review authors encourage formal preoperative dysphagia screening for patients undergoing OCF to ensure appropriate counseling. Since postoperative dysphagia after OCF is mechanical in etiology, the consensus recommended management is early revision surgery with a focus on increasing the O-C2 angle with extension, which tends to be curative [60].

Other Complications of OCF Malalignment

Similarly, a significant reduction in the O-C2 angle also generates local airway stenosis and can induce sleep apnea or even persistent dyspnea in severe cases [56]. In rheumatoid arthritis patients, for example, it has been observed that planned extension of the O-C2 angle can improve chronic sleep apnea symptoms [61]. Notably, postoperative dyspnea after OCF accordingly tends to be more frequently seen in rheumatoid arthritis patients; a more informed understanding of its multifactorial predictors in patients with other CVJ pathologies, namely tumors, requires further investigation. Lastly, fixation of the O-C2 angle in an overextended position can also have long-term consequences in the form of compensatory subaxial kyphosis to maintain horizontal gaze and subsequent early development of degenerative disease in the lower cervical spine [8]. Intraoperative fluoroscopy both during positioning and at the time of instrumentation remains a crucial component of surgical planning, and technique in OCF and careful attention to optimizing the O-C2 angle for each patient are advised.

Conclusions

Indications for OCF after skull base tumor resection in particular are driven by either or both the degree of condylar resection and disruption of the anterior or lateral atlantoaxial joints. When necessary, reliable rigid occipitocervical fixation can be achieved with the modern occipital plate and rod constructs with good long-term fusion rates and function outcomes reported in contemporary series. Optimizing the O-C2 angle is critical to ensure maintenance of horizontal gaze with minimal strain on the subaxial spine and the potential for compensatory subaxial kyphotic degeneration. Additionally, surgeons must take care not to establish a small O-C2 angle in excessive flexion, which can promote dysphagia or, in severe cases, dyspnea from airway obstruction.

References

1. Ottenhausen M, Greco E, Bertolini G et al (2023) Craniovertebral junction instability after oncological resection: a narrative review. Diagnostics (Basel) 13(8)
2. Shin H, Barrenechea IJ, Lesser J, Sen C, Perin NI (2006) Occipitocervical fusion after resection of craniovertebral junction tumors. J Neurosurg Spine 4(2):137–144
3. Kooshkabadi A, Choi PA, Koutourousiou M et al (2015) Atlanto-occipital instability following endoscopic endonasal approach for lower clival lesions: experience with 212 cases. Neurosurgery 77(6):888–897
4. Lu DC, Roeser AC, Mummaneni VP, Mummaneni PV (2010) Nuances of occipitocervical fixation. Neurosurgery 66(3):A141–A146
5. Choi D, Melcher R, Harms J, Crockard A (2010) Outcome of 132 operations in 97 patients with chordomas of the craniocervical junction and upper cervical spine. Neurosurgery 66(1):59–65
6. Nockels RP, Shaffrey CI, Kanter AS, Azeem S, York JE (2007) Occipitocervical fusion with rigid internal fixation: long-term follow-up data in 69 patients. J Neurosurg Spine 7(2):117–123
7. Deutsch H, Haid RW Jr, Rodts GE Jr, Mummaneni PV (2005) Occipitocervical fixation: long-term results. Spine 30(5):530–535
8. Shimizu T, Fujibayashi S, Otsuki B, Takemoto M, Murata K, Matsuda S (2021) Long-term radiographic outcome of occipitocervical fixation: an analysis of fusion rate and spontaneous subaxial alignment change at an average 7-year follow-up. Spine 46(3):152–159
9. Panjabi M, Dvorak J, Crisco J 3rd, Oda T, Hilibrand A, Grob D (1991) Flexion, extension, and lateral bending of the upper cervical spine in response to alar ligament transections. J Spinal Disord 4(2):157–167
10. Dvorak J, Panjabi M, Gerber M, Wichmann W (1987) CT-functional diagnostics of the rotatory instability of upper cervical spine. 1. An experimental study on cadavers. Spine 12(3):197–205
11. Wolfla CE (2006) Anatomical, biomechanical, and practical considerations in posterior occipitocervical instrumentation. Spine J 6(6 Suppl):225s–232s
12. Cardoso AC, Fontes RB, Tan LA, Rhoton AL Jr, Roh SW, Fessler RG (2015) Biomechanical effects of the transcondylar approach on the craniovertebral junction. Clin Anat 28(5):683–689
13. Little AS, Perez-Orribo L, Rodriguez-Martinez NG et al (2013) Biomechanical evaluation of the craniovertebral junction after inferior-third clivectomy and intradural exposure of the foramen magnum: implications for endoscopic endonasal approaches to the cranial base. J Neurosurg Spine 18(4):327–332
14. Harris MB, Duval MJ, Davis JA Jr, Bernini PM (1993) Anatomical and roentgenographic features of atlantooccipital instability. J Spinal Disord 6(1):5–10
15. Golub D, Kuffer AF, Garrel S et al (2024) Anatomic determinants of occipitocervical fusion in skull base chordoma resection: a systematic review of the literature with illustrative cases. Neurosurg Focus
16. Foerster O (1927) Die Leitungsbahnen des Schmerzgefühls: und die chirurgische Behandlung der Schmerzzustände. Urban & Schwarzenberg, Berlin
17. Vender JR, Rekito AJ, Harrison SJ, McDonnell DE (2004) The evolution of posterior cervical and occipitocervical fusion and instrumentation. Neurosurg Focus 16(1):E9

18. Cone W, Turner W (1937) The treatment of fracture-dislocations of the cervical vertebrae by skeletal traction and fusion. J Bone Joint Surg 19:584–602
19. Hamblen D (1967) Occipito-cervical fusion: indications, technique and results. J Bone Joint Surg Br 49:33–45
20. Luque E (1982) The anatomic basis and development of segmental spinal instrumentation. Spine 7:256–259
21. Sonntag V, Dickman C (1993) Craniocervical stabilization. Clin Neurosurg 40:243–272
22. Sasso RC, Jeanneret B, Fischer K, Magerl F (1994) Occipitocervical fusion with posterior plate and screw instrumentation. A long-term follow-up study. Spine 19(20):2364–2368
23. Garrido BJ, Sasso RC (2012) Occipitocervical fusion. Orthop Clin North Am 43(1):1–9
24. Macki M, Hamilton T, Pawloski J, Chang V (2020) Occipital fixation techniques and complications. J Spine Surg 6(1):145–155
25. Joaquim AF, Osorio JA, Riew KD (2020) Occipitocervical fixation: general considerations and surgical technique. Global Spine J 10(5):647–656
26. Ahmadian A, Dakwar E, Vale FL, Uribe JS (2014) Occipitocervical fusion via occipital condylar fixation: a clinical case series. J Spinal Disord Tech 27(4):232–236
27. Sutterlin CE 3rd, Bianchi JR, Kunz DN, Zdeblick TA, Johnson WM, Rapoff AJ (2001) Biomechanical evaluation of occipitocervical fixation devices. J Spinal Disord 14(3):185–192
28. Garrido BJ, Myo GK, Sasso RC (2011) Rigid versus nonrigid occipitocervical fusion: a clinical comparison of short-term outcomes. J Spinal Disord Tech 24(1):20–23
29. Winegar CD, Lawrence JP, Friel BC et al (2010) A systematic review of occipital cervical fusion: techniques and outcomes. J Neurosurg Spine 13(1):5–16
30. Kisinde S, Hu X, Hesselbacher S, Satin AM, Lieberman IH (2022) Robotic-guided placement of cervical pedicle screws: feasibility and accuracy. Eur Spine J 31(3):693–701
31. Jing L, Sun Z, Zhang P, Wang J, Wang G (2018) Accuracy of screw placement and clinical outcomes after O-arm-navigated occipitocervical fusion. World Neurosurg 117:e653–e659
32. Abode-Iyamah KO, Dlouhy BJ, Lopez AJ, Menezes AH, Hitchon PW, Dahdaleh NS (2016) Comparison of hinged and contoured rods for occipitocervical arthrodesis in adults: a clinical study. J Craniovertebr Junction Spine 7(3):171–175
33. Neal MT, Richards AE, Curley KL et al (2021) Carbon fiber-reinforced PEEK instrumentation in the spinal oncology population: a retrospective series demonstrating technique, feasibility, and clinical outcomes. Neurosurg Focus 50(5):E13
34. Perez-Roman RJ, Boddu JV, Bashti M et al (2023) The use of carbon fiber-reinforced instrumentation in patients with spinal oncologic tumors: a systematic review of literature and future directions. World Neurosurg 173:13–22
35. Khan HA, Ber R, Neifert SN et al (2023) Carbon fiber-reinforced PEEK spinal implants for primary and metastatic spine tumors: a systematic review on implant complications and radiotherapy benefits. J Neurosurg Spine 39(4):534–547
36. Pan J, Huang D, Hao D et al (2014) Occipitocervical fusion: fix to C2 or C3? Clin Neurol Neurosurg 127:134–139
37. Martin MD, Bruner HJ, Wolfla CE, Yoganandan N (2010) Biomechanical implications of extending occipitocervical instrumentation to include the subaxial spine. Neurosurgery 66(6):1148–1152. discussion 1152
38. Park HH, Park JY, Chin DK, Lee KS, Hong CK (2020) The timing of fusion surgery for clival chordoma with occipito-cervical joint instability: before or after tumor resection? Neurosurg Rev 43(1):119–129
39. Shkarubo AN, Andreev DN, Konovalov NA et al (2017) Surgical treatment of skull base tumors, extending to craniovertebral junction. World Neurosurg 99:47–58
40. Champagne PO, Voormolen EH, Mammar H et al (2020) Delayed instrumentation following removal of cranio-vertebral junction chordomas: a technical note. J Neurol Surg B Skull Base 81(6):694–700

41. Rupp R, Ebraheim NA, Savolaine ER, Jackson WT (1993) Magnetic resonance imaging evaluation of the spine with metal implants. General safety and superior imaging with titanium. Spine 18(3):379–385
42. Son SH, Kang YN, Ryu MR (2012) The effect of metallic implants on radiation therapy in spinal tumor patients with metallic spinal implants. Med Dosim 37(1):98–107
43. Mastella E, Molinelli S, Magro G et al (2017) Dosimetric characterization of carbon fiber stabilization devices for post-operative particle therapy. Phys Med 44:18–25
44. Takayanagi A, Siddiqi I, Ghanchi H et al (2021) Radiolucent carbon fiber-reinforced implants for treatment of spinal tumors-clinical, radiographic, and dosimetric considerations. World Neurosurg 152:61–70
45. Li J, Yan L, Wang J, Cai L, Hu D (2015) Influence of internal fixation systems on radiation therapy for spinal tumor. J Appl Clin Med Phys 16(4):279–289
46. Cofano F, Di Perna G, Monticelli M et al (2020) Carbon fiber reinforced vs titanium implants for fixation in spinal metastases: a comparative clinical study about safety and effectiveness of the new "carbon-strategy". J Clin Neurosci 75:106–111
47. Lee SH, Kim KT, Seo EM, Suk KS, Kwack YH, Son ES (2012) The influence of thoracic inlet alignment on the craniocervical sagittal balance in asymptomatic adults. J Spinal Disord Tech 25(2):E41–E47
48. Shoda N, Takeshita K, Seichi A et al (2004) Measurement of occipitocervical angle. Spine 29(10):E204–E208
49. Matsubayashi Y, Shimizu T, Chikuda H, Takeshita K, Oshima Y, Tanaka S (2016) Correlations of cervical sagittal alignment before and after occipitocervical fusion. Global Spine J. 6(4):362–369
50. Gore DR, Sepic SB, Gardner GM (1986) Roentgenographic findings of the cervical spine in asymptomatic people. Spine 11(6):521–524
51. Diebo BG, Challier V, Henry JK et al (2016) Predicting cervical alignment required to maintain horizontal gaze based on global spinal alignment. Spine 41(23):1795–1800
52. Le Huec JC, Demezon H, Aunoble S (2015) Sagittal parameters of global cervical balance using EOS imaging: normative values from a prospective cohort of asymptomatic volunteers. Eur Spine J 24(1):63–71
53. Protopsaltis TS, Lafage R, Vira S et al (2017) Novel angular measures of cervical deformity account for upper cervical compensation and sagittal alignment. Clin Spine Surg 30(7):E959–e967
54. Passias PG, Wang S, Kozanek M, Wang S, Wang C (2013) Relationship between the alignment of the occipitoaxial and subaxial cervical spine in patients with congenital atlantoxial dislocations. J Spinal Disord Tech 26(1):15–21
55. Tatter C, El-Hajj VG, Fletcher-Sandersjöö A, Edström E, Elmi-Terander A (2023) Radiographic measurements for the prediction of dysphagia after occipitocervical fusion: a systematic review. Acta Neurochir 165(5):1161–1170
56. Miyata M, Neo M, Fujibayashi S, Ito H, Takemoto M, Nakamura T (2009) O-C2 angle as a predictor of dyspnea and/or dysphagia after occipitocervical fusion. Spine 34(2):184–188
57. Ota M, Neo M, Aoyama T et al (2011) Impact of the O-C2 angle on the oropharyngeal space in normal patients. Spine 36(11):E720–E726
58. Meng Y, Wu T, Liu Z et al (2018) The impact of the difference in O-C2 angle in the development of dysphagia after occipitocervical fusion: a simulation study in normal volunteers combined with a case-control study. Spine J 18(8):1388–1397
59. Wang X, Chou D, Jian F (2018) Influence of postoperative O-C2 angle on the development of dysphagia after occipitocervical fusion surgery: results from a retrospective analysis and prospective validation. World Neurosurg 116:e595–e601

60. Izeki M, Neo M, Takemoto M et al (2014) The O-C2 angle established at occipito-cervical fusion dictates the patient's destiny in terms of postoperative dyspnea and/or dysphagia. Eur Spine J 23(2):328–336
61. Ataka H, Tanno T, Miyashita T, Isono S, Yamazaki M (2010) Occipitocervical fusion has potential to improve sleep apnea in patients with rheumatoid arthritis and upper cervical lesions. Spine 35(19):E971–E975

Index

D. M. Sciubba (ed.), *Spinal Tumor Associated Deformity*, https://doi.org/10.1007/978-3-031-87939-5

GPSR Compliance

The European Union's (EU) General Product Safety Regulation (GPSR) is a set of rules that requires consumer products to be safe and our obligations to ensure this.

If you have any concerns about our products, you can contact us on ProductSafety@springernature.com

In case Publisher is established outside the EU, the EU authorized representative is:

Springer Nature Customer Service Center GmbH
Europaplatz 3
69115 Heidelberg, Germany

Batch number: 10732090

Printed by Printforce, the Netherlands